The
24-Hour
Turnaround

The 24-Hour Turnaround

The Formula for Permanent

Weight Loss, Antiaging, and

Optimal Health—Starting Today

JAY WILLIAMS, PH.D.

with Debra Fulghum Bruce

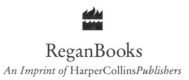

ReganBooks
An Imprint of HarperCollins*Publishers*

To Michael, Riley, Dustin, and R.J.,
the most incredible family on planet Earth

The material on pages 148–149 and 151 is excerpted from *The Food Revolution* by John Robbins. Copyright © 2001 by John Robbins, by permission of Conari Press.

HarperCollins books may be purchased for educational, business, or sales promotional use. For information please write: Special Markets Department, HarperCollins Publishers Inc., 10 East 53rd Street, New York, NY 10022.

FIRST EDITION

Designed by Katy Riegel

Printed on acid-free paper

Library of Congress Cataloging-in-Publication Data
Williams, Jay, Ph.D.
    The 24-hour turnaround : the formula for permanent weight loss, antiaging, and optimal health—starting today / Jay Williams, with Debra Fulghum Bruce.—1st ed.
        p. cm.
Includes bibliographical references.
ISBN 0-06-039431-5
    1. Health. 2. Physical fitness. 3. Nutrition. I. Title: Twenty-four hour turnaround. II. Bruce, Debra Fulghum, 1951– . III. Title.
RA776.W6858 2002
613—dc21   2002022108

02 03 04 05 06 WB/RRD 10 9 8 7 6 5 4 3 2 1

Contents

PREFACE   vii

INTRODUCTION
Your 24-Hour Turnaround Prescription   1

DARE TO BE DIFFERENT—
in Just 24 Hours   15

TOTAL LIFE CHANGE 1
Mood, Belief, and Mastering Motivation   44

TOTAL LIFE CHANGE 2
Your H.E.A.R.T. Workout Formula   75

TOTAL LIFE CHANGE 3
The ABC's of the Definition Diet   125

TOTAL LIFE CHANGE 4
Healing Hydration   193

TOTAL LIFE CHANGE 5
Alcohol and the Myth of Moderation   217

TOTAL LIFE CHANGE 6
Sweet Dreams   236

TOTAL LIFE CHANGE 7
Balancing Hormones   264

TOTAL LIFE CHANGE 8
Destress with Mind-Body Innercise   295

YOU *CAN* TURN BACK THE CLOCK
Rewriting the Rules on Aging   328

SPA SECRETS   342

RECIPES FOR YOUR 24-HOUR TURNAROUND   369

SOURCES   399

ACKNOWLEDGMENTS   407

Preface

BETWEEN MY aesthetic surgery practice in Santa Barbara and my post as clinical assistant professor and codirector of the facial plastic surgery fellowship at UCLA, I have seen and observed (often with a cynical eye) most approaches to people's quest to look and feel younger. I have, for instance, participated in the development of minimally invasive and nonablative lasers, and I was a pioneer in many noninvasive and endoscopic techniques for facial rejuvenation.

No longer satisfied with the outward illusion of the fountain of youth, more and more of my patients have been seeking a total approach to their health as they head toward maturity. Jay Williams first came to my attention over a decade ago when her revolutionary ideas and techniques began to capture the awareness of many of my aesthetic surgery patients. Rapidly my medical vocabulary started to include terms like H.E.A.R.T. training, Definition Diet, and hormone-friendly environment. It didn't take me long to realize that my own specialized work in antiaging, cell rejuvenation, and minimally invasive cosmetic approaches was destined to marry with Jay's extraordinary and intuitive approach to the total health and well-being of the mind-body complex.

Jay's selfless commitment to helping others achieve near freedom from the degenerative effects of time has resulted in a tremendous, worldwide following of devotees. I am constantly amazed at the number of people who attribute their success to this extraordinary human being. Perhaps what I admire about Jay the most is that she is her own laboratory. Nothing that she expounds or prescribes has not been thoroughly tested on herself. Clearly the fitness and antiaging buzzword of the new millennium is *Jay*.

—Gregory Keller, M.D., F.A.C.S.

Your 24-Hour Turnaround Prescription

ALOHA from the beautiful Kona coast of the Big Island of Hawaii. As an exercise physiologist and spa health consultant who has prescribed diet, exercise, and personal health programs for tens of thousands of men, women, and families, I want to tell you about an exciting program that gives you the benefits of antiaging, permanent weight loss, *and* total fitness and that starts to work *immediately*.

No matter what your age or health status, I know that you can become *different* in just 24 hours—with increased energy, stamina, and libido, elevated mood, more fat-burning enzymes, and youthful vitality. Although a "24-hour turnaround" may sound unbelievable, I have the professional background, experience, and facts to convince you that it is true and that it can happen to you. Let me explain.

Your Personalized Turnaround

My clients come here because they have the utmost confidence in me and the 24-Hour Turnaround. Through the years they have seen my program work for friends or colleagues. Or they've heard about it through one of my regular corporate seminars, and they want to know if it can help them improve their own bodies and personal health. At the resort, I work one-on-one with clients, counsel couples, and help entire families to upgrade their nutrition, implement fitness programs, and make lifestyle changes, even helping them find alternative medicine practitioners. Often they fly me to their homes to work with their chefs and to introduce healthy lifestyle changes within their families' busy schedules. In most cases, my clients take my advice seriously and follow my instructions with diligence. The majority of my clients are not interested in the clinical research or the journal articles that back up the various recommendations I make. They usually say, "Please, just tell me what works."

Because I have thousands of people who rely on me for up-to-date, cutting-edge information about antiaging, weight loss, and health, my practice has always been somewhat ahead of the times, particularly when it comes to using clinical studies in the program. It often takes years for medical research to be approved and make it through all the bureaucratic red tape. By the time you read about a breakthrough study in the media, it could have been in a testing lab or clinical trial for five or ten years or longer. I find it's hard to be patient and wait on published journal results when you know that the outcome could help someone lose weight, get fit, or prevent a disease right now.

Throughout the book I have included the scientific studies and the supporting references that apply to my recommendations. But sometimes the life-changing results clients achieve come from the specialized, time-tested diet and fitness techniques I have developed through years of helping men and women to achieve lean, healthy, and youthful bodies. Some of these strategies are based on intuition, faith, and a commonsense philosophy of good health. These are all life practices I strongly believe in. Whether grounded in conventional science or common sense, the bottom line is that this program works time and again for the clients who come to my office, and it will work for you.

I am writing this book as if you *are* my client, sitting across from me in my office or on the telephone during a phone consultation. No, I can't see your face, gauge your reaction, or track your progress. But I am going to tell you the same things I tell my clients, and I know you will have the same success if you stay focused and motivated. You see, for the past twenty-six years, I have had a passion for knowledge about the human body. I've read literally hundreds of medical journal studies searching for the keys to optimal health and longevity. I've interviewed renowned researchers, prominent doctors, alternative medicine practitioners, and other health-care professionals who are experts in their fields.

I've also talked with people like you who are desperate for answers to their diet and health questions and are suffering needlessly because of inaccurate information. My personal and professional quest motivates me to go beyond what conventional medical studies confirm as "truth" and seek known and little-known breakthroughs to help people get lean, feel younger and more energetic, and virtually halt or even reverse the degenerative aging process.

Making Total Life Changes (TLCs)

Until I see you in Hawaii, I want to do the next best thing to consulting with you in person. I'll give you eight Total Life Changes (what I call TLCs) that are vital to staying lean, looking and feeling young, and living an active life—for the rest of your life.

These following eight TLCs will help transform your body, mind, and emotions as you make simple changes in the way you eat, think, sleep, and exercise each day.

- **TLC 1: Master your mood and motivation.** You will prepare for your 24-Hour Turnaround by gaining new insight into how motivation, mood, and belief are essential components in achieving optimal health. You'll call upon these fundamentals to keep you focused even when you don't feel like staying with the program. I have witnessed clients who were chronically tired or even depressed and had a dramatic turnaround in energy, mood, and productivity in just hours by using the motivational strategies in TLC 1.

  When we have the right motivational tools, we can immediately change our lifestyle, including poor eating habits, sleep problems, sedentary behavior, and how we cope with stress. The specific motivational steps offered here will give you the tools to feel healthier, change a negative thought process, and achieve weight loss and optimal fitness. In doing so, your relationships, career, and other aspects of your life that depend on positive communication will greatly benefit starting today!

- **TLC 2: Become your own personal trainer with the H.E.A.R.T. workout.** I developed *Heart-rate-specific Exercise with Aerobic Resistance Training* (the H.E.A.R.T. workout) as a unique and effective way to promote and sustain weight loss without overstressing the body. Exercising at the wrong intensity ages your body unnecessarily; raises your blood sugar level; alters the hormonal environment in your body, making it difficult to burn fat for the rest of the day; and compromises your immune system, which increases your risk of disease—not to mention that it hurts. Training at a specific heart rate (what I call your Zone One) personalizes the H.E.A.R.T. workout to your fitness level, ability, and body type. Aerobic resistance training is also far more effective and timesaving than the conventional approach to aerobics and weight training. The H.E.A.R.T. workout stimulates endorphins, natural "opiate" hormones that elevate mood and change chemicals in the brain, similar to the way some antidepressants like Prozac work. Exercising in your personal Zone One guarantees that you will develop the fat-burning enzymes you need to lose weight and, more important, speed up your metabolism to maintain that weight loss. You can increase those enzymes *in the next 24 hours* and be on your way to a lean and healthy new you.

● **TLC 3**: **Learn the ABC's of the Definition Diet.** In TLC 3, I will teach you to nourish and *feed* (not starve!) your hormones, your bones, your cardiovascular system, your muscles, and your brain—so you lose weight, balance raging hormones, have fewer mood swings, and remain youthful and strong at any age. My Definition Diet will give you a complete understanding of why the foods you choose must provide optimal nutrition. The array of natural, whole foods in the Definition Diet can speed up your metabolism and weight loss and slow down your biological aging today. I believe that *food is medicine* and can be used to keep your body balanced, healthy, and satisfied. No matter what you eat, from the moment you ingest it your body's chemistry changes. Food can *immediately* alter your mood, affect the widening of the arteries and blood flow to the brain and sexual organs, improve the symptoms of menopause, and help you sleep more soundly at night (or . . . keep you wide awake).

● **TLC 4**: **Quench your body's thirst with healing hydration.** There's one more step you must take to function at an optimal level and to look and feel great: drink water, and lots of it. Drinking water may sound like an oversimplified Total Life Change, but it is necessary to stop the negative effects of aging. Nearly two-thirds of the human body is made up of water and fluid. This includes 90 percent of the blood, 80 percent of the brain, 73 percent of the muscle tissue, 60 percent of the skin, and 22 percent of the bone. When you go for only a few hours without replenishing the water in your body, it affects all your body's processes, even causing dehydration, characterized by headaches, fatigue, a feeling of extreme hunger, and foggy memory.

As we get older, we begin to dry out, leading to flaky and wrinkled skin, constipation, reduced saliva, and even joint aches and pains. With age we also lose sensitivity in our thirst mechanism—which is why we must follow a regular schedule to drink water each day. I will give you a hydration schedule, along with the facts about fluids and your health that will affect your life (and your family's life). The following are just some of the benefits you will gain *in the next 24 hours* by increasing water in your daily diet:

- More efficient digestion
- Reduced hunger between meals
- Hydrated skin cells
- More energy and an improved mood
- Increased ability of muscles to burn fat
- Increased removal of toxins
- Reduced chance of constipation

TLC 5: **Learn about the myth of alcohol moderation.** In this Total Life Change, we will evaluate the effect of alcohol on weight loss, aging, optimal health, and sleep. Chemically, alcohol acts as a diuretic and causes dehydration—just what you want to avoid to look and feel young. While the accepted wisdom for most people is that a glass of wine every evening is good for your heart, it may, in fact, be packing on the pounds and contributing to wrinkled skin. More research confirms that just one glass of wine inhibits your body's ability to burn fat for the next 48 hours. But here you will learn how to turn this fat-burning condition around *in the next 24 hours.*

In TLC 5, I'll also unravel the "French paradox" and give strong evidence revealing that alcohol is linked to some types of cancer, as well as age-related diseases.

TLC 6: **Extend your life with antiaging deep sleep.** In TLC 6, I show how healing sleep can extend your life, boost your immune function, prevent aging, and even help you drop unwanted pounds. It's no news that most Americans are sleep deprived. Nearly one in three people surveyed by the National Sleep Foundation reported getting six hours or less of sleep each

SLEEP AND HEALTH ARE INTIMATELY RELATED

If you ignore your body's natural clock by working and playing at any time of the day or night, you could be setting yourself up for illness, injury, and even death, according to sleep experts. The price of ignoring your natural sleep patterns can range from aches and pains to heart disease to chronic fatigue syndrome. A regular bedtime can be as important to your health as stopping smoking or cutting back on saturated fat.

night during the week—although 98 percent of those surveyed said sleep was as important to them as exercise and good nutrition.

New studies confirm that sleep affects *more* than just alertness: it influences your memory, your productivity, and your reflexes. Cellular regeneration takes place primarily during sleep, and the amount of deep sleep and dream sleep you get every night may be a fair indicator of your life span. Research confirms that lack of deep sleep can tear down your immune system, making you more susceptible to viral and bacterial infections, and greatly affect your youthful good looks and how you relate to those around you. So TLC 6 is important to decreasing your biological (as compared with your chronological) age.

But what about those who have difficulty getting to sleep or even maintaining restful sleep? TLC 6 will help you incorporate important sleep steps in your daily routine so that you feel younger and more alert, energetic, and productive *in the next 24 hours.*

● **TLC 7: Balance your hormones—naturally.** While hormone replacement therapy (HRT) used to be the gold standard when a woman entered menopause, many recent studies are now waving a red flag when it comes to introducing foreign hormones into the body. Not only do prescriptive hormones increase your risk of breast and uterine cancer, we now know that women who have heart disease may further increase their risk of a second heart attack by taking HRT. Heart disease is the number one cause of death for women, so this is a topic we all must take seriously.

In TLC 7, I help you understand the hormone fluctuations of perimenopause, a normal period of change leading up to menopause that usually lasts four to five years, as well as the decline of estrogen during menopause and how this can affect your physical and emotional state. I will give you some natural remedies, including hormone-friendly whole foods, increased cellular hydration, antiaging exercise, and natural hormone balancers that can give you amazing relief from perimenopausal and menopausal symptoms. I will give you the opportunity to feel young and alive again—*each and every 24 hours of your life.*

- **TLC 8**: **Destress and halt aging with mind-body techniques.** You won't miss the calming benefit of alcohol once you learn how to destress naturally, using the relaxation response, meditation and deep breathing, yoga, or biofeedback. When confronted with life's stress, your body produces adrenaline. The release of adrenaline is like sending a thousand messages to various key parts of the body at once, resulting in a racing heart, increased blood pressure, and a system on red alert. These messages prepare your body to deal with the stress.

The problem with high levels of stress is that they can weaken the body, reducing the number of T-cells—the killer cells in our immune system that help to ward off diseases. This effect happens immediately and can last for days. Ongoing stress can also result in unresolved muscle tension, increased blood pressure, rapid heartbeat, and general arousal—as if we couldn't get out of passing gear (as opposed to normal or low gear). Eventually the tension, arousal, and tightness seem normal, and we find ourselves more vulnerable to illness and poor self-care habits. Chronic tension can lead to weight gain, skin problems, knotted muscles, lower mobility, degenerative joint and spine problems, and sheer exhaustion.

Meditation and deep breathing induce the relaxation response, which can slow down your heart rate, reduce blood pressure, and calm the feel-

BENEFITS OF TOTAL LIFE CHANGES

Lean and toned body
Younger biological age
Reduced risk of short and long-term diseases
Support for bone, breast, and cardiovascular health
Reduced blood pressure and blood fat ratio
Increased energy, stamina, and libido
Mental clarity
Boost in productivity

ings of anxiety that you experience during chronic stress. You will learn how to change a highly charged moment into a period of calm (I call it "relaxation on demand") and protect your body from the ravages of increased stress hormones today and every other day.

One Size Does *Not* Fit All

Unlike many authors of more trendy diet and exercise books, I am not an advocate of the "one size fits all" health philosophy. Instead, I believe there are many turnaround options, depending on your age, fitness level, and specific health and weight-loss needs.

There are thousands of competing health books in the bookstore about diets, exercise, motivation, hormones, relaxation, yoga, and meditation, all offering conflicting information. Perhaps that's why clients always ask me, "Can't you recommend *one book* that combines proven information that really works for total life change?" My answer to that is *The 24-Hour Turnaround*. To give you added insight, throughout this book I will relate personal experiences, anecdotes, and comments from clients and seminar attendees who did a complete turnaround and reclaimed lean bodies, increased vitality, and a new outlook on life.

Sure, I could have given you a book exclusively about quick weight loss. I have a strong background in nutrition and fat metabolism, and diet books sell. But I'm here to tell you that good health and defying aging are not just a matter of counting calories and eating carrot sticks: everyone has already done that at least once. One client, Mira, told me that she had lost more than 300 pounds over a period of two decades on a low-calorie diet—losing and gaining the same 15 pounds twenty times. Can you imagine the sense of failure and frustration she experienced? And she is not alone with her years of yo-yo dieting. Most clients come to me with lengthy histories of eating disorders, diet deprivation, and sedentary lifestyles. Many have hit middle age tilting the scales at the highest number to date and have experienced immune dysfunction, chronic health problems, and lack of motivation. Sadly, they also have a biological age that is greater than their chronological age.

My Story

I too have experienced the consequences of not always taking care of myself during times of great stress and know firsthand how quickly life's interruptions can age you and add pounds.

Let me share a personal story. When I separated from my first husband in 1984, the stress was incredible. No one could have prepared me for the unending court battles, followed by emotional custody decisions over our son, Dustin. Not only did the divorce deplete my energy and self-esteem, it was financially draining. Here I was a single mom with no financial or emotional support; I felt hopeless.

Trying to play the role of both mom and dad, along with working to pay the rent, I had no time or energy to take care of my body, mind, or spirit. Despite my belief in a healthy lifestyle, I found myself eating on the run—sometimes convenience and fast foods that I normally would never eat. Dinners for my son were quick and easy—the typical "busy family" fare. I found myself skipping exercise, particularly on days when I needed it the most. And I was moody, even depressed, as I saw the reality of my life with no reprieve in sight and no time to take care of me.

One day as I was sitting in the car waiting for Dustin's soccer practice to end, I glanced in the rearview mirror and was shocked. The woman I saw in the mirror could not be me! My skin looked horrible from lack of a healthy diet, good sleep, and exercise; I had put on an extra 20 pounds; I had dark circles under my eyes. As I stared at this tired older woman in the mirror, I realized that while I might be talking the talk, I was not walking the walk.

I decided at that moment to turn my life around and begin to take care of myself so I could be a happier, healthier person and a better mom.

I knew which negative habits had to be changed. I just had to motivate myself to change them—and believing you can accomplish something is half the battle, as I will explain later. I was determined to take responsibility for my health and well-being and devise a schedule that would include time to exercise, quiet time to meditate, and a bedtime that allowed the sleep needed to feel young and energetic again. I threw out the boxes and cans in my kitchen and returned to the "real" whole foods that had always kept me lean and healthy. I woke up the next day (without the alarm clock!) ready to take on my busy schedule with a completely different attitude toward life.

Today I'm remarried, but this time to the man of my dreams. My life is still incredibly busy, as my family has grown from one to three children. My career is demanding but rewarding, and I love it all because I feel young, lean, healthy, and energetic even though I'm now over fifty.

Reliable Information Is the Key

I've been there, and I want to teach you—once and for all—that no matter what your life circumstances may be, you can take crucial steps to regain control of the way you take care of yourself—for an immediate change. Even if you've never had a major crisis but have simply neglected yourself, *The 24-Hour Turnaround* will help you see dramatic changes. In this book I will show you how the 8 TLCs can affect you today, tomorrow—and in years to come.

Not long ago, one of my clients, Kim, came into my office with a look of frustration and announced, "I've eaten virtually nothing for the past two weeks but salad, and I'm starving. The scale has not budged, and I can't take it one more day. I have no energy and am so irritable that I have to drink several glasses of wine after work so I don't snap at my husband or kids. I need help!"

I calmly asked, "Well, what if I told you that just one glass of wine stops your body's ability to burn fat for forty-eight hours? And no matter how much you diet, exercise is the key to burning fat and building muscle?" Kim responded with surprise, saying, "Wine causes you to stop burning fat? My doctor told me a glass or two of wine may help me relax, and I've read that wine is good for your heart. I really need to lose weight and increase my energy. How can I turn this around?"

Now you too, just like Kim, can have the answer to this question. I will give you the most up-to-date health information—and information is the foundation for a belief system. A significant reason for eating food that is not beneficial to health or weight loss is having a weak belief or grave misunderstanding about the need for eating nutritious food. A typical reason for living an inactive life is a weak belief or, again, misunderstanding about the body's ability to affect the mind and the emotions. And most people have very little belief or knowledge about the effect water can have on the aging process. Through my years of diet and health counseling, I've seen that lack of credible information is the reason most people fail when they begin a new diet or health plan. Knowledge is power, and information is how you get it.

So where do you turn for credible health information? Most of us get health information from our doctors, health or diet books, TV commercials, magazines, celebrities, and the Internet. But problems arise because this information is often incomplete, ineffective, outdated, and only occasionally tested on humans, if at all.

While there are a few doctors, including Dr. Dean Ornish, who have provided extremely valuable studies and information in their books, most of the popular diet and health books that I've reviewed are based on a theoretical nutritional premise or on clinical experience limited to a particular disease condition. Very few authors of modern diet books actually work with people on a daily basis, tracking their progress and listening to their problems.

CELEBRITY DIETS: PRIME TIME OR WASTE OF TIME?

Not only are popular diet and health books presenting inaccurate or slanted information to readers, books written by celebrities may be setting you up for failure as well. These highly marketed books usually prescribe a celebrity's glitzy fad diet or health gimmick rather than a practical lifestyle plan that really works. In my opinion, most celebrities have the *least* experience at solving problems of weight loss or degenerative medical conditions. I know this because I work with celebrities! The truth is, many people (especially young people) are infatuated with what celebrities say and do and therefore are influenced by their opinions. But when it comes to your health, following a celebrity's advice could be a grave mistake—especially when you see that the same public figure who is promoting a diet book or miraculous health cure also recently endorsed a cigarette company.

BRINGING EXERCISE UP TO DATE

Unfortunately, the exercise industry, like the medical industry, tends to wait until studies are complete to implement new and effective changes. Therefore, trends in training are somewhat behind the latest information, and it's not always easy to locate a fitness professional who is current with all the latest findings. The industry as a whole has not been successful in painting a complete picture of how profoundly a single hour of exercise can impact the other 23 hours of your day, and they have failed to adequately describe—at least in the popular press—how exercise interacts with your weight, your hormones, and ultimately with how quickly or slowly your body ages. There are many manufacturers of so-called wellness and fitness products that are more concerned with their profits than your health or weight loss. I find this irresponsible, especially with new reports that some 300,000 Americans die each year from illnesses caused or worsened by obesity, a condition that may soon overtake cigarette smoking as the chief cause of preventable deaths—and one that could be halted with the 24-Hour Turnaround.

What's Holding You Back?

Before you can make any lifestyle change, including breaking negative habits, you need to look inside yourself to see what's holding you back. I have heard all the excuses people have for not losing weight, for not exercising, and for not doing something about their health. From my experience, I have identified the following four main stumbling blocks that keep men and women from sticking with a diet and fitness program. The good news is that all of these can be resolved to allow you to become different—healthier, leaner, and younger looking—starting today.

Check the statements that apply to your situation, and then keep reading to find ways you can use the Total Life Changes to get past your stumbling blocks or negative habits.

- BOREDOM

    ___The exercise routine gets old after a week or two.

    ___I get sick of eating just lettuce, carrots, and apples.

    ___I fall asleep when I meditate.

    ___I never lose weight fast enough, so eventually I stop dieting.

- STRESS

    ___I have problems in my marriage (or other relationship).

    ___I have too many deadlines at work to stick with a plan.

___I have an important event in a few weeks and feel overwhelmed.

___Having to prepare a special diet makes me anxious since I'm not a cook.

⬤ A V O I D A N C E

___I gained 20 pounds after my divorce, and a new diet won't help now.

___I broke my ankle a few years ago, and I'm hesitant to start exercising again.

___I've always been overweight. Both my parents were overweight. It just runs in our family.

___I don't feel good while I'm exercising or when I'm finished.

⬤ H A B I T

___I always watch the news after dinner and then read in bed. I couldn't start a new routine at this age.

___We always have pizza on Thursday night and Chinese food on Friday night. I'd hate to change this.

___When I get up in the morning, I immediately drink coffee. There's no way I could force a glass or two of water down first.

___I religiously have a glass of wine with dinner every night. I can't substitute water or tea.

_____

Taking Charge of Your Health

No one can resolve your personal weight and fitness issues but *you;* each of us must take personal responsibility for our own health. But we all know that no matter how good our intentions are, the people we love can either support us or undermine our actions. I will show you how to deal with family members and friends so they do not sabotage your 24-Hour Turnaround.

Forty-two-year-old Vivian said that after starting the 24-Hour Turnaround, losing 20 pounds, and meeting a new man, her friends acted thrilled and sent her a bottle of expensive champagne. "They knew I made the 'no alcohol' pledge because drinking packs on the pounds and is unhealthy. I felt like they were trying to sabotage my efforts. So I took the champagne to a birthday luncheon a few weeks later and watched my girlfriends drink it all. The temptation was gone for me, and I wasn't interested in adding any more toxins to my body."

Keep in mind that you are doing the 24-Hour Turnaround for you—not for your husband, children, mother, sister, doctor, or best friends. Let your motivation to start the 24-Hour Turnaround come from within and then watch how it changes you into a completely different, more contented person. If family members and friends try to discourage you and get you off track, reread the chapter on Total Life Change 1 to reevaluate why *you* are doing the program and motivate *you* to recommit to good health. Within each chapter I'll also give you a few surefire tips on how to include family members in your healthy antiaging program so they can reap positive health benefits too.

I invite you to come to Hawaii, check into the spa, and take time for you. There are so many actions, large and small, that you can take to lose weight and reduce problems associated with aging. I want you to learn these techniques that have successfully changed so many lives. In the meantime, I offer you the same effective program in *The 24-Hour Turnaround*. By tomorrow, I know that you will be well on your way to a leaner, stronger, and healthier body—and a totally different you!

Dare to Be Different
—in Just 24 Hours

YOU MAY BE THINKING, "I'm not sure I'm ready to start another diet." Or, "Everyone likes me just the way I am." The 24-Hour Turnaround is *not* a diet, and *you* may like yourself a whole lot better once you begin!

As you start your Turnaround, you will increase your body's reserves and enhance its ability to heal itself at the cellular level. Techniques from your Turnaround will also facilitate dramatic changes in your body to promote youthfulness at a physiological, emotional, and mental level. Within 24 hours of starting your program, you will notice increased energy, alertness, and vitality. Within hours of starting your Definition Diet, your blood chemistry will change. Within hours of increasing your fluid intake, your cells will be hydrated and performing at increased levels. Within minutes of starting a meditation exercise, your blood pressure will change. During and after your H.E.A.R.T. workout, you will increase your fat-burning enzymes. And—in case I forget to mention it—within 24 hours of increasing blood flow to your sexual organs, your romantic life will be exciting and fulfilling again.

I'll never forget Julia, a vivacious forty-two-year-old attorney from Manhattan who came to Hawaii one summer to check out the spa. Julia had gained almost 20 pounds since law school, and while it didn't affect her activity level, it was a red flag for problems she might face with increased age—being overweight influences high blood pressure and diabetes, and both ran in her family. Yet when I consulted with Julia and started to explain my 24-Hour Turnaround, she immediately assured me that it was not for her, saying, "I feel fine! I love to eat, and I'm not going to train for a marathon. I just want to enjoy the here and now, and I'm not really concerned about when I am going to die."

I'm *all* about enjoying my life too. And the here and now is great if you are young and healthy—but most people over forty with that attitude are like ticking time bombs just waiting to explode. I asked Julia to consider the following before she went back to New York and settled back into her couch potato lifestyle:

- What if the blood flow to your brain were increased? What if you could think more clearly, feel more alert, and have greater concentration? Wouldn't you get greater benefits from life?

- What if the blood flow to your heart were improved? What if increased oxygen in your muscles allowed you to burn more fat and have a thinner body? Wouldn't you be more active and enjoy life even more?

- What if the blood flow to your sexual organs were increased and your sexual potency improved? No matter what your age, wouldn't your life be more sensual and pleasurable?

- What if the nutrient-dense whole foods you ate were delicious and satisfying? What if the Definition Diet increased your energy and productivity and also helped you look young again? Wouldn't your life become more fulfilling than ever before?

After attending a meditation class at the spa and listening to other women's experiences, Julia was finally convinced to start the Turnaround. Interestingly, her biggest fear was that the whole foods prescribed by the Definition Diet would not fill her up or taste good! She was surprised that the chef's vegetable lasagna (made with soy) tasted like the "real thing." Julia even began to enjoy her H.E.A.R.T. workout before she left to go home. Last I heard, Julia had dropped 16 pounds, had more energy than she did in college, and was planning to visit the spa during the holidays.

Getting Organized

As you start your Turnaround, here are some necessary tools you will need to gather or purchase and some helpful Turnaround Tips that will make the program easier to implement.

Turnaround Tip 1. Start a daily journal. An integral part of your Turnaround includes keeping a daily journal. I am a huge believer in journaling, as it allows you to experience an in-depth awareness of your life. I like the discipline of keeping track of my exercise hours, daily food choices, and personal stats, such as weight, energy levels, and mood. Journaling also helps me identify my deepest concerns or destructive emotions as I write about personal insights, relationships, and even vivid dreams that may, in fact, affect my daily behavior, including what I eat, how much I exercise, and even my outlook on life.

Research shows that keeping a written record of your life is a powerful way to identify your barriers—stumbling blocks you may not normally see. The data-gathering is not just about keeping track of your weight or food choices. Rather, it's about tracking the processes that affect your weight and overall health and also about measuring your progress every day. Once you've gathered enough information, use your problem-solving skills to analyze it, and then brainstorm ways to overcome personal barriers.

For instance, you may find that your weight stays the same for three weeks in a row. I know that can be frustrating, especially for those who have set a weight-loss goal and worked hard to monitor their food choices and exercise diligently. Yet after you read through your daily journal, you may see some emotional stumbling blocks that occurred, such as an argument with your child or coworker. You may read that you ate a few (or many!) servings of that favorite Italian dish and some homemade chocolate chip cookies while visiting your relatives. And you may note that your water intake was greatly reduced one week, and you had several alcoholic drinks after work with friends. While none of these are earth-shattering problems, they alert you to the exact factors that sabotaged your weight loss, helping you become more focused on your Turnaround, follow the Definition Diet more mindfully, and be keenly aware that emotions and stress are linked with snacking or overeating. I remind my clients who have a sweet tooth that *stressed* spelled backward is *desserts*. They get the message quickly!

Make a copy of the page from my favorite journal (see page 19). Or purchase a three-ring notebook or Day-Timer to use as your journal. Keep your journal on your desk or in your purse, so you have easy access to it throughout the day. If you are too busy during the day to take time for journaling, then set a time, such as after dinner, to record in your journal. Some clients do a daily journal on their computer by starting a file called Turnaround or Total Life Changes. Any method is acceptable, as long as you can access this information for daily updates. Find what method works best for you and stay committed to it.

Turnaround Tip 2: Schedule time for exercise, grocery shopping, and meditation. Many clients ask, "How can I find time for exercise and meditation if I am already overly committed with my career, family, and community obligations?" You find time for yourself by making yourself a top priority in your life. I'm sure that if your child wanted to take gymnastics, you'd make the time to take her to classes each week. Or if your spouse asked for more time alone with you, you'd find a way to ensure time for R&R (relaxation and romance!).

I want you to do the same for yourself. I want you to set aside time each week for exercise, meditation, and food shopping, and I want you to keep those "you" appointments—they're mandatory! You will also need to allow for a couple of hours at a natural food store before you start the Definition Diet, to stock up on natural and organic whole foods. This could be an educational weekend activity for you and any family member who will join in.

Hint: Use an on-line calendar—you fill in the dates and times, and the program alerts you to these commitments at a future date. Check with your Internet service provider to see if such a calendar is available.

Turnaround Tip 3: Collect the necessary equipment to begin the TLCs. Make sure you have the following available:

- *Tape measure.* Any inexpensive tape measure will do.

- *Athletic shoes.* Get a good running or cross-training shoe with a sturdy arch support and wide base for stabilization.

- *Heart-rate monitor.* The heart-rate monitor is the secret to the success of your H.E.A.R.T. workout. I encourage you to purchase or borrow one before you

	Prioritize To Do Today A, B, or C	Attitude P or N	Stress Level 1–10	Vitamin Times	Water Times	Water Ounces	Fiber Grams	Fat Grams
Exercise A								

Day _____ Date _____

Warm water (lemon optional) _____

Breakfast _____

Snack _____

Lunch _____

Snack _____

Dinner _____

Snack _____

Other? _____

Totals

Exercise Minutes _____

Hours of Waking Inactivity _____

Total Hours of Sleep Last Night _____

Perceived Effort _____

Mood Today _____

Quality of Sleep _____

Heart Rate _____

Time to Bed _____

Notes:

begin the program. You can use a basic heart-rate monitor with a transmitter chest strap and a wrist receiver that displays your heart rate. (You wear it like a watch.) Many sporting goods stores or bike shops offer heart-rate monitors for around $49 to $79, or check my website at www.24hourturnaround.com for recommendations. This is the price of a dinner, a pair of shoes, or a doctor's visit. Once you start to exercise with a monitor, you will never leave home without it. Monitoring your heart rate is the only way to guarantee reduction of body fat if you are a woman. You'll also learn a lifesaving stress-reduction technique with your new "personal trainer" on your wrist.

- *Water bottle to use during H.E.A.R.T. exercise.* Keep your water bottle filled when you exercise, and use it frequently to stay hydrated. You may need two bottles if you are going to be away from home and there is no source of bottled water. Clean the bottle out each night with warm water and soap, and let it air dry.

- *Nutrient counter.* Purchase a paperback book that lists all foods and their fat and fiber content. Two of my favorites are *The Complete Book of Food Counts* by Corinne Netzer and *The Most Complete Food Counter* by Annette B. Natow and Jo-Ann Heslin. There are also options on line that offer this information. Check with our website.

Turnaround Tip 4: Take your body measurements. Before you start your Turnaround, you need to weigh and measure yourself and write the stats in your journal. Time to break out the tape measure!

Biceps: Measure halfway between your shoulder and elbow at the widest part of your upper arm.

Waist: Measure the smallest part of your waistline, which should be close to belly button level.

Hips: Measure the widest part of your hips and buttocks. Don't worry, that number is going to get smaller!

Top of thigh: Go for the largest number on the top of your leg. (Yes, this will shrink too.)

Weight: Weigh yourself in the morning with your clothes off. Pick a time that you can replicate on other mornings.

After twenty-one days, take these body measurements again and record them in your journal. Fat takes up more room than muscle, so taking your measurements is a more reliable way of knowing that your body is changing than getting on a scale. If a body composition test is available at your gym or local university, take advantage of it; it's also an accurate way to measure your progress. Schedule a test this week and again in three months.

Turnaround Tip 5: Find your resting heart rate. You will need your resting heart rate to calculate your Zone One, which is discussed in TLC 2, the chapter on exercise. You can do this by strapping the heart-rate monitor on your chest immediately upon awakening. Place it by the side of the bed the evening before so you don't have to get out of bed. Now lie back in bed and relax. Write down the lowest heart rate you observe on the monitor.

If you do not have a heart-rate monitor, take your pulse manually for an entire 60 seconds. Remember to have a watch or a clock with a second hand by the side of the bed so you do not have to get up before taking your pulse. Write this number in your journal. I show you how to use this number in TLC 2.

Turnaround Tip 6: Bookmark www.24hourturnaround.com on your computer. Throughout the program, I will give you information on specific books, products, and other tools that will be helpful for your Turnaround.

Let's Start—Right Now!

If you were sitting in my office for this consultation, I would pour you a glass of water (not wine!) and say, "Okay, this is exciting! Let's start right now." The eight Total Life Changes I explain in this book will help you break old lifestyle habits and form new ones. Because it will take some time to read the entire book thoroughly, digesting all the new information about the TLCs and implementing them in your routine, I'm going to give you some ways to turn around your life right now. Start all of these Turnaround strategies *today*.

TLC 1: MAKE UP THREE POSITIVE "I AM" STATEMENTS

Think of three positive statements that describe the new you—the healthier, leaner, and younger-looking you that will come as a result of your Turnaround.

A host of studies confirm that among hospital patients, those who have positive expectations of their outcome tend to heal faster than those who are less hopeful about reaching their goals. It may be because positive expectations trigger a physical healing response while they motivate patients to be compliant and stick with prescribed therapies. In one review of the literature, researchers concluded that the association between positive expectations and reaching a health goal was the greatest in studies of parents who were trying to lose weight.

As you identify positive expectations for your Turnaround, I don't want to hear statements that describe what you *were* ("an overweight, middle-aged woman" or "a junk food addict whose hobby is watching television"). Rather, I now give you permission to become the person you want to be. Think of what you personally hope to accomplish with this program, and make it into a positive descriptive statement in the present tense. Some examples are:

"I am an incredibly healthy person who eats nutritious, whole foods."
"I am an athlete. I thrive on exercise, especially walking and swimming."
"I am a nondrinker. My body functions much better without toxic chemicals."
"I get plenty of sleep, going to bed early and waking up at least eight hours later."
"I crave water and what it does for my body and skin."
"I enjoy trying whole foods, substituting them for packaged or prepared foods."
"I practice self-care and set aside time to meditate and practice deep abdominal breathing each afternoon."

Keep the following Turnaround definitions in mind as you write your statements and become the new you:

Body. Noun. The whole material or physical structure of the living person.
Mind. Noun. The part of an individual that knows, thinks, reasons, wills. Awareness.
Spirit. Noun. The breath, the immaterial part of an individual, our religious or emotional nature. Energy.

Regimen. Noun. Set of habits of diet, exercise, or manner of living intended to improve health, reduce weight.

Write your three "I am" statements here:

1. _____

2. _____

3. _____

Remember to write positive statements in the present tense. I don't want to hear about what you won't or cannot do today or in the upcoming weeks. Your past is just that—past! In the following chapter on mastering motivation, TLC 1, I explain why positive thinking can keep you motivated to stay with your 24-Hour Turnaround. For now, write down your three statements, and then read them aloud. Memorize them, and say them as you fall asleep tonight, and then again upon awakening before you get out of bed.

THE 24-HOUR PAYBACK

The word *motivation* comes from the Latin word *movere*, "to move." Motivation is not something you have or do not have but more like a throttle that has a low, medium, and high gear. Highly motivated people know how to rev up this mechanism every day. In the chapter on TLC 1, you will acquire the motivational skills to keep you on the path to a lean body, good health, and an extended life span.

TLC 2: GET PHYSICAL

Start moving today—even if you only take a short, moderate-intensity walk around your neighborhood (see Determining Intensity of Exercise). Go ahead and tie up your shoelaces now, and start using your muscles to elevate your heart rate.

If I could recommend one cure-all to help you lose weight, get lean muscles, and halt or even reverse the signs of aging, it would be *exercise*. Too bad this remedy does not come in a bottle at your pharmacy! As I explain in the chapter on TLC 2, exercise has been proved to keep you lean, fit, and younger looking and feeling, and it's available to anyone. Oh! And it's free.

If you're a beginner and are more than thirty pounds overweight, I want you to enjoy a 15-minute walk at an easy to moderate pace. Try to walk outdoors, if possible, so you can benefit from the sun and nature. If you can't walk outside, use an indoor treadmill. Or walk inside your local mall, but skip the window-shopping and focus more on your breathing and movement. Just remember to stay at a moderate pace and not overdo it. More is not better when it comes to beginning a regular exercise program, particularly if you have spent the last ten years sitting in your BarcaLounger, exercising your wrist with your remote control. (If you are over forty, check with your doctor before you start the exercise program.)

While you are walking, I want you to feel your entire body working—your legs tightening, hips moving, muscles pulling. Tighten your buns and abs; make a fist and swing your arms with determination. Hold your head up and shoulders back; bend your knees, and use a long stride. Ask your muscles to move you. Connect your mind with your muscles, and your workout will be more effective.

If you are fit and already in an exercise program, I want you to upgrade your current workout today by taking the following two steps:

1. *Engage as many muscles as you can to do the workout movement.* I always tell my clients to judge the quality of their aerobic workout by how many muscles they use to elevate the heart rate. For instance, if you normally run for exercise, I want you to walk uphill instead, using arm and ab resistance, making deliberate arm movements, and holding a slight pelvic tuck to engage your abs and buns. If you do aerobic classes, choose a low-impact aerobic class or a sculpt class that focuses on the upper body and incorporates standing or functional ab exercises. If you regularly spin, slow down and stand, or include an upper-body segment in your spinning regimen.

2. *Go for an hour (or longer if you can).* I want you to lower—yes, lower—your heart rate and increase the length of your workout. Unfortunately, many fit women have forgotten what *moderate intensity* feels like. So use this guideline: work at an intensity that allows you to say aloud "I could do this for hours." (If you have difficulty talking, slow down until you can easily speak.) Trust me, your workout will feel much better both during and afterward.

DETERMINING INTENSITY OF EXERCISE

You'll need a heart-rate monitor to get the most out of TLC 2, but in the meantime there are some other easy ways to determine the intensity of your exercise. Using a scale of 1 to 10, where 10 represents high exertion and 1 stands for low exertion, I want you to use a perceived exertion of 5. One way to determine this is to make sure you can still sing a few lines of your favorite song. Go ahead, don't be shy! I want you to be able to talk (or sing) during exercise. If you have difficulty doing either, you're pushing it way too hard and need to slow down.

After 12 minutes at a good pace, try to find your pulse on your neck or wrist, and once you've found it, count for six seconds and remember that number. If you have trouble finding it, don't worry—your heart-rate monitor will make the job simple and efficient. If you were successful in tracking your pulse for six seconds, write that number down.

If you do have a heart-rate monitor, do exactly the same as above, walking at a perceived exertion of 5 and making a mental note of the number on your monitor so you can write it down after you finish exercising. You'll use that number to evaluate your fitness level after you learn about Zone training. If you are injured or if it is uncomfortable to walk, use a bicycle (stationary or open road) or swim.

If you're tempted to go for the burn, watch out. It may show on your face and in your hormone balance in the next 24 hours. It's a known fact among exercise experts that high-intensity exercise ages you. It greatly increases your appetite for carbohydrates, dehydrates you, and will not give you the fat loss you are probably looking for.

Wear your new heart-rate monitor, if you have it, and write down the heart rate numbers observed during your workout. They'll come in handy when we delve further into TLC 2.

THE 24-HOUR PAYBACK

- Increased blood flow to the muscles, skin, brain, and sex organs
- A burst of energizing hormones
- Increased stimulation to the nervous system to produce chemicals called

endorphins that elevate mood and produce feelings of well-being and self-confidence

- Greater production of the enzymes that make you a better fat-burner for the next 24 hours and give an immediate boost to your sluggish metabolism

TLC 3: PLAN YOUR MENU TODAY

I want you to make plans now—*on paper*—for what you will eat today. I'll give you detailed information on the Definition Diet in the chapter on TLC 3, but for now, here's a Turnaround challenge to get you started: *Eat whole food today.*

What is whole food? Whole food is "nature's own"—in its natural state, unprocessed, and not packaged. Pretend that you are the first person on earth and are searching for food. You can't eat anything that comes in a bag, can, or box—and certainly nothing processed or prepared. The food has to come from a tree or bush. Or you have to pull it out of the ground. Check your refrigerator for those foods that prehistoric people may have eaten. Include your children in the game. Suggest that they pretend to be prehistoric children and see if they can figure out what whole foods to eat. If there are none in your refrigerator, consider it a wake-up call to get to the grocery store ASAP. Some whole food choices for today might include the following:

Apples	Cauliflower	Mushrooms
Apricots	Chard	Onions
Artichokes	Eggplants	Pears
Asparagus	Grains (only whole)	Peas
Avocados	Grapefruit	Peppers (green, red, yellow,
Bananas	Grapes	orange)
Beans (green, wax)	Greens (collard, turnip)	Potatoes (white, sweet)
Beets	Kale	Raspberries
Blueberries	Kiwi	Soybeans
Broccoli	Legumes (dried)	Spinach
Brussels sprouts	Lentils	Squash (summer, winter)
Cabbage (red, green)	Melons (cantaloupe,	Strawberries
Carrots	honeydew)	Tomatoes

Menu Tip 1. Eliminate red meat and anything white (white bread, flour, white rice).

Menu Tip 2. If you eat animal products, choose tuna, salmon, chicken breast, or turkey (white meat only, cooked without the skin); use only nonfat dairy products.

Menu Tip 3. Watch for sugar in hidden places. If you think your diet has been relatively low in sugar, I challenge you to read the packaging labels on foods you commonly ate to see how sugar is used (look for sugar, glucose, sucrose, dextrose, fructose, crystalline fructose, high-fructose corn syrup, corn syrup, molasses, malt sugar, malitol, sorbitol, and mannitol, among others). On the Definition Diet, you can use a little honey or fruit spread on your toast.

Make your choices. Now review the following ten food choices and select three that you will enjoy for today's menu. In TLC 3, the Definition Diet chapter, you will learn how these whole foods can help accelerate weight loss, give you 24-hour energy, and keep you satisfied, young looking, and healthy.

1. *Beans, lentils, or peas.* Have lentil/split pea soup, garbanzo beans on your salad, or a veggie burrito.
2. *Nuts.* Have ½ ounce or about 10 to 12 nuts only (nuts are high in calories) as a snack or on salads or veggies.
3. *Dried fruit.* Choose an ounce of raisins, peaches, apples, prunes, apricots, cranberries, or pears. Dried fruits are easy to pack and carry with you for quick and nutritious snacks away from home. (The Hunzas of eastern Pakistan eat dried apricots, among other dried fruits, and live to be well over a hundred.)
4. *Whole grain.* Choose barley, bran, brown rice, bulgur, couscous, millet, oats, polenta, or quinoa as a cooked cereal or grain with your dinner.
5. *Tomatoes.* Eat at least 4 slices per serving.
6. *Soy.* Choose 1 cup (8 ounces) of light soy milk or a serving of edamame, tempeh, or tofu.
7. *Peppers (green, yellow, orange, or red), carrots, or cabbage.* Use sliced, diced, chopped, or whole. Put in salads, soups, or sandwiches. Or use for dipping. Remember, raw is best!

8. *Broccoli.* Use raw florets and chopped stems in your dinner salads or eat them steamed crisp (lightly steamed).
9. *Two pieces of fruit.* Choose citrus fruits, apples, bananas, blueberries, grapes, guavas, mangoes, melons, papayas, pears, strawberries, or others. One serving size is ½ cup berries, 12 grapes, or a medium-size piece of fruit.
10. *Nonfat dairy.* If you choose to eat dairy, select skim or nonfat milk, low-fat or nonfat yogurt, cheese, or cottage cheese. Organic is best.

Eat more frequently. "Students, you must always eat three balanced meals each day, and no snacks." I can still hear my high school home economics teacher telling us that eating three meals with no between-meal snacks was the "proven way" to stay lean and healthy. Three decades ago, most experts did promote eating three meals a day and no snacks. But times have changed, and now nutritionists know that minimeals (more frequent, smaller meals) can keep your blood sugar level stable and your energy level up, keep you from binge eating, and help you lose weight. Eat minimeals by taking your total food for the day and splitting it into five or six portions.

Try not to go more than 3 hours without some form of nutrition. If it has been 3 hours since lunch, then snack on a piece of fruit, ½ ounce nuts, a piece of dried fruit, or a nonfat organic yogurt. Have dinner 2 or 3 hours later. If you have dinner after 7 P.M., make sure it totals less than 500 calories. Heavy eating before bedtime makes it difficult to maintain deep sleep, as your body is focused on digesting food instead of revitalizing itself. And how many times have you been awakened with heartburn after eating a heavy meal before bedtime?

We have many facts to sort out, some shopping to do, and some decisions to make to personalize your 24-hour strategy. We also have to decide what to do about friends, husband, and/or family—those well-meaning people whom you adore yet who seem to sabotage your efforts to be healthy. I know that making radical changes in your diet can be difficult—or it can be challenging and fun. And if you like to eat as much as I do, you probably look forward to trying some new and delicious foods, perhaps recipes you've seen but never tried. Now it will be even more exciting, because those same foods will be a part of your Definition Diet, defining the course of your health and longevity, defining your physiological age, and defining those lean, strong muscles that are hiding under a layer of body fat.

THE 24-HOUR PAYBACK

- Improved body chemistry
- Increased metabolism
- Greater blood volume available to your brain, your sexual organs, and your muscles
- Increased satiety and more energy
- Deep, healing sleep and improved attitude
- More effective and efficient fat-burning during your training tomorrow
- Happier hormones

Take your vitamins. I also want you to take your vitamins. Don't worry too much about what kind of vitamins they are, just take some of whatever you have on hand. I want you to establish a pattern of behavior—to have a specific place for your vitamins and a certain time of day at which you take them. If you're out of vitamins, have a glass of water instead. In TLC 3, the chapter on the Definition Diet, we will sort through the most important ways to use whole food supplements for weight loss, antiaging, and good health, including which supplements to buy and when to take them for the greatest benefit.

As you will learn in TLC 3, the most important nutrients come from whole plant foods. I do not want you to rely on a pill for optimal health—and never, ever rely on a pill for weight loss. The best vitamins you can take are better described as specialized food concentrates, which are included in the whole foods that you eat.

THE 24-HOUR PAYBACK

Certain vitamins and minerals are not made by the body and have to be replaced at least once a day. Vitamin C is one of those. Raising levels of these health-boosting substances immediately begins to protect you from the oxidative damage that causes aging and disease. Increasing the levels of missing nutrients also helps to bring your body into balance. It takes a healthy and balanced body to lose weight and to keep it off for a lifetime, and your Turnaround will help you meet this harmonious goal.

TLC 4: HYDRATE

I want you to start hydrating your body today by drinking at least 10 glasses of water by bedtime. It's no news that most of us, even the most health-conscious people, forget one of the most life-supporting substances: water. Water cleanses your system, detoxifies your cells, carries oxygen and nutrients to all cells, and acts as a giant cooling system to regulate your body temperature.

Starting right now, I want you to drink a tall glass of water. If you'd like, keep fresh lemon slices in the refrigerator to use for added flavor in your water. (Bonus: lemon has proven antiviral and antibacterial properties.) In 1 hour, have another glass of water. You are now well on your way to healing your dehydrated body.

Every day, every waking hour on the hour, drink a *minimum* of 8 ounces (1 cup) of water. Drink more if you can. If you are reading this chapter in the middle of the day, have 16 ounces (2 cups) right now. Aim for 8 ounces (1 cup) every hour until bedtime. Keep drinking until your urine is clear.

RED FLAG

Beware! By the time you are thirsty, you are already 1 to 2 percent dehydrated and aging your cells at a rapid rate. Drink water by a schedule, not by your body's thirst.

If you still have a thirst indicator, you are lucky—most of us don't. A lifetime of *not* drinking enough water has desensitized us to our actual level of need. Learn to reactivate your sensitive thirst detector, and drink *before* you think you are thirsty. In the chapter on TLC 4 we will calculate your personal hydration goals.

THE 24-HOUR PAYBACK

- Fully hydrated cells that age at a slower pace
- Increased fat-burning
- Improved digestion and elimination
- Hydrated brain cells for improved mood and concentration
- Healthy, hydrated skin

TLC 5: HAVE AN ALCOHOL-FREE 24 HOURS

Do *not* have another glass of alcohol until you've read TLC 5, "Alcohol and the Myth of Moderation." One of the first questions on my client profile form is "Do you drink alcohol?" It's ironic that I usually get the answer "No. I only have wine or beer with dinner."

Read my lips: wine and beer are alcoholic drinks! A critical part of the interview process when a new client comes to me is determining whether she or he can give up alcohol on their Turnaround. If the answer is no, then I ask these clients to rethink their health priority and resolve the need for alcohol or I will not be much help to them.

Not only are there life-threatening consequences associated with drinking alcohol, but that one little glass of wine is guaranteed to disrupt your deep, antiaging sleep and slow down your fat-burning mechanism. Alcohol's empty calories also replace whole foods that have beneficial nutrients. And alcohol is known to be toxic in relationships and cause even the most cautious people to say things or act in ways that are out of character and that they will later regret.

THE 24-HOUR PAYBACK

- Improved body chemistry within the first 24 hours
- Prevention of cancerous tumor growth
- More efficient fat-burning

- Balanced hormones
- Immediate overall health upgrade
- Hydrated skin cells that instantly look better

TLC 6: GO TO BED 15 MINUTES EARLIER

Plan to get into bed 15 minutes earlier than normal tonight—even if you don't immediately fall asleep. Whatever you normally do during that last 15 minutes of the day can be done the next morning. Unless you are an extreme night owl, you are probably more efficient in the morning than at midnight anyway. Set your alarm 15 minutes earlier tomorrow morning to help you recapture that extra bit of time and reset your body clock. In TLC 6 you will learn how quality sleep will keep you leaner, younger, and healthier.

RED FLAG

Not only does sleep deprivation make you fatigued, unable to concentrate, and irritable, losing sleep over a long period of time can reduce your functioning capacity. A surprising study published on October 23, 1999, in *The Lancet* revealed that the young adults in the trial who cut sleep from 8 hours to 4 hours each night had striking changes in glucose tolerance and endocrine function, representing the effects of advanced age or even the early stages of diabetes. These changes were reversed when the volunteers spent 12 hours in bed.

I'm not asking you to spend 12 hours in bed. But I do want to educate you on the importance of sleep and how getting 8 hours or more each night can reverse some of the key markers of aging.

THE 24-HOUR PAYBACK

- Increased tissue and cell regeneration and rejuvenation for antiaging results
- Improved quantity and quality of sleep that increases antiaging hormones

- Boost in immune function
- Reduced mood swings and greater optimism
- Increased alertness
- Boost in productivity
- Production of weight-loss hormones

TLC 7: EAT SOY FOODS TO BALANCE HORMONES

New research continues to point to soy foods high in phytoestrogens for reducing or erasing the symptoms of perimenopause and menopause. Phytoestrogens occur naturally in plants and mimic the role of estrogen in the body without the harmful side effects. The most common phytoestrogens are isoflavones, flavones, and lignins.

I include two servings of soy in my daily diet. It is inexpensive, dairy-free, and low in saturated fat. But even more, soy is a complete protein source that can help keep your hormones stable. Soy helps reduce your rate of heart disease, breast cancer, and osteoporosis. The rates of these diseases are much lower for Asian women, who traditionally have a diet high in soy, than for Americans.

Today, choose one serving from the following list:

Roasted soy nuts	¼ cup
Tempeh	½ cup
Tofu	½ cup
Edamame (soybeans)	½ cup
Low-fat soy milk	1 cup

TLC 8: TAKE A 2-MINUTE BREAK

Stress is synonymous with aging, disease, and weight gain. In TLC 8 you will learn how innercise can reverse the effects of stress. For today, schedule a 2-minute rejuvenation break between 12 and 2 P.M. Scientists know that our thoughts and feelings influence our body through the nervous system and the circulatory system, particularly through the heart. These are the pathways of communication between the brain and the rest of the body. Although you cannot control the intrusions of

> "Only the person who is relaxed can create, and to that mind ideas flow like lightning."
>
> —Cicero

daily life, you can find 2 minutes to meditate or to do deep breathing or biofeedback. These mind-body exercises solicit the relaxation response, producing a feeling of calmness and a sense of control that comes from within.

Studies have shown that meditation can have an amazing effect on you in the first minute and have lasting effects during the day. Choose one of the following activities for your stress-reducing break. If you have time, do this relaxation activity again around 4 P.M. for at least 2 minutes.

2-MINUTE DEEP BREATHING WITH VISUALIZATION

1. Either lying on your back or sitting straight in your chair, close your eyes, tune out all distractions, and focus on the present moment.

2. Slowly inhale, focusing on your breathing as you do so, and then slowly exhale; repeat three times.

3. Now imagine that you are a strong swimmer, lying on your back and freely floating faceup in the clear water. Feel how the water surrounds your body— your legs, back, shoulders, and head, holding you afloat without effort.

4. Slowly inhale and exhale, twice. Again focus on your breath and how it calms all your senses. Notice how your heart rate is slowing down and your muscle tension is easing.

5. Now envision that you are an eagle with full wingspread, soaring high above the earth. Sense how the air holds you as if you were a feather.

6. Slowly inhale and exhale, twice.

7. See yourself in a slow and graceful free fall, surrounded by warm, bright light. Now open your eyes, and celebrate the calmer you.

2-MINUTE MEDITATION OR PRAYER

1. Go to a quiet place, so you can meditate or pray without distraction. Get away from the telephone, computer, television, or any other intrusion.

2. Sit in a chair or lie down on the floor. Relax your body, and then close your eyes. Slowly inhale and exhale three times, paying attention to your breathing, as it is life itself.

3. Now close your eyes and use this quiet time for a 2-minute prayer to God or your Higher Power, acknowledging the sanctity of life and love not created by human hands. Or meditate for 2 minutes using a simple sound like "om," or "one," saying this repeatedly and focusing on your breath instead of on the worries of the day.

THE 24-HOUR PAYBACK

- Reduced heart rate
- Lower blood pressure
- Increase in antiaging hormones
- Reduced levels of cortisol, a stress hormone
- Improved mood
- Decreased appetite
- Greater ability to focus
- Increased antiaging oxygen to the cells

——

A Review of the 24-Hour Turnaround: Eight Total Life Changes to Start Right Now!

TLC 1: Make up three positive "I am" statements.
TLC 2: Get physical.
TLC 3: Plan your menu today.
TLC 4: Hydrate.
TLC 5: Have an alcohol-free 24 hours.

TLC 6: Go to bed 15 minutes earlier.

TLC 7: Eat soy foods to balance hormones.

TLC 8: Take a 2-minute break.

Just Do It! Five Easy Ways to Stop Procrastinating

"These Total Life Changes sound great in theory, but I still have some hurdles to overcome to make them work for me." Mira, age fifty-three, is the woman I spoke about in the Introduction who had lost 300 pounds (the same 15 pounds gained back twenty times). She did have a lot to overcome. She craved red meat, loved to drink wine in the evening while watching old movies, and lived a stressful and sedentary life as a magazine editor.

If all you have just read sounds good in theory but you are having trouble getting past a personal problem area, I know how to help. I've had many clients who were slow starters, but once they got going they made up for lost time. The following client problems are typical when undertaking a life-changing program, particularly one as dramatic as the 24-Hour Turnaround. Read each problem, then consider how you can apply the action to your own situation.

PROBLEM: CONFUSION

"The 24-Hour Turnaround is just what I need, but it seems so overwhelming. I honestly don't know how to find a starting point."

—Jenny, 39

ACTION: MAKE MOLEHILLS OUT OF MOUNTAINS

If the entire program seems overwhelming, then realize that the simple Turnaround strategies in this chapter are easy to incorporate into your daily routine. Once you've accepted these changes as healthy new habits, then slowly work in more specific lifestyle changes that are detailed in the chapters on TLCs 1 through 8. Perhaps one day you can make some changes in your diet, as outlined in TLC 3. Once this becomes a habit, make another change, such as adding some mind-body

DETOX YOUR BODY—STOP SMOKING TODAY

f you smoke, stop. Smoking makes you look old; it damages your skin, causing deep wrinkles; and it triggers an early menopause. It will also keep you from realizing the total health benefits of your Turnaround.

America spends more than $50 billion each year in health care costs for ailments that are attributable to smoking, including cancer, heart disease, atherosclerosis, stroke, lung disease, diabetes, and peptic ulcer. And each year more than 400,000 people die of the direct effects of cigarette smoking. Perhaps even more disturbing, more than one-third of all high school students currently smoke cigarettes.

Cigarette smoke contains thousands of chemicals—and two hundred of them are known to be poisonous. The chemical nicotine is addictive, and it takes only 10 seconds to be absorbed in the bloodstream and reach the brain. Once in the body, nicotine "hits" brain cell receptors and stimulates the release of neurotransmitters—the brain's chemical messengers. These messengers—acetylcholine, dopamine, serotonin, and beta-endorphin—affect how we pay attention, think, eat, deal with stress, and feel pleasure. If you smoke, now you know why you anxiously reach for a cigarette when you are faced with life's stressors—or even boredom.

Though smoking increases the risk of serious health problems, it is one harmful habit you can turn around today as you take charge of your health, longevity, and good looks. Talk to your doctor or call your local chapter of the American Lung Association or the American Cancer Society for ways to stop smoking.

innercise like deep breathing or a yoga position. If you break up the Turnaround program into small chunks, you will find that it is easy to learn and manage. Work on tips given in this chapter that you can do in a day, and focus on the changes you've made. Once you feel confident, begin adding more TLC changes outlined in this book.

Speaking of making changes in your daily routine, it's important to flex your "flexibility muscles" in your new program. By that I mean, do something different today, such as take a walk after dinner or have breakfast foods for dinner instead of your usual fare. You never know what changes you might enjoy, and breaking routine will help you get out of some bad habits that feel comfortable (like lying on the couch and watching TV all night!).

PROBLEM: FEAR OF RISK-TAKING

"I've been eating and sleeping this way for almost fifty years. I'm so afraid of changing my lifestyle for fear it won't work."

—Teresa, 48

ACTION: LEARN TO RELISH RISK

Many successful people face new situations and realize that they may make mistakes. Yet they also know that they'll gather new and valuable information along the way. The negative outcomes of your current habits are probably more devastating than making a few mistakes as you turn around your life and change your habits to increase health and longevity.

PROBLEM: LACK OF TIME, CAN'T PRIORITIZE

"How can I add one more activity to my day? As a single working mom, I never even finish the household chores or bill paying, much less have time to exercise."

—Candace, 53

ACTION: LEARN TO PLAN AHEAD

You can easily find time to include exercise and activity, as well as a 2-minute meditation or other stress reducer, if you plan ahead. Make a list of things that need to be accomplished today, including your exercise and 2-minute breaks. Use the following ABC method to determine your priorities. Then stick with your list.

Priority A—Absolutely must do. For example, exercise is a daily "must do." As you will soon learn, exercise always gets priority A.
Priority B—Better do. This task is a high priority, but not mandatory. Perhaps someone else could help.
Priority C—Could do. You can go to bed at night with no guilt if you haven't accomplished a priority C.

Write your daily "to do" list in your journal. Read the list aloud and ask how each action, commitment, or task relates to your life goals and objectives. (And the absolute truth is that these tasks won't be accomplished unless you have good health.) Assess the urgency of the task, and then ask yourself if you can delegate it to a family member, friend, or coworker.

They say that nothing is certain in life but change. Realize that change is inevitable, and begin to embrace it.

Learn to say no—and mean it. Failing to say no or set limits in your life will put you in overload and add to your already rising stress level, which can interfere with your food choices, exercise, and sleep. As you evaluate your daily "to do" list, surely there are many B and C level tasks or commitments. Cross these tasks out for the day or week if you are feeling overwhelmed. There are many shortcuts you can take during the day, but the amount of time you have to exercise (45 minutes or more) and the amount of sleep you need (about 7½ to 8½ hours) cannot be compromised.

PROBLEM: DIFFICULTY BEING "GOOD"

"I always wake up ready to go with the 24-Hour Turnaround. I tell myself that I *can* succeed and be 'good'! I drink my water followed by a healthy breakfast of fruits and grains. I eat yogurt for a midmorning snack. Then I have my lunch—usually tuna fish on whole-wheat bread with tomato slices, an apple, and carrots. I leave for a 45-minute walk after lunch—then destruction hits. When I get back to my office, everyone's having dessert—cookies, candy, and someone's homemade chocolate cake. Without fail, I go to the vending machine to buy a Snickers bar and practically inhale the chocolate-coated no-no, and it's downhill from there. Once I've been 'bad,' I give up and figure I'll start tomorrow. Help."

—Paula, 62

ACTION: FOCUS ON THE BIG PICTURE

While it's great to have daily goals, perfectionism can stop you in your tracks! If you do indulge in a candy bar or even if you eat a high-calorie lunch, consider that action in the past. And by the way, a bad person is not someone who eats a candy bar; I happen to know many good people who have horrible diets. Don't go there with the bad and good routine; it can be destructive and can lead to a host of unhealthy behaviors such as eating disorders. Move forward by completing the rest of the day with as many of the Total Life Changes as possible. Your daily journal will help you stay on track. If you accomplished one TLC that day, record it. Try for two the next day, and three the day after that. Soon the rewards of the Turnaround program will exceed any temptations you may have to cheat.

PROBLEM: FOOD CRAVINGS

"I can stay on the program for about two weeks. Then suddenly all I think about are the things I should not eat. How do I stop these cravings?"
—Rosemary, 45

ACTION: CRAVINGS ARE NORMAL. GIVE IN SOMETIMES!

You will have cravings—almost everyone does. But cravings often represent deficiencies, and once you address the deficiencies, you will use your natural motivation to transform these cravings back into positive habits, such as replacing the craved food with another whole food or even eating some of the craved food to satisfy the craving. Some tips I share with my clients on how to deal with cravings include:

1. Make sure you are doing your H.E.A.R.T. workout, as it regulates blood sugar levels and certain nerve chemicals that stimulate cravings.
2. Don't skip meals—ever. It's especially important to eat a healthy breakfast. Eating a satisfying breakfast can reduce cravings for the rest of the day.
3. Consider trying biofeedback, which has been shown to reduce cravings if they are related to emotional stress, boredom, or habit. Biofeedback is based on the idea that when people are given information about their bodies' internal processes, they can use this information to learn to control those processes. This type of therapy has been shown to bring about improvement in stress management as well as stress-related problems, including smoking and overeating.

I teach you an easy biofeedback technique using your heart-rate monitor in TLC 8, the chapter on destressing. In the meantime, try meditation and deep breathing to stop cravings when they surface—and, equally important, keep drinking water. It's hard to crave a fudge brownie when your stomach is filled with 3 glasses of water.

> "It is within our power to use the intelligence of our head and the intuition of our heart to live a more balanced, healthy, and effective life."
>
> —Anonymous

Finding What Works for You

Sorting through all the latest research isn't always an easy task. One problem we consumers face is what I call "science by press release." This means using attention-grabbing news headlines as your source of health information. STOP!

As you begin your Turnaround, you might become more aware of the latest front-page news item with alluring headlines about the benefit of a new diet drug or a certain wonder food that will keep you young and lean. More often than not, this information is based on a small study or is misinterpreted by an anxious journalist seeking to get the public's attention and an editor's approval. Also, powerful public relations firms represent the major drug companies, and clever firms representing new pharmaceuticals can be very convincing—their *job* is to sell drugs! Responsible scientists and careful journalists report research within the context of other studies. And one study rarely changes the accepted opinion.

For instance, you've probably read in the newspaper or on the Internet that estrogen replacement therapy helps to prevent Alzheimer's disease. But when you thoroughly read all the research, you will see the facts: one study found a protective effect; another study did not; and a third had inconclusive results. If we choose to follow the first study promoting estrogen replacement to prevent short-term memory loss, does that mean that when we develop breast or uterine cancer (from synthetic hormones), we will remember our pain and misery better? A curious thought.

It is only natural for the media to report on what's new and controversial. Hundreds of studies show that a diet high in fat and animal protein is unhealthful, fattening, and accelerates aging. Yet if a new study comes out suggesting that a high-protein diet may be healthy, it makes headlines, no matter how poorly

DO YOU REALLY WANT TO BE AVERAGE?

Science has now taken us to a place where processed food and pharmaceuticals are an accepted way of life. That's a scary thought, isn't it? Sadly, with all our modern groundbreaking scientific research, the United States has the highest rate of chronic diseases, the highest health-care costs, and the most overweight people (including children) of any country. We are no longer on the list of the top ten countries based on longevity, even with our superdrugs. The statistics are disturbing:

- *The average American consumes in a lifetime:*
  Two 3,000-pound cows
  6 pigs
  3,000 chickens and birds
  30,000 quarts of milk
  2,000 gallons of alcohol

- *The average American consumes annually in junk food:*
  300 soft drinks
  400 candy bars
  500 doughnuts
  170 pounds of sugar (over a fourth of the average caloric intake)

- *The average American consumes over a lifetime in medication:*
  30,000 aspirin
  20,000 other over-the-counter meds
  Untold prescription meds

- *Changes the average American made between 1900 and 1980:*
  Decreased whole-grain consumption by 50 percent
  Increased beef consumption by 75 percent
  Increased cheese consumption by 400 percent
  Increased food coloring consumption by 90 percent

The bottom line? Don't be an average person!

designed the study might be. This is true about the recent reports touting the health benefits of a daily glass of wine or beer, despite massive (and often unreported) evidence to the contrary.

If you take the time to weigh all the unbiased and credible scientific information, you will find that it is extremely consistent and less controversial than you might have thought.

Turnaround Time

You can't change your genetic makeup and the unknown environmental factors that affect your health each day. You cannot change your gender, age, or the fact that you are short or tall or have a large or small frame. And there is no point in grieving over the decades when you abused your body, mind, and spirit with bad health habits. There is no benefit to be gained from focusing on what you can't control. Instead, direct your energy and your attitude toward turning around the everyday functions that you can control.

As you read the following eight chapters, I want you to know that no matter how out of shape, overweight, unhealthy, or tired you are, you can *dare to be different*. All of us have been given a profound gift: the capability to be lean, strong, healthy, and creative—to think fast and be active. It is your choice *not* to be that person!

Mood, Belief, and Mastering Motivation

NO MATTER WHAT YOUR DIET or exercise history, to succeed with your Turnaround, you need the right information and exact tools to conquer negative moods, strengthen your personal beliefs, and increase motivation. In this first TLC, I'll teach you how to replace destructive thoughts and habits with healthy lifestyle behaviors so that you can finally look and feel young, enjoy optimal health, and lose that weight once and for all—no matter what your age.

"Just the thought of another diet and exercise program puts me in a bad mood," said Jane, who started dieting about forty years ago at the age of twelve, the same time her adolescent hormones began to go haywire. Since that time she has weighed as little as 112 pounds (on her wedding day) and as much as 187 pounds (after the birth of her second baby; she topped the scales at 220 on delivery day). "I've memorized all the diets and have a lifetime membership to almost every health club in town. Not only do I lack motivation, but when I think of starting a self-improvement program, I get confused and focus on my failures."

Modulate Mood

Jane's not the only one who gets moody when she contemplates her personal health and fitness. Over the years I've consulted with many women who become downright depressed when challenged to change their poor eating habits or to move around more. "It's too time-consuming, it's too confusing, and I've had too many failed attempts to think about making healthy changes," they claim.

More than nineteen million Americans suffer from chronic mood disorders, some serious enough to warrant medical treatment or psychological therapy. Not only can your mood affect how you perceive life and your relationships, it can also influence your lifestyle choices such as the foods you eat (or don't eat), your exercise routine, whether you smoke cigarettes or drink alcohol, and many other habits.

But we have a chicken and an egg here. Just as mood affects your lifestyle choices, so do your lifestyle choices affect your mood. You can wake up in the morning in a great mood and with good intentions, and it all goes down the drain when you skip breakfast, have a glass of wine for lunch, or forget to drink ample water.

There is hope, however. Your 24-Hour Turnaround is a natural, whole-life approach to helping you lose weight, replace flabby cellulite with taut, lean muscles, and improve your overall health and well-being. But in order to undertake the lifestyle challenges I present in this book, you first have to evaluate the internal or emotional you—how you feel on the inside about undergoing a major life change. You need to assess your mood stumbling blocks—those situations that cause you to feel irritable, sad, lonely, or even angry. The following questions will provide some insight into the challenge of training your emotions, willpower, and motivation so that you will succeed in your makeover of body, mind, and soul.

MOOD-BUSTERS QUIZ

Respond to the following questions and see which ones are negatively affecting your mood and motivation:

TRUE OR FALSE

____1. Just thinking about changing the foods I eat seems overwhelming.

____2. When I reflect upon all the weight I've lost and gained during adulthood, I get depressed.

____3. I am contented with my body until I see myself in a mirror without clothes on. Then I feel ashamed and embarrassed.

____4. My family life is out of control, which causes me to feel anxious and eat from stress.

____5. The only time I'm in a good mood is on weekends, when I don't have job responsibilities.

____6. If I don't get enough sleep at night, I find myself in a bad mood the next day.

____7. My mood plummets during the long, cold winter months.

____8. When I look through fashion magazines, I feel depressed knowing that I could never look like the models.

____9. I obsess about sweets, and after dieting for a week I usually binge on cookies, candy, or cake.

____10. In the past ten years my metabolism has dropped, and I feel lethargic and sluggish most of the time.

How did you respond? If you found even one statement that was true of you, then you need this Total Life Change to help you turn around your attitude. The reality is that our mood or emotional state plays a key role in our lifestyle habits, and often a bad mood will cause us to give up habits that can improve health and increase longevity.

This chapter is not about me trying to motivate you; it is about giving you the skills to wake up each day and motivate yourself. It is also about learning to believe in yourself again—the young, healthy you. Let's look at how the following five *Super Mood-Boosters* will change your attitude throughout your Turnaround.

SUPER MOOD-BOOSTER 1: EXERCISE

Your irritable mood will do an upswing as soon as you begin your H.E.A.R.T. (Heart-rate-specific Exercise with Aerobic Resistance Training) workout regimen, outlined in the following chapter. Unlike the mood boost you get from an expensive pharmaceutical, the mood elevation you get from exercise is immediate and without harmful side effects. Exercise spontaneously increases blood flow to the muscles and the brain, energizing your body and your mind.

Your H.E.A.R.T. workout gives you innovative and effective choices for developing lean muscles and releasing those feel-good endorphins—the "happy" hormones in the body. Not only does physical activity increase alpha waves in the brain, which are associated with relaxation and meditation, but it acts as a displacement defense mechanism for those who are stressed out and habitually in a bad mood. How does this work? Well, if you have ever walked several miles, you know how your mind becomes focused on the activity, not the problems you face each day. That's because you have displaced your ruminating, anxiety-ridden thoughts with a new, healthier focus. It's not easy to work your body and continue to dwell on problems at the same time.

Many therapists now prescribe exercise or movement therapy to combat depression, stress, or anxiety. For those who are simply in a bad mood, regular exercise provides the same benefit. But here's the catch: All exercise is *not* the same when it comes to altering mood. High-intensity exercise is stressful. Not only does an intense workout leave you feeling exhausted, your body is also filled with lactic acid, which sometimes causes that burning sensation in muscles and also prevents your muscles from burning fat. Lactic acid causes bad moods and irritability. In contrast, your H.E.A.R.T. workout is "heart-rate-specific training" that stimulates the brain chemicals that increase alertness. Training at a specific intensity also raises levels of serotonin, a brain chemical that boosts mood in much the same way as Prozac and other popular antidepressants. And as levels of serotonin increase, the levels of stress hormones like cortisol decrease. (I tell my clients they get two for the price of one with the H.E.A.R.T. workout.)

The H.E.A.R.T. workout also gives you an "exercise high" that is caused by the release of endorphins, your body's natural morphine-like chemicals. Having adequate endorphins in the body helps to regulate food intake, again ultimately affecting mood. This daily boost of endorphins from exercise increases a sense of well-being and triggers enthusiasm for life.

Do you see how muscle tone and body fat are no longer the only rewards for a fitness program? While personal and even spiritual growth are not the primary goals of exercise, these benefits may be part of your unique experience with the H.E.A.R.T. workout.

SUPER MOOD-BOOSTER 2: SUNLIGHT

I encourage all my Turnaround clients to get outside each day, preferably in the early morning light, to exercise or meditate. If free morning time is limited, enjoy a cup of tea at an open window or walk your children into school. Studies show that light entering the eyes stimulates the brain just as Prozac or any other psychotropic drug does. And while substantial evidence supports the idea that light boosts brain serotonin, it is clear that other body neurochemistry is affected as well.

Some interesting research indicates that even though humans' innate biological clocks change according to the four seasons, this only occurs in half of all people—the female half. In a study in the May–June 1999 issue of *Comprehensive Psychiatry,* researchers concluded that men appear to be more sensitive to artificial light than women are, yet they react less to seasonal changes. This finding could explain why more women suffer from seasonal affective disorder (SAD), a type of depression that occurs during the long winter months and that often results in binge eating. SAD is thought to be associated with changes in the production of melatonin, a neurotransmitter in the brain that gives rise to serotonin. SAD causes feelings of sadness, fatigue, and social withdrawal, a decrease in energy, and an increase in appetite that can lead to weight gain. Symptoms appear to worsen the farther one moves from the equator. Some studies show that exposure to early morning sunlight and artificial light can help reduce these symptoms.

WHY YOU EAT WHAT YOU EAT

To see how food can work to change your mood, increase alertness, and boost energy, it's important to understand *why* you feel the need to eat. There are three factors that regulate your food intake:

1. *The hunger center,* which is located in the hypothalamus section of the brain, stimulates you to eat.
2. *The appetite control mechanism,* which is found in the brain stem, is influenced by the time of day and by the smell and sight of food. It also triggers the need to eat and helps you decide which foods to choose, as well as the balance and quantity of food.
3. *The satiety center,* which is connected to the hunger center and the appetite through neurological "wiring," helps control whether you feel full or satisfied after eating.

If getting outside more to capture some early morning sunlight is not an option, you can look into buying or renting a light box for your home or office. According to some studies, winter depression can be greatly improved with light therapy, and in one study published in the November–December 1999 issue of *Comprehensive Psychiatry,* bright light therapy decreased winter bingeing in women with eating disorders.

SUPER MOOD-BOOSTER 3: FOOD

There are powerful chemicals in food that affect your mood, motivation, cognitive ability, intelligence, and energy. In fact, we know that most brain neurotransmitters are manufactured directly from food, and you can manipulate their levels by eating certain foods at certain times. For example, carbohydrate-rich foods increase the production of serotonin in the brain and produce a calming or drowsy response after eating. Likewise, foods high in protein trigger the production of

INTERNALLY SPEAKING

Carbohydrates are broken down to glucose in the liver and are then sent out to the rest of the body for use as energy. Glucose is the only source of energy the brain can use. A drop in brain glucose due to insufficient carb intake will result in slow reflexes and reduced concentration. You may also experience a gnawing hunger, dizziness, lethargy, and irritability. If you do not satisfy your body's need for whole carbohydrates at your first meal of the day, you may pay the price later on with decreased productivity and increased grouchiness.

dopamine and norepinephrine, two brain chemicals that give you a feeling of alertness, increased ability to concentrate, and a quick reaction time—all important for boosting productivity. You can use the food-mood link to your advantage by choosing the foods you need to boost you up or calm you down, depending on the time of day and situation at hand.

Sarah Leibowitz, Ph.D., of Rockefeller University has done a significant amount of research on food and the brain and believes that what we put in our mouths and when we do it is profoundly influenced by a group of neurotransmitters located in the appetite control center of the brain. These neurotransmitters not only guide our selection of foods at breakfast, lunch, and dinner but also determine individual differences in appetite and weight gain. Two of these neurotransmitters are neuropeptide Y, a chemical that is active in turning our carbohydrate cravings off and on, and galanin, which is associated with fat intake. Leibowitz found that the stress hormone cortisol stimulates production of neuropeptide Y. And when we are tense and irritable, we produce more cortisol. Now you know why you head for the cookie jar or bag of salty chips when life's stressors seem overwhelming. Leibowitz also revealed that neuropeptide Y urges your body to hold on to stored fat, making it even harder to lose weight when you get *all stressed up with no place to go!*

"So this explains why I crave carbohydrates. I was beginning to think I was abnormal and destined to be fat the rest of my life," said Shelly. She certainly isn't abnormal— craving carbs is perfectly normal for all of us. The media have led many of my clients like Shelly to believe they are afflicted with some kind of disease if they crave carbs. Dr. Atkins and other high-protein diet gurus may promote a high-protein, high-fat diet as the cure for carbohydrate addiction, but listen carefully: it won't work. Without carbohydrates, your brain would literally die. The brain relies exclusively on carbohydrate calories (and water) for fuel, and that's the real reason you crave carbs. So be careful. Following a high-protein, low-carb diet may defeat your Turnaround response and result in decreased energy, increased moodiness and irritability, and even some physical problems such as kidney damage.

WHICH BREAKFAST FOODS ENHANCE MOOD?

WHAT WORKS	WHAT DOESN'T
Ezekiel Bread*	Pastry
Angelika's Cereal[†]	Cheerios
Alvarado St. Bakery sprouted-grain bagel*	Doughnut
Veggie omelet	Scrambled eggs
McCann's steel-cut oatmeal	Instant oatmeal
Tofu scramble	McDonald's "happy breakfast"
Smoothie with soy milk and fruit[†]	Orange juice

*Available at most health-food stores.

[†]See the chapter "Recipes for Your 24-Hour Turnaround," page 369.

GET A JUMP START ON THE DAY

Eating a high-carbohydrate breakfast like a sprouted-grain or whole-grain bagel and fruit starts your day with optimal serotonin levels. Later in the day, if you eat a tuna sandwich, which has plenty of protein, you boost production of dopamine and norepinephrine, which increase alertness and concentration.

HOW TO MAKE BRAIN CHEMICALS (INSTEAD OF TAKING PROZAC)

SEROTONIN
Action: feelings of calmness, mood elevation, and a sense of well-being
Sources: nonfat organic milk, turkey breast, legumes, whole-grain breads and cereals, high-fiber carb snacks (see Zip-Lock Snacks, in "Recipes for Your 24-Hour Turnaround," page 392)

DOPAMINE
Action: feelings of excitement, increased energy, coordinated motor ability, and mental alertness
Sources: beans, legumes, tofu, tempeh, lean turkey, tuna

NOREPINEPHRINE
Action: increased memory, quick reaction time, mental energy, alertness, goal seeking, and sexual activity
Sources: salmon, oatmeal (not instant), legumes

ACETYLCHOLINE
Action: increased memory, verbal behavior, and concentration; decreased aging
Sources: egg whites, soybeans, wheat germ, peanuts, salmon, chicken breast

24 HOURS TO A BETTER MOOD

MOOD-BUSTER	MOOD-BOOSTER
Skipping meals	Small but frequent minimeals will correct a neurotransmitter imbalance immediately.
Eating sugar	Eliminating sugar for just 24 hours will have a dramatic effect on those who feel tired or depressed for no apparent reason.
Drinking caffeine	Reducing your intake of caffeine will help you sleep sounder tonight, and within 24 hours you will be more alert and have a better attitude.

Mood-Buster	Mood-Booster
Drinking alcohol	This is a definite no-brainer. Even eliminating that one glass of wine will change your chemistry and improve your mood today.
Eating high-fat foods	Saying no to potato chips, ice cream, and chocolate, will result in improved mood within 24 hours.

SUPER MOOD-BOOSTER 4: LAUGH

It may come as no surprise that the average adult laughs only about 17 times a day whereas a six-year-old child laughs as many as 300 times. Laughter cannot make your problems diminish, but it can help to relieve anxiety and allow you to regain a healthy outlook on life.

There is a growing body of evidence that links laughter with a strengthened immune system, findings that could point to humor as your Turnaround defense against stress-related ailments. In 1994 researcher H. M. Lefcourt found that laughter resulted in higher natural killer cell activity. Natural killer cells protect your health by attacking foreign cells, virus-infected cells, and cancer cells without prior exposure. Since Lefcourt's findings on laughter and immunity, other studies have shown that laughter strengthens the body's ability to fight disease by increasing production of salivary immunoglobulin A (sIgA), the body's first-line defense against the harmful infections to which we expose ourselves with every breath. In one study done at the University of Waterloo in Ontario, Canada, researchers divided volunteers into two groups: one group normally

ATTITUDE CHECK

Many recent studies have added to the body of evidence associating positive feelings with improved health. People who are happy or optimistic have a lower risk of stroke than people who are generally sad or depressed. The stroke-reducing benefits of a positive attitude are as important as weight, blood pressure, or smoking habits.

used humor to cope with stress, and the other group did not. After both groups viewed a comedy routine, the group that relied on laughter to fight stress had higher sIgA levels than the other group.

We know that laughter also increases energy levels. Try this the next time you're feeling run-down or fatigued: instead of pouring another cup of java, give a hearty belly laugh. If you don't feel like laughing, call a funny friend, watch a humorous video, or go on-line and check out some joke websites. Laughter will help reduce your pent-up emotional tension and allow you to breathe normally, which helps to decrease signs of stress. And by the way, laughter is good exercise, too. Now I don't want you to substitute a funny video for your daily H.E.A.R.T. workout, but we know that laughing a hundred times has the same effect on the body as exercising on a rowing machine for 10 minutes or a stationary bike for 15 minutes.

SUPER MOOD-BOOSTER 5: SOCIAL SUPPORT

It's becoming increasingly clear that a strong social network of friends, family members, coworkers, and others helps us feel secure and positive, no matter what stressors we may face. In fact, it's not the quantity but the *quality* of your social network that's important. After all, not everyone who knows you really cares that when your stock portfolio dropped, your weight soared.

Social support occurs when we really connect with other men and women in our social network. This interaction allows us to nourish our hungry souls and recharge, especially after giving all to careers, kids, and community. When we are tied emotionally to those in our social network, we can express our feelings of fear, insecurity, and guilt and receive comfort from people who accept us just as we are, with no strings attached. If we have no place that feels safe enough to let down our emotional defenses, we tend to keep our guard up all the time—a negative, cynical, and sometimes defensive attitude that masks the very problems we are facing.

You know how stress can cause a positive day to suddenly take a nosedive. In contrast, social support has a complex healing effect on mood and well-being. Social support may change your assessment of a stressful event, or it may prevent you from reacting to stress in damaging behavioral or physiological ways. For example, in a study reported in the February 2000 issue of *Preventative Med-*

While men tend to react to stress with the primitive "fight or flight" response, women are more likely to "tend and befriend" during hard times. This makes some scientists conclude that women simply handle life's stressors better. (I'm sure you may question this conclusion when you binge eat after a long day at work.) In a study done at UCLA, researchers found that when women are under stress, they typically reach out for social support through friends and family, or they may pour themselves into nurturing their children or others. These researchers concluded that the different responses to stress may help to explain why women generally have lower rates of alcohol and drug abuse as well as a reduced tendency toward stress-related disorders such as hypertension. The female hormone oxytocin appears to play a lead role in this "tend and befriend" coping skill. Although this hormone is present in both sexes, scientists believe that oxytocin is enhanced by the female hormone estrogen and turned off by the male hormone testosterone.

icine, researchers from the Centers for Disease Control and Prevention concluded that the more people participated in group social activities, the more likely they were to exercise, have their cholesterol and blood pressure checked at regular intervals, and eat sufficient amounts of vegetables and fruits. In another study published in the May–June 1995 issue of the *American Journal of Health Promotion,* findings suggested that friendships that involved exercising together and the social contacts that result from exercising in public places, such as health clubs, may motivate exercise behavior and increase compliance with exercise programs.

Strengthening Belief

Our personal beliefs, or what we know to be true in life, are crucial to staying well and can be incorporated into our daily lives as functional healing powers. Beliefs support every decision and choice we make—including those choices that affect

MUST-DO YOGA POSE TO BOOST MOOD

Yoga can stabilize your mood by releasing the brain chemicals endorphin and serotonin. This pose can also calm you in the middle of a stressful day. Lie down with your legs resting straight up against a wall. Your buttocks should touch the wall, and your arms should be at your side with palms up. Breathe deeply through your nose. Hold this pose for at least 2 minutes.

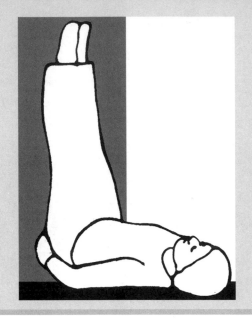

our health. Our belief system is formed during early childhood (from birth to age twelve), and it is influenced by many in our social network—parents, friends, religious leaders, teachers, and doctors—as well as the media. The problem is that most of us were not given the right information during this developmental period to form healthy beliefs about food, exercise, and taking care of our bodies. (Don't blame Mom: she probably did the best she could with the information that was available.)

As adults we must realize that our eating habits reflect our deepest beliefs about life. In order to change those habits, we must first learn how to decode our behavior and uncover our real beliefs. For instance, we may say we believe in the health benefit of a low-fat diet. Yet when we buy groceries, we stock up on high-fat snacks, pastries, and animal products. Our choices indicate our real belief: we are not totally convinced that eating low-fat foods will yield enough benefit to justify the change.

EXTRINSIC OR INTRINSIC BELIEF?

Some revealing research has distinguished a key difference between people who make a lifestyle change for extrinsic reasons (for someone or something else)

and those who do so for an intrinsic reason (a strong personal belief). Those who change for extrinsic reasons, such as that their doctor tells them to exercise to reduce the risk of heart disease, or that they want to look good for their daughter's wedding next month, usually start out enthusiastically. Yet while the need for change remains in their minds, it is never realized in their heart or emotions. Some studies show that 70 percent of those who make a lifestyle change for extrinsic reasons do not stick with it after a short period of time. In contrast, those people who make lifestyle changes for intrinsic reasons usually stick with the program and see a dramatic improvement in health and emotional well-being. For instance, when you believe in the health benefit of exercise and you enjoy and are grateful for the time you spend exercising, your belief can spark a profound commitment that keeps you focused and on track.

I have witnessed this over and over with my clients. Once they claim personal ownership of their Turnaround, believing in the health benefits and enjoying every aspect of the program, they become committed to their program and realize greater results.

How do you know if you are an intrinsic exerciser? If you can say to yourself during exercise, "I love to exercise, this feels so good," then you are *in*. Doing the H.E.A.R.T. workout that's outlined for you in TLC 2 will guarantee a level of effort that will feel good and produce those "happy" brain chemicals.

FAITH INCREASES COMPLIANCE

Deepak Chopra, M.D., author of *Ageless Body, Timeless Mind,* has said that at every stage of spiritual growth, the greatest ally you have is your body. Does this surprise you? Many of us assume that our body and our spirit stand at opposite ends of the spectrum. But Chopra contends that "a spiritual person is one who lives fully in the present moment, which means living fully in the body."

In the past two decades I have counseled literally thousands of clients about their health. I have also observed what appears to be a major component of motivation to adhere to weight loss and fitness plans. It seems that those clients who are more successful in following dietary and exercise recommendations are the ones who are faithful, who live "fully in the present moment and in their body," to paraphrase Chopra. By faithful, I mean they are by choice and disposition spiritual beings who profess a belief in a power greater than themselves.

Recently a doctor I consult with confided that he had observed the same phenomenon throughout his years of practice: that the human body has a strong spiritual dimension to it and that those patients who acknowledged this with a solid faith—a body-soul connectedness—were the patients who stuck with their treatment programs and saw improvement in their health, whether they had a chronic disease or wanted to lose 10 pounds.

FAITH IS A VITAL KEY TO WEIGHT MANAGEMENT

In Greek, the word for faith is *pistis,* which means "the act of giving one's trust." I believe that *pistis,* trust or faith, is a vital key to weight management that has been ignored by nutritionists, health-care professionals, and weight-loss programs. You see, the very act of trusting something greater than ourselves permits us to trust and commit to proven medical, nutritional, or exercise regimes we know will benefit us. Researchers are now studying the effects of spirituality and religion on health and have made some revealing conclusions thus far. For example:

- People who actively practice a religious belief have fewer mental and physical disorders than those who don't.
- Religious people need to see the doctor less frequently than nonreligious people.
- People who go to church/temple/synagogue regularly are healthier than those who don't.
- Israelis who live in a religious kibbutz have half the death rate of those who live in a nonreligious kibbutz.
- It is not uncommon for retired nuns to live past one hundred.
- When people pray, they engage in a type of meditative relaxation experience.

So does this mean that if you don't go to church or temple you will have major health problems? Of course not. A spiritual person isn't always a religious person, and vice versa. But it does show that we are just on the edge of understanding how belief and personal faith can help us experience optimal health for years to come.

Master Motivation in the Next 24 Hours

Now that you understand how your Turnaround can "bust a bad mood" and you're enlightened about the importance of belief in staying committed to a health and fitness program, let's talk about mastering motivation. For years I have consulted with my good friend and colleague John Zulli, Ph.D., to find ways to help clients boost motivation. Zulli, a master motivator and renowned mind-muscle seminar leader and author, has developed a technique to help you harness the power of your own natural "motivational response" to achieve success in your life Turnarounds. Before we unravel the mystery of where our motivation lies, we should first correct a serious misconception: *the belief that you cannot exercise or eat well because you lack motivation.*

I have good news: you are loaded with motivation right now! Like a knee-jerk reflex, motivation is a *natural, inherent process* that governs every action we take and each decision we make. According to Zulli, this motivational response is activated by your focus of attention. When you focus on the comfort of lying on the couch, your desire to exercise decreases and your desire to take a nap increases. When you focus your attention on the high you get from running, you create a compulsion to exercise. When you perceive your workouts as unpleasant or painful, you become *motivated to avoid them.* The same process that generates interest and desire also produces feelings of lethargy and inertia.

Let me be very clear. There is nothing wrong with you. You are not lazy. You are not broken and don't need to be fixed. You do not lack motivation. What you are experiencing is perfectly natural. The very same energy you have been using to hold yourself back can be transformed into a force that catapults you forward toward your dreams. You simply need to put this remarkable resource to work *for* you. Let's look at how John Zulli perceives the motivation response, and the suggestions he has for boosting this response.

For most people, the motivation response seems to disappear in a blinding blur. One minute you are doing well on your diet, and suddenly you find yourself face-down in a half-gallon of rocky road ice cream. However, if you slow the motivational response down, you can see that it has four distinct phases, represented by the letters *CVEA*.

CVEA stands for Conceptualization, Visualization, Emotionalization, and Actualization. It is through CVEA that thoughts take form as physical reactions, emotional responses, and finally actions. You can experience the CVEA response for yourself right now by imagining that you have a cutting board, a kitchen knife, and a large yellow lemon. The lemon is very sour and juicy. As you slice the fruit in quarters, the tart lemon juice oozes out of the lemon and onto the cutting board. Imagine that you are bringing one of the lemon slices to your mouth and sucking on the juice.

Mouth watering? If so, congratulations! You have begun to consciously *direct* your motivation. If you did not respond, close your eyes, relax, and concentrate on the thought of sucking on a lemon wedge. If that *still* doesn't work, reach over to your wrist and make sure you have a pulse. It is your body's natural reaction to salivate when you hold the image of a cut lemon in your mind. Here is how this reaction works.

Phase 1: Conceptualization. When you think of a lemon, your mind, like a computer, searches its database for experiences associated with lemons. From one thought, a series of related ideas merges together to form a concept. Individual thoughts gain power as they fuse together in this process of conceptualization. Once the conceptualization process hits "critical mass" it engages your imagination and moves to phase two of the CVEA response.

Phase 2: Visualization. You may be familiar with a relatively new phrase in the American vernacular: "Don't go there!" The *there* that people are talking about is this *movement from conceptualizing into the act of visualizing.* During the visualization, your creative imagination springs forward in the form of internal visual images, perceptions, and self-talk. These internal images, sounds, and experiences breathe life into your emerging thoughts and ideas. They energize and animate your concepts. Just as digital data create pictures that come alive on the monitor, the ideas and thoughts you have about lemons become the images you hold in the visual centers of your brain. Your creative imagination then takes the concept of *interactive* to a whole new level by mobilizing the body to process lemon juice.

Phase 3: Emotionalization. Your visualizations are "living ideas" to which you react emotionally. Sometimes, if the concepts and images have strong personal significance, you will explode with feeling. Welcome to phase three of the motivational response: *emotionalization*. Emotionalization works like a supercharger to amplify your thoughts and internal communication to a level you can literally feel and experience—to the physical embodiment of your ideas. It is this emotionally charged energy that moves you to action.

Phase 4: Actualization. Actualization is the culmination of the motivational response process. It is the outward expression of the energy accumulated from the combined actions of conceptualization, visualization, and emotionalization. Actualization results in behavior or in physical changes. You thought of biting into a lemon, visualized it in detail, reacted emotionally, and your mouth responded by salivating. You consciously activated your peripheral nervous system, directed blood flow to major organs, and changed the biochemical composition of your body. Not bad for a novice. CVEA transformed your thoughts into physical change.

ZULLI'S CVEA RESPONSE TRAINING

Great change starts with conceptualization. Conceptual change, which means "to integrate new ideas into our models of the world," takes place on two levels: the conscious and the subconscious. Now don't let the term *subconscious* intimidate you. Think of your mind as a computer and imagine the subconscious as the programmable part where software and memory are stored. Just as you can add or delete programs from your personal computer, you can disable, integrate, or upgrade your internal subconscious software.

The best way to upgrade your internal software is to write a script. More than just words on the page or simple affirmations, the CVEA script embodies the very ideas that you want to transform into action. The script changes concepts at the subconscious level and gives direction and inspiration to the mind. Using a simple set of guidelines, you can create a body of work that speaks directly to your motivational response in a language it understands.

According to Zulli, to fire up your imagination and accelerate the CVEA process, you must pick a change that is meaningful to you. These must be *your* goals, *your* dreams, and *your* desires. Use this process to quit smoking, but do so because it is essential to *you* and not because you want to get your family and friends off your back. Get into shape because you like the way you feel in that little black dress, not because that certain someone thinks you are getting heavy. Pick a change that is important to *you*.

The next step is to narrow the scope of the change you want to make. When dealing with the deeper mind it is best to be specific. Isolate the specific area of change you *want* to make, and condense it into one or two sentences. Write them in the space below.

My important change is:

_____

_____

EXAMPLE

Wrong: I want to become a brain surgeon, overcome my chocolate addiction, and win the Nobel Peace Prize so that I can finally get the respect and admiration from my friends and family that I've always deserved but have never received.

Right: I want to lose weight, get healthy, look and feel younger, and have more energy. I also want to feel more confident and be more positive.

CREATING YOUR CVEA SCRIPT

Zulli explains that the CVEA script doesn't have to be long or complicated to be effective. One or two paragraphs of bold ideas that jump-start your imagination are better than three pages of vague ideas that are void of feelings. Simple concepts filled with emotional content and visual imagery reach and energize the subconscious mind. While your directions to your subconscious need to be clear and complete, it is best to keep the script short and straight to the heart. Here are a few guidelines for creating a great script.

Start with positive concepts. Right now, think of any animal you choose except monkeys. Do *not* think of a monkey. Do *not* think of the little organ grinder's monkey in his little fez and red vest. And please do *not* think of barrels of monkeys. Get the picture? Focusing your attention on what you don't want starts the CVEA cycle working against you. You can't think of what you don't want without conjuring up that very image and corresponding emotions. Word modifiers such as *don't, no, never,* and *not* are neutral words to the subconscious. The deeper mind reacts to the actual word, not the modifier. Talk show diva Oprah Winfrey tells an enlightening story about going to a hypnotist for weight loss. During her session the hypnotist kept repeating over and over to her, "You will *not* eat french fries, you will *not* eat french fries. . . ." As soon as the session ended, Oprah said, she went out and ate, you guessed it, french fries.

Once you understand how CVEA works, Oprah's actions are completely understandable. If your goal is to eat healthier foods, then start your script with "I now choose foods that give me long life and great health. As I learn more about the healthy food choices that are available to me, I find wholesome and nutritious food that I love to eat." In all your script writing and editing, make an effort to eliminate every negative word and replace it with a positive one. Focus on what you want to have happen.

Create powerful imagery. Positive words create positive images. Your script should generate positive mental pictures and give you something to hang your visualization hat on. "When I work out, my body feels strong and my movements are smooth and graceful. I become more flexible, toned, and vibrant each time I exercise. I recognize my progress by the sleek fit of my clothes and my smiling face in the mirror!"

Integrate the environment and all five of your senses into your imagery. To develop better eating habits, incorporate the aromas of wholesome foods as they cook, the attractive colors of fresh vegetables, and the clean taste of unprocessed foods into your script.

When it comes to visualizing, don't just be positive, *be perfect*. The smallest dress in your closet now fits. You look and feel twenty years younger than your chronological age. Smaller food portions turn you on. While that may not be the way it is in real life, we are not dealing with the part of your mind that is reality-based. We are programming your subconscious computer with what you truly want to have happen, and perfect visualization creates peak performance.

Emotionalize your ideas. If you have ever copied or cut a quote out of a magazine and carried it with you in your wallet or purse, then you understand the basic concept of emotionalization. When we emotionalize an idea, we feel it in our bodies. Spontaneously jumping to your feet and cheering for your team at a sporting event—or feeling crippling panic and draining anxiety from watching a disaster on the news—both are graphic illustrations of highly emotionalized ideas.

Your CVEA script should contain *power words* that invoke strong, positive emotional reactions. Power words can be any words (or sounds) that have deep emotional significance to you. *Proud, beautiful, radiant, vibrant, triumphant, wise, remarkable, muscular, lean,* and *loving* are all power words that excite the imagination. Power words are the language of motivation to the subconscious mind. As you actualize your dreams and goals, do you want to feel fine, or would you rather feel elated, excited, and electrified? Fill your CVEA script with words and phrases that are inspiring and meaningful to you.

Actualize real potential. Perfect visualization may lead to peak performance, but telling yourself that you will "think only positive thoughts" or "always be enthusiastic" is counterproductive. To avoid setting yourself up for failure, avoid using absolute terms such as *never, always, everyone,* and *all* in your script. Be specific and detailed when it comes to describing the actions you want to take.

EXAMPLE

Wrong: "When I play tennis I ace every serve. I easily win every game I play. I will never be beaten."

Right: "I love to play tennis. My serve is strong, fast, and deadly. When I play tennis I am focused and energized. I read my opponent's intentions quickly and I respond with power, speed, and accuracy."

Stay in the present tense. The subconscious mind lives in the moment. The ideas in your script must be presented to the subconscious as if they were occurring in the present. Avoid *I will be* and *I am going to* and use *I am, I now feel,* or *today* to get an instantaneous response from the subconscious.

WRITING YOUR PERSONAL CVEA SCRIPT

To write a successful CVEA script, John Zulli recommends finding a place where you can concentrate and taking 10 minutes to write out the first draft. Then come back and review it against the preceding guidelines and the sample script below. Work with the draft until you have eliminated all the negative ideas, vague directions, and hazy images. Allow your ideas and concepts to take shape and become more solid with each reading or revision. Here is a sample script to follow:

Goal: I want to lose weight and learn to love exercise

I am a powerful and innovative person. Today I put the full power of my resources to work sculpting and designing my physical body. My goals are to build beautiful lean muscles, increase my energy levels, and create radiant health. I sense positive changes taking place in my body with each positive choice that I make.

I enjoy eating wholesome foods that are clean and healthy for me. I buy wonderful and nutritious foods and prepare them with loving care. I easily eat only what my body needs to maintain fabulous health and great strength.

I relax and eat slowly. I chew thoroughly and enjoy every bite. My body easily digests my food, absorbs the nutrients, and eliminates what is not needed. By eating the right amounts of the most nutritious foods, I feel my body growing slender, stronger, and younger. Making the right food choices immediately gives me greater energy, vitality, and health.

I love to exercise. I look forward to working out. Each time I work out I move closer to my fitness goals. My workouts leave me energized and revitalized. As I go through my regular daily activities I feel stronger, more flexible, and more powerful. As I look into the mirror I like what I see. I see my slender, stronger, younger self emerging.

CREATING THE CVEA SYMBOL

Once you have a working copy of your CVEA script, it's time to give it a title. According to Zulli, you should think of your title as a symbol that stands for everything contained in your script. Look for a symbol that brings vivid images to your mind and strong feelings to your heart.

Your title can be a single word or an entire phrase. One athlete preparing for the grueling Hawaiian Ironman Triathlon titled his script "Unshakable Confidence," while a dancer once symbolized her entire performance using three powerful words: "I Can Fly." A woman looking to lose weight and improve her love life found that the title "Little Black Dress" said it all.

Once you have decided on a title, add this line to the end of your script: "The ideas, images, emotions, and actions contained in this script are all symbolized in the phrase/word _____ (fill in your title)." You have now created your subconscious software. Now it's time to install it.

INSTALLING YOUR CVEA SOFTWARE

The process I am about to teach you has been designed by John Zulli to minimize the amount of effort you must consciously make while maximizing your CVEA response. Our culture has a tendency to underestimate what we perceive as simple. Please resist the temptation to equate ease of use with ineffectiveness; not everything needs to be complicated to be powerful. Remember, before we put astronauts on the moon, performed open-heart surgery, or split the atom, all we had were some ideas and a little imagination.

There is a rule of the mind that states: "Once an idea has been accepted into the subconscious mind, it remains until it is replaced by another idea." You have written the script that contains the replacement ideas. Now you must get the subconscious mind to accept them. Reading the script to yourself over and over might produce some benefits, but the process is tedious and boring. If consciously reviewing our wish list over and

> "Imagination is everything."
> —Albert Einstein

over were the way to create dynamic change, we would all be masters of motivation. The key to installing your CVEA software is timing.

Accelerated learning and near-sleep states. It's been said that American philosopher Henry David Thoreau would lie in bed for a few minutes each morning and think positive thoughts. He would remind himself that he was healthy, that his mind was alert, that his work was interesting, that the future looked bright. When he got out of bed, he entered a world filled with the kind of positive people and opportunities that he expected—a kind of self-fulfilling prophecy.

Thoreau never knew that he was making use of a very special state of consciousness called the *hypnopompic state*—the time between being asleep and being fully awake. It is a time when our subconscious mind is accessible to us. Have you noticed how easy it is to remember a dream in vivid detail when you first wake up, only to find that it has completely vanished just a few minutes after getting up? Dreaming is a subconscious process. When you had access to the dream, you were in the hypnopompic state and your subconscious was open to you. You were also conscious enough to think about the content of the dream. When the dream left your mind, your subconscious submerged and your conscious mind took over.

The hypnopompic state is an important time because the subconscious mind is open while you are conscious enough to give it direction. Thoreau wasn't just practicing wishful thinking; he was filling his subconscious mind with powerful and positive ideas at a time when it was open and ready to accept this information.

There is a nighttime version of the hypnopompic state called the *hypnagogic state,* which is the time between wakefulness and sleep. Once again the balance of power shifts, this time from conscious dominance to subconscious control. In fact, in order to go to sleep at all you must allow this shift to occur (as you know if you've ever spent a sleepless night because your thoughts were racing).

Near-sleep states are naturally occurring opportunities for accelerated learning and growth. When you learn to work with these special states of consciousness, you get all the amazing benefits of hypnosis without having to go to a hypnotist.

CVEA before sleep. About half an hour before going to bed, read your CVEA script aloud to yourself. The act of reading the words and vocalizing the sounds causes the subconscious to become involved. If you find it is too embarrassing to read your script out loud, read it silently. After you have read your script, get into bed and allow your mind to focus on the script's symbol or title. Make no effort to remember what you have written. Focus your attention on the symbol, and allow your mind to absorb the images, ideas, and feelings that are generated. As your subconscious comes to meet you at the threshold of sleep, it connects with the symbol and all it represents. Message delivered, you drift off into the sleep state and let the subconscious take it from there.

CVEA upon waking. Start your day by taking a few moments before getting out of bed to think about your symbol. Make no conscious effort, just allow yourself to connect with what the symbol represents. As your conscious mind becomes more active, read your script again. Be creative; find ways to integrate the actions contained in your script into your upcoming day. Let these powerful ideas, images, and emotions energize you and create a sense of forward momentum. Now let it go. Go to work, go play, go live your life, and trust your natural CVEA response to take over.

The mind-muscle connection. Your H.E.A.R.T. workout, described in the next chapter, is an excellent time to work with your script and symbol. Workouts give us time to integrate ideas and concepts directly into our subconscious. Physical activity such as playing a sport, running, walking, and sex all require conscious critical functions to release control and allow the subconscious mind to come forward and run the body. (You would be hard-pressed to solve an involved math problem while dancing the tango, or recite the Gettysburg Address from memory while making love.)

To take advantage of this subconscious opportunity, simply read your script before you start your workout, and think about your symbol once you're into your routine. Stay focused on your breathing, and periodically repeat the symbol silently to yourself.

Actions speak louder than words. Once again, the word *motivation* comes from Latin and literally means "to move," which brings us to one last point. *All true motivation culminates in action.* Period. You get zero points for "feeling motivated." You get no points for "trying" or "thinking about it" or saying, "I'm going to." Like every other aspect of life, it's what we *do* that counts, not what we think, say, or feel. When you have truly mastered motivation, you'll know because you will be *behaving differently.* As the great mythological sage Master Yoda said, "Do or do not. There is no try."

Eight Turnaround Tips to Boost Mood and Motivation

Turnaround Tip 1. Drink water. Always start your morning with at least 8 ounces of lukewarm water, preferably with lemon. Getting the toxins out of your body and starting with a clean slate is first on your agenda. Additionally, the smell of the lemon is incredibly energizing and uplifting. Make sure you continue drinking water every hour on the hour. Because your brain is 80 percent water, when you are dehydrated, your mood is crippled. Bonus: by drinking enough water, you will not mistake a food craving for an actual need to hydrate.

Turnaround Tip 2. Eat breakfast. Make sure you include high-fiber foods. For instance, try for one or two fruits and a slice of whole-grain bread with some nuts or nut butter. (Nothing out of a box, please!) Even if you have to make breakfast and take it on the run, your metabolism will get a boost, your mood will improve, and your family members and coworkers will thank you. If you feel you need it, add a small amount of protein from nonfat organic dairy or egg whites.

Turnaround Tip 3. Look to the light. Make sure you have early exposure to natural light at the beginning of your day. An hour would be great, but if your schedule does not permit it, just 10 minutes can make a big difference in how you feel and your outlook on life. (Early morning light also helps to reset your circadian rhythm, making it easier to fall asleep and stay asleep at night—a definite perk for your Turnaround.) When you get to work, hang outside your building to enjoy the sunshine. Or return business or personal calls on your cell phone while you bask in the sun. Be sure to wear sunblock or cover yourself if you burn easily.

Turnaround Tip 4. Exercise. Even a light walk after lunch will help to increase endorphins. Exercise is one of the best ways to improve mood and overcome fatigue as it increases blood flow to the muscles and the brain, energizing mind, body, and spirit.

Turnaround Tip 5. Meditate. Take a 2-minute "meditation break" at 10 A.M., a peak time in your morning cycle. Taking a brief time-out will not only improve your mood but give you added energy for the next 4 hours.

Turnaround Tip 6. Eat hormone-friendly foods. I have gotten so many calls from clients who have fallen off their path because of hormone imbalances. Sunflower seeds, pumpkin seeds, and almonds are rich in essential fatty acids, which help balance hormones. Eat a half ounce of nuts as your snack (see Zip-Lock Snacks in the recipe chapter).

Turnaround Tip 7. Snack smartly. If your inner mood craves sweets or high-fat foods, ignore it. Instead choose nutrient-dense foods from the Zip-Lock list, like fresh fruit, raisins, or Ezekiel Bread with almond butter. If you crave carbs, it's a must to plan ahead and have fiber-rich snacks available to keep you out of the office sweets or the junk food shelves in the grocery store. Choose nutritional superstars at lunch, including thiamin-rich foods like acorn squash, asparagus, and black beans— all shown to improve cognitive functioning. Plan for a low-fat meal that contains a mixture of carbs with a small amount of protein to keep you on track for the day.

Turnaround Tip 8. Eliminate alcohol. Many studies have shown a relationship between depressive symptoms, anxiety, and alcohol consumption.

Just Believe It

A significant reason for eating food that is not beneficial to health or weight loss is having a weak belief in the need for eating nutritious food. This results in succumbing to the distractions and temptations that get in the way of a healthy diet. Educate yourself by reading the nutrition ABC's in the chapter on TLC 3. This will help you sort out the facts and give you the basis for your new belief system. I know from experience that at the very least you can look at two food choices and have a reasonable idea as to which is more nutritious. Given the choice between broccoli and M&M's, even kids know that the "yucky green stuff" is better for you, yet they invariably choose the candy.

Knowledge empowers you. Ignorance is probably the greatest risk factor for obesity, poor fitness, and a shorter life span. As you read "Total Life Change 2: Your H.E.A.R.T. Workout Formula," seek knowledge to strengthen your belief system about aerobic and resistance exercise, and then make appropriate choices that reinforce it. Then learn all you can about the healing benefits of whole foods and the Definition Diet in TLC 3. Read the journal studies and client stories that I present regarding the need for healing hydration, saying no to alcohol, getting healing sleep to boost immune function, balancing hormones for energy and youthful looks, and destressing for longevity. Use this information to form your new belief system (or reinforce your old one). "Own" this belief system in your mind, emotions, and body, and use it now to lose weight, look young, and stay healthy.

In the next 24 hours, and every 24 hours after that, accessing a strong belief system is fundamental to nurturing yourself and your loved ones. Believing in yourself is just the beginning.

FOR YOUR KIDS

Many years ago when my oldest son, Dustin, was in grade school, I took home the recipe book from our school cafeteria, and what I found was horrifying. Almost every recipe listed ingredients such as white sugar, white flour, and canned meats, vegetables, and fruits. I immediately sat down in the principal's office and informed her that the school was contributing to the increased risk of the children becoming obese or getting cancer and heart disease at a young age. After offering my assistance, I was told that they had a budget, and the local food distributor had bid on the job and was awarded the contract. Since that eye-opening encounter, bag lunches have been a way of life for my kids, and teaching my kids the facts about healing foods and staying fit has been a number one parenting goal.

I can tell you from twenty-six years of experience as a mom and as a counselor to children of other families that kids are too smart to believe something about nutrition or health simply because you say so. Remember, knowledge is what empowers you to accept an idea as true. This holds true for your kids too. Give them some actual facts from a credible source, and you might be surprised at how much they already know about their bodies and nutrition, especially if they are ten or older. Always preface everything you say to them about the Total Life Changes with "because I love you, I want you to be healthy and feel good." Don't be discouraged if they say something negative or act as if they don't care. The information went in. In my opinion, two of the greatest gifts you can give your children are love and the right tools and foundation to be as healthy as possible.

EATING DISORDERS AND MOOD

Studies estimate that more than *seven million* American adolescent girls and young women have eating disorders. Although once considered a "female obsession," with the new emphasis on men's fashion, more stress is put on the way men look, and now teenage boys are becoming subjected to the same body image concerns. In fact, it is estimated that more than one million adolescent boys and men have eating disorders. Recent studies show that anorexia, bulimia, and binge eating are not separate diseases but varying manifestations of using eating (or not eating) as a way to cope with moods, problems, and pain. In fact, new findings suggest that "average dieting" and eating disorders are not different behaviors at all—just points along a continuum. (Which confirms my long-held belief that most people have an "eating disorder" of some kind—even if it's as innocent as "I can't pass on the licorice grape vines at the movies, even if I am trying to avoid sugar.")

The general signs and symptoms of eating disorders appear to be the same for both men and women:

- Extreme weight change
- Insomnia
- Constipation
- Skin rash or dry skin
- Thinning or loss of hair
- Poor nail quality
- Unusual eating habits like binge eating
- Skipping meals
- Hyperactivity and high interest in exercise
- Denial
- Changes in personality

The problem arises when parents are not aware of these symptoms because the teen keeps them hidden—just like the trauma, insecurities, depression, or low self-esteem that initially triggers the disorder.

If you suspect any type of eating disorder in your teenage daughter (or, less commonly, in your son), realize that this condition can stem from mood or belief. Eating disorders are not physical conditions, yet they manifest as such. The physical condition is a consequence of whatever is going on emotionally in the teen's mind. There is hope! Cognitive behavioral therapy, sleep, and small amounts of the proper food will help. Above all, counseling is mandatory (usually for both parents and child). Ask your doctor to refer you to a specialist. I have had tremendous success with clients who have eating disorders and adopt a healthy approach to being lean. Combining the Definition Diet's minimeals with Zone One exercise and quality sleep allows the body to maintain a lean look without sacrificing health or emotional well-being.

Experts say that *5 percent* of American women are bulimic. This emotional disorder usually starts in late adolescence and early adulthood and manifests itself in cycles of bingeing or rapid consumption of foods followed by purging, vomiting or laxative use, use of diuretics, or hours of aerobic exercise. Warning signs include extreme preoccupation with weight, strict dieting followed by high-calorie eating binges, overeating when distressed, feeling out of control, disappearing after a meal, depressive moods, alcohol or drug abuse, frequent use of laxatives or diuretics, excessive exercising, and irregularities in menstrual cycle.

Bulimia is not the only serious eating disorder; anorexia nervosa affects about 1 percent of American women. One twenty-year study showed that only half of all anorexics recover; there is a death rate of 20 percent for chronic sufferers.

Anorexia (self-starvation) usually appears between the ages of fourteen and eighteen. It manifests itself in avoiding food and in extreme weight loss, although the person is usually below an average weight to begin with. Symptoms include having a distorted body image, skipping meals, unusual eating patterns, oversensitivity to criticism, perfectionistic behavior (excellent grades or performance), absence of menstrual cycle (amenorrhea), withdrawal from friends or unusual immersion in activities, inflexibility, and frequent weighing.

Binge eating, another very common eating disorder, is characterized by eating unusually large amounts of food. Binge eaters eat until they are full and uncomfortable and eat very quickly during these binges. Sometimes binge eaters eat alone to hide the massive quantities of food they eat. Someone with bulimia would purge or vomit after binge eating to get rid of the food and try to avoid weight gain.

FOR YOUR HUSBAND

If your husband is too busy to get motivated, he may also be too busy to make a few changes in his daily diet. My husband is grateful that I make time to shop for nutritious food and prepare healthy meals. If you take time early on in your Turn-around to prepare the recipes in this book, your husband may enjoy the new tastes, begin to feel more energetic, and start the program with you.

My observation about men is this: if it's their idea, it's a good idea. Instead of lecturing about good health and longevity, give your husband his own copy of *The 24-Hour Turnaround*, and let him read it himself!

TOTAL LIFE CHANGE 2

Your H.E.A.R.T. Workout Formula

THE ONLY 24-HOUR CHANGE I would get with this new exercise regimen would be exhaustion, sore muscles, and stiff joints." Kerri's honest assessment was based on her past exercise experience—but it was totally inaccurate. I explained to Kerri that the H.E.A.R.T. workout would do just the opposite, giving her a boost of energy and helping her easily achieve her weight-loss goal.

What Is the H.E.A.R.T. Workout?

The H.E.A.R.T. workout is a controlled-intensity, total fitness program that is a synchronized combination of aerobics, resistance training, and core training, building all aspects of fitness—the formula for endurance, strength, balance, posture, overall coordination, and fat-burning enzyme production. This workout focuses on specific intensity, duration, frequency, and movement, and all exercise components influence a multitude of hormones, including insulin-like growth factor, testosterone, insulin, estrogen, and human growth hormone (HGH).

As you train using your H.E.A.R.T. workout, you'll combine an aerobic workout with a resistance workout to increase the effectiveness of each one. For instance, if you walk on a treadmill (aerobic), you will also use an isometric rope* or circuit training for resistance exercise. Or if your favorite exercise is swimming (aerobic), you'll use swim gloves and a kickboard for resistance training. In this way, with each H.E.A.R.T. workout session you will use your muscles to elevate your heart rate instead of using high-intensity exercise and momentum movements.

This moderate-intensity exercise method has been proved to burn more fat and total calories than other conventional exercise regimens because it increases the body's metabolic rate (number of calories burned in a day). For instance, depending on how much muscle you have and how fit you are, the average woman burns from 400 to 800 calories in 1 hour of exercise. But with the H.E.A.R.T. formula's unique combination of aerobic exercise and resistance training, you burn calories from fat during exercise, and this high rate of fat-burning continues for the other 23 hours of the day (even during sleep). Because the H.E.A.R.T. workout is a moderate-intensity workout, it creates the enzymes in your muscles to burn fat efficiently. This residual effect, not the exercise itself, is the H.E.A.R.T. workout's greatest benefit for burning calories and losing weight. In fact, researchers at West Virginia University found that women who exercised four days a week or more at the proper heart rate lowered their percentage of body fat without even cutting calories. Their cravings for fatty foods also decreased as their bodies developed a taste for the right complex carbohydrates to fuel their workouts.

H.E.A.R.T. formula: aerobics + resistance = increased calories burned = weight loss

A Heart-to-Heart Chat

Before I teach you the basics of the H.E.A.R.T. workout, let's have a serious talk about why we *all* must take exercise seriously—and why we *all* must start today. According to the U.S. Surgeon General's Report on Physical Activity and Health

---

*The isometric rope (iso-rope) is an exercise rope that is about 28 inches long and has handles. It allows an entire upper-body workout with the treadmill, power walk, stationary bike, or swimming pool. The isometric rope is used similarly to exercise bands, but it gives a benefit for both heart and muscles. It can be ordered from 800-529-9080 or from my website.

(1996), only 22 percent of adults in the United States are active enough to receive health benefits from physical activity; 53 percent are somewhat active, but not at a level to benefit health; and 25 percent are sedentary. Other credible studies show that only one in nine adults exercises regularly. And by the age of seventy-five, most men and women don't exercise at all. That is very frightening considering that millions of men and women over sixty-five have osteoporosis, which can lead to painful, debilitating fractures. Exercise is the one remedy that guarantees strong bones and a reduced risk of fractures.

We must commit to exercise because inactive lifestyles contribute to weight gain, elevated blood fats, cardiovascular disease, cancer, reduced blood sugar regulation, and increased depression, memory loss, cognitive dysfunction, fatigue, and a host of other emotional and physical problems. Exercise is also vital because it dictates your biological age—no matter how old you are chronologically. Did you know that if you're a woman over twenty-one (twenty-five for men), your chronological age is not nearly as important as the physical condition of your body? That means that if you are forty and haven't exercised in years, your biological age could actually be fifty or even higher. Scary, isn't it? Aging doesn't just happen with the passing of time but is more a product of how you take care of yourself, including whether or not you exercise and how fit you are. This helps to explain why a fit fifty-year-old has a longer life expectancy than someone ten years younger who leads a sedentary life. The Surgeon General's report qualified this by stating that physical inactivity and low levels of cardiovascular fitness are among the greatest risk factors for death, more so than cigarette smoking, high blood pressure, elevated cholesterol, and obesity. Go ahead and read that last sentence again. Exercise is not just about looking good. Sedentary lifestyles are responsible for one-third of all coronary heart disease, colon cancer, and diabetes deaths each year. You hold the key to avoiding *all* of these problems *if* you start your H.E.A.R.T. workout today.

Another reason we must start to exercise is that we cannot possibly use all the calories we eat with our sedentary lifestyles. And extra calories mean added weight—even if you are relatively conscientious about what you eat. The H.E.A.R.T. workout helps you burn those extra calories with its 24-7 increase in the body's metabolic rate.

I always like to take a step back in time and learn from our past. Research has shown that our ancestors, who were incredibly lean, walked and ran often, built their dwellings themselves, and spent about 20 hours each week just gathering food. Imagine all the energy required for hunting, digging, picking, and gathering.

A 150-pound person probably used about 1,400 calories a day just gathering food for survival. This active lifestyle is one reason why those who did live beyond their eighties remained active, lean, and relatively disease-free.

In the past two decades, I've heard every excuse imaginable for not exercising, from "I'm not motivated" to "I don't have time" to "I get bored when I even think of exercising." Perhaps the reason you don't enjoy exercise is that it was presented as work—as one more duty or obligation you had if you wanted to stay healthy and maintain a normal weight. Your H.E.A.R.T. workout is different. I'm going to teach you how to be your own personal trainer with the H.E.A.R.T. workout so that you end up with more energy and a better attitude about allowing time for exercise in your busy life.

Benefits of Your H.E.A.R.T. Workout

Heart-rate-specific
Exercise with
Aerobic
Resistance
Training

Your H.E.A.R.T. formula incorporates heart-rate-specific exercise that is targeted at the exact intensity your body needs. Can the H.E.A.R.T. workout produce results within 24 hours? You bet! Here are some of its key benefits:

- *It regulates your appetite and reduces cravings for sugar (carbs).* Some people believe that exercise increases your appetite to the point where you crave extra food. This is not so. Once your muscles begin to use fat, more sugar (carbs) becomes available to the brain. In response, the brain stops sending out the "feed me sugar" signal that causes the craving for sweets. As you incorporate the H.E.A.R.T. workout in your daily schedule, the pH of your blood will change slightly after your workout, helping to reduce hunger and squelch cravings. These blood chemistry changes also release endorphins in the brain, elevating mood and indirectly modifying hunger by affecting your attitude. If you feel healthier, you will make better choices in what you feed your body.

- *It has an antiaging effect.* The H.E.A.R.T. workout will change key markers of aging, boosting aerobic capacity, muscle mass, and hormone production, for example, to help you look and feel ten to twenty years younger. With the H.E.A.R.T. workout, increased delivery of oxygen and nutrients will improve the health of your skin, reversing the hands on that clock today! This dual workout has been shown to result in a 30 percent reduction in chronic illness, helping to increase life span as well as letting you live your life with optimal health, doing the activities that are important to you.

- *It increases fat-burning enzymes.* Your muscles need very specific enzymes to burn fat. These enzymes are different from and harder to come by than carbohydrate-burning enzymes. Some new research has shown that people who exercise at the proper intensity (what I call "Zone One") have far more fat-burning enzymes in their muscles than people who exercise at the wrong intensity or don't exercise at all. The more you use your muscles in Zone One, the more fat-burning enzymes your muscles develop, allowing them to burn fat 24 hours a day. In other words, you "earn" fat-burning enzymes by doing your Zone One training.

- *It lowers resting blood pressure.* If you've been concerned about increasing blood pressure, the H.E.A.R.T. workout may help you control it without medication. Just a single H.E.A.R.T. session lowers systolic blood pressure by 18 to 20 points and diastolic blood pressure by 7 to 9 points, letting you turn around your blood pressure reading today. In one study performed on sedentary, overweight, and hypertensive adults, researchers found that just 45 minutes of Zone One treadmill exercise reduced blood pressure enough to result in a significantly lower reading 24 hours later.

- *It increases your core body temperature.* Another marker of aging that appears to be universal is lack of temperature regulation. As we lose the ability to produce heat, we convert increasing numbers of calories into fat. Your ability to produce heat is directly related to your state of fitness. To a great extent, this lack of temperature regulation is controlled by the diameter of the vascular system in your skin.

- *It improves your cardiovascular response.* During your H.E.A.R.T. workout, your muscles will demand more energy and oxygen due to the increased workload. This means that your heart and respiratory rates must increase in order to get the additional fuel to your muscles. As the heart muscle responds to exercise, it becomes stronger and more efficient. In addition, the entire circulatory system begins to work more efficiently because of vascular dilation, reduced blood pressure, and the lowering of overall blood fats.

- *It boosts aerobic capacity.* Aerobic capacity, an important marker of aging, is the ability to deliver adequate levels of oxygen to the muscles so that lactic acid doesn't build up, causing the muscle to stop working. Your aerobic capacity generally decreases by about 1 percent per year after age twenty. With exercise, this decrease is actually reversed, giving you back years of endurance, strength, and vitality. Turning back the "aerobic capacity clock" can happen at any age.

- *It lowers total cholesterol.* While the body's blood lipids are complex, we do know that exercise has an extremely positive effect on total cholesterol levels, helping to reduce the bad—low-density lipoprotein (LDL)—cholesterol and triglycerides while boosting the good—high-density lipoprotein (HDL)—cholesterol to help protect you from heart disease. Even after a single session of the H.E.A.R.T. workout, there is strong evidence that acute changes in levels of serum triglycerides and HDL cholesterol occur. Imagine what six months of the H.E.A.R.T. workout will do to your cholesterol profile!

- *It strengthens the skeleton.* Exercise not only prevents bone calcium loss, but with the H.E.A.R.T. workout bone calcium actually increases, reducing your risk of osteoporosis. Did you know that hip fractures are *not* the most common injury of women with osteoporosis? The most common injury is vertebral compression fracture, in which the weakened bones of the spine virtually collapse. This can cause acute or chronic pain, loss of height, and poor posture. But results of a study published in the April 2001 issue of *Medicine and Science in Sports and Exercise* confirm that aerobic and resistance workouts like H.E.A.R.T. have a positive effect on bone mineral density (BMD). BMD is also influenced by hormonal status and nutrition.

It influences healthy hormonal changes. The endocrine system is the chemical regulator of the body. The glands react to aerobic stimulation by secreting hormones that have specific effects on parts of our bodies. One hormone reduces cholesterol, others elevate mood, and another suppresses the appetite. Your H.E.A.R.T. workout in Zone One results in estrogen-like effects on the body, resulting in reduced hot flashes, younger-looking skin, and lower lipid levels. The positive regulation of estrogen also results in a reduction in estrogen-dependent cancers, especially uterine and breast cancers. Zone One exercise positively affects a number of hormones in your body that are related to fat storage, such as insulin, adrenaline, and cortisol. Endorphins, small morphinelike chemicals, are also secreted with exercise and can help reduce fat storage. For a 24-hour hormonal turnaround, put on your shoes, turn on your heart-rate monitor, and get moving!

And there are a host of other amazing benefits with your H.E.A.R.T. workout:

- Increased neural stimulation
- Increased muscular stimulation
- Increased function and flexibility of joints and reduced inflammation associated with arthritis
- Improved digestion
- Improved lymphatic flow
- Reduced stress
- Decreased insulin sensitivity
- Reduced risk of developing non–insulin dependent diabetes
- Increased immune system resistance
- Improved sexual function
- Increased desire to lose weight and eat healthfully
- Increased quality of life and independent living in older adults
- Reduced risk of developing cancer
- Improved sleep patterns
- Increased energy
- Improved mental alertness and IQ
- Improved self-esteem and self-confidence
- Reduced chance for depression, anxiety, and stress

Five Important Benefits

My clients are always looking for an effective, timesaving approach to their health and fitness regimes. The benefits they appreciate most about the H.E.A.R.T. workout include the following:

Benefit 1: Saves time. The benefit most of my clients put at the top of their list was timesaving. When you combine aerobic and resistance training, you really do get two for the price of one—the exercises are done simultaneously, which saves time. Although it's true that the longer you exercise, the more fat you'll burn, keep in mind that exercise that uses more muscles takes less time to burn the same amount of fat than exercise that uses fewer muscles.

Benefit 2: Safe, efficient, and natural. You get a much more efficient workout because your heart rate increases as a result of "natural overload"—muscle contraction. You want your heart rate to be elevated for the right reason—not as a unhealthy result of stress, dehydration, heat, or lack of oxygen.

Benefit 3: Prevents aging side effects. When muscles contract, they demand a large amount of oxygen from the blood. When you sit on a bench in the gym and press a heavy weight, after a number of reps the muscle says "no oxygen," and it fails or starts to burn. That's your internal alarm letting you know that you're headed for accelerated aging and possible hormonal side effects. Alternately, when you are moving around with the H.E.A.R.T. workout and your heart rate is elevated (sending life-giving blood to your arms and legs), the muscles you are strengthening have a blood and oxygen supply. The bottom line—your resistance workout is better.

Benefit 4: Functional. Your H.E.A.R.T. workout is functional exercise that trains the whole body to be stronger for "real-life" movement. Isolating a muscle group (such as with a biceps curl) is not as effective as using your entire upper body (including the biceps), as you naturally do during daily activity.

Benefit 5: Improves coordination and balance. Your H.E.A.R.T. workout combines movements of balance and coordination, which involve the body and the brain. The simultaneous use of the upper and lower body muscles stimulates the central nervous system (the interaction of the nerves and muscles or neuromuscular connection) to become more efficient. This improved interaction between different parts of the body results in better coordination and performance during exercise and everyday activity. Doing activities that require balance also stimulates our nervous system to activate reflexes in our posture muscles.

All About Your Amazing Fat-Burning Capability

Now that you have an idea of some of the health benefits you'll gain from your H.E.A.R.T. workout, let's talk about what most of you are really concerned about—burning fat and calories and losing weight. In case you are wondering how this fat-burning process occurs and where all those calories go when you burn them up with exercise, here's an easy explanation. A calorie is burned in the mitochondria (cells) of the muscle. It's a basic fact that the more muscle you have, the more calories you can burn both during exercise and at rest. Now get this: a pound of muscle can burn anywhere from *50 to 100 calories* a day. That's why muscle is called metabolically active tissue. On a down note, a pound of fat burns only *2 to 3 calories* a day.

Muscle accounts for 90 percent of your metabolism. Because the H.E.A.R.T. workout combines aerobics with resistance training and builds lean muscle, it lets you lose weight much faster than friends who focus on aerobic exercise alone (or who do no exercise at all).

Note that because most men have more muscle mass than women, they naturally tend to lose weight faster than women. The good news is that there's *equality* when it comes to building new muscle. Women who do the H.E.A.R.T. workout daily can stay lean, muscular, and strong and boost their calorie-burning ability.

By the way, I'm sure you or a friend has experienced a 5- to 7-pound weight loss in just one week using a "quick weight loss" diet plan. The bad news about those plans is that the 7 pounds is mostly water and muscle (not fat)—and you *will* gain it back. The human body is capable of losing two pounds of fat a week—no more. When you use the H.E.A.R.T. workout to reduce your body fat, you will lower your set point (see page 92), helping to maintain your new body weight.

The Honest Truth About Your Metabolism

Whether you are a rapid or slow calorie-burner is determined by how much muscle you have. The basic ability to burn calories is called your *basal metabolic rate*. As you increase your amount of muscle through the H.E.A.R.T. workout, you will naturally increase your basal metabolic rate. In fact, just 3 pounds of muscle, which you can put on in as little as two weeks if you are consistent with TLC 2, will boost your basal metabolic rate by at least 1,050 calories a week. I think building muscle should be considered the miracle cure for obesity!

The energy that the body uses for digestion is called the *thermic effect* of food digestion. This energy is used to digest, absorb, transport, and store nutrients in your body. What's exciting is that this thermic effect can be increased by 50 percent following the *3/500 Rule* explained in more detail in the chapter on TLC 3. With the 3/500 Rule, you eat regularly (every 3 hours) so you stay full and energized, yet no meal has more than 500 total calories. By exercising for 1 hour using the H.E.A.R.T. workout and following the 3/500 Rule, you are guaranteed to burn at least 600 more calories today than you normally would. This can translate into a 1½-pound loss per week without even dieting. Hmmm! I don't know of many diets that can make that claim, do you?

If you want to boost that weight loss, upgrade your daily diet to include additional servings of nutritious raw foods, which actually increase the "thermic effect" in the body, burning even more calories for a total loss of about 2 pounds a week.

Here's how it works. The elements of energy expenditure (metabolism) are basal metabolic rate, daily physical activity (including exercise), and the thermic effect of food digestion. Basal metabolic rate uses from 60 to 80 percent of your daily calories, activity uses an additional 10 to 25 percent, and food digestion another 10 to 15 percent.

Elements of energy expenditure (metabolism)
All these factors can be altered to burn more calories in the next 24 hours.

Basal metabolic rate	60 to 80 percent of total daily calories
Daily physical activity and exercise	10 to 25 percent of total daily calories
Thermic effect of food digestion	10 to 15 percent of total daily calories

This example shows the same client (let's call her Jane)—before the Turn-around, after 24 hours on the Turnaround, and six months later after she had lost weight, gained muscle, and was following her Turnaround program regularly.

Jane: a sedentary 160-pound woman (no muscles, high body fat, eats twice a day)

Basal metabolic rate	80 percent (1,120 calories)
Daily activity	10 percent (140 calories)
Food digestion	10 percent (140 calories)
Total calories burned for the day	1,400

Jane, 24 hours after starting her Turnaround

Basal metabolic rate	60 percent (1,200 calories)
Daily activity and H.E.A.R.T. workout	25 percent (500 calories)
Food digestion	15 percent (300 calories)
Total calories burned for the day	2,000

Jane, 6 months into her Turnaround, now weighs 140 pounds, eats nutritious food every 3 hours, and does the H.E.A.R.T. workout five times a week

Basal metabolic rate	60 percent (1,500 calories)
Daily activity and exercise	25 percent (625 calories)
Food digestion	15 percent (375 calories)
Total calories burned for the day	2,500

How to Boost Your Fat-Burning Enzymes

Now that you understand the simple way calories are burned, let's talk about burning fat calories with your H.E.A.R.T. workout. In the body there are special enzymes, existing only in the muscles, that actually increase calorie-burning fiftyfold during exercise. That's why your muscles are so important to keeping you lean. Some of the enzymes, such as the sugar-burning anaerobic (without oxygen) enzymes in the muscles, are very stable and easy to access. Even if you haven't exercised for years, your muscles keep producing those enzymes, because burning sugar is essential to the stress response and to keep your brain functioning normally.

On the other hand, your fat-burning enzymes disappear quickly if you don't exercise for a while. To make matters worse, as you age your fat stores receive less blood circulation unless you exercise. Therefore the fat in your fat cells has a much harder time making it to the muscles to be converted to energy by the enzymes. As you can see, aging and inactivity do *not* make a good combination.

When you use your muscles moderately (with oxygen), they metabolize fat that you have recently eaten and stored fat for use as energy. To accomplish this, the muscles activate a fat-breaking enzyme called *hormone-sensitive lipase*. In a host of comprehensive blood tests, researchers have shown that this enzyme's activity is seen after just 1 hour of walking, and it retains its fat-breaking activity for 12 hours. With the proper-intensity exercise, the fat-breaking enzymes increase in both number and activity. When this fat-breaking enzyme is circulated in the blood, it cleans blood vessel walls of fatty plaques and deposits. The bottom line? You need to exercise at a specific intensity to "earn" these incredible fat-burning enzymes. That intensity is called your Zone One.

METABOLISM BOOSTER

Here's an easy way to boost your metabolism: *watch less TV.* Researchers at Memphis State University monitored thirty-two girls as they watched a half-hour television program. They found that the metabolic rates dropped as much as 16 percent below resting metabolic rate. In other words, they burned fewer calories watching television than they did by just sitting.

In another recent study, researchers reported that cutting TV viewing could help children avoid obesity. In the United States the number of hours children watch television jumped from about 2 hours per day in 1969 to more than 5 in 1990. Meanwhile, obesity among adolescents had tripled, and it doubled in younger children between 1980 and 1994. Limiting television (and commercials) may help control how children perceive food as well as give more time for activity and exercise.

RESTING MUSCLES

As you sit in a chair reading this book, you burn about 1 calorie per minute. At rest, muscles burn a higher percentage of fat than sugar. That's because inactivity requires little muscular action, so the muscles have a lot of oxygen available. Unfortunately, the total amount of fat burned is low during inactivity. For instance, if you read for an hour, you burn 60 calories, and about 40 of those calories are from fat. Big deal.

MOVING MUSCLES

When you put down this book and start to move around, the number of calories you burn per minute will increase. Now, if you break into a full run the number of calories you burn will go up. But it may surprise you to know that the percentage of calories burned from fat will start to go down. The harder and more intensely you exercise, the harder it is for your muscles to burn fat. While it's true that the muscles use more calories, these are mostly sugar calories. The secret to burning both calories *and* fat is to maintain a specific heart rate that is high enough to burn a lot of calories yet moderate enough to continue to burn fat. Again, that intensity is called Zone One. When a sedentary, overweight person's muscles become anaerobic (without oxygen) during high-intensity exercise, her fat-burning ability literally goes to zero. Even if she increases her speed to increase the calorie burn, she's not burning more fat calories, only sugar calories. The more fit you are, the more efficiently your muscles burn fat. Your H.E.A.R.T. workout will help you become fit—and lean.

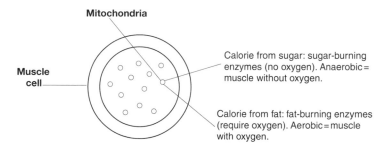

A calorie is burned at the mitochondria of the muscle cell. How can you tell your cells to burn fat? Make sure you exercise *with oxygen*—in your Zone One.

Low Intensity vs. High Intensity:
Which Is Better for Your Health?

Many fitness professionals continue to encourage people to train at higher heart rates, claiming that it's the *total calories* that make a difference. They may claim that the amount of fat burned in a high-intensity workout will end up being the same as in a moderate-intensity Zone One workout. That's not true.

1. This claim is based on the way a professional athlete's body performs—not the way your body will perform.
2. A higher-intensity workout does not allow you to "earn" the fat-burning enzymes necessary to burn the fat, during exercise or, more important, during the other 23 hours of the day.

HIGH-INTENSITY EXERCISE = AGING

What if I told you that high-intensity exercise actually accelerates aging? This statement always gets the audience's attention in my seminars—especially those men and women who believe in "no pain, no gain." While we once believed that high-impact power aerobics or sprinting uphill was the key to weight loss, we now know that high-intensity exercise actually causes oxidative and mechanical damage. This injury is followed by an inflammatory response that leads to excessive *apoptosis,* a process of cell death involved in aging. Simply put, cell death in high-intensity exercise replicates aging! In one particular study published in January 1998 in *Medicine and Science in Sports and Exercise,* researchers tested adults exercising on a treadmill until they were exhausted, and found DNA strand damage in lymphocytes immediately after exercise. The scientists concluded that this damage might explain the greater incidence of upper respiratory infections in highly trained athletes following exhaustive training periods. In contrast, researchers believe that moderate-intensity exercise over a lifetime may increase resistance to upper respiratory tract infections.

I think you would agree that a "no pain, no gain" exercise philosophy has dominated the fitness industry for decades. This philosophy is due in part to the research done in the sixties and seventies on competitive athletes, not on the general population. In spite of recent public health recommendations encouraging Americans to engage in moderate-intensity activity on most days of the week, the "go for the burn" mentality still exists in many of the fitness clubs in America. Many fitness enthusiasts have been training at high heart rates for so many years that they have a distorted sense of what moderate training feels like. For most, it seems that unless a workout is "heart-pounding and sweat-producing," it doesn't really qualify as a "good workout." Wrong. Competitive athletes have known for years that too high a heart rate leaves you with less fitness, not more. That's the very reason they wear a heart-rate monitor that gives them instant feedback and keeps them in a productive zone.

Exercise physiologists are becoming increasingly concerned about overtraining, because it can also set you up for serious injury. Don't make the mistake of trying to mimic a professional athlete's workout that you read about in a book, or going for Mr. America's workout, as described in one of the muscle magazines. Remember, it took them many years of work to get in that condition. If you have the well-rounded goals of optimal weight loss, antiaging, and wellness, your H.E.A.R.T. workout in Zone One is a more effective form of exercise.

HIGH-INTENSITY EXERCISE COMPROMISES THE IMMUNE SYSTEM

Because the body cannot differentiate between types of trauma, a high-intensity heart rate and "going for the burn" are both considered physical trauma by the body's intelligence. In fact, due to this stress many components of the immune system show adverse change after intense exertion. During this "open window" of impaired immunity, which may last from 3 to 72 hours, viruses and bacteria can gain a foothold, increasing the risk for subclinical and clinical infections. High-intensity exercise is also associated with an extensive disturbance of white blood cell counts. (Your white blood cells fight infection. Very high or very low white blood cell counts may indicate a severe disorder.)

In recent tests, scientists found that following a running episode at high intensity, the concentration of serum cortisol, one of the stress hormones, was significantly elevated above control levels for several hours. This high elevation of cortisol has been related to many of the immunosuppressive changes experienced during recovery from intense exercise. Also during high-intensity exercise, substances released from injured muscle cells initiate an inflammatory response in the body, and natural killer cell activity is decreased 40 to 60 percent for at least 6 hours. The changes are similar to those that occur in response to physical trauma such as a car accident or a heart episode.

In contrast, during moderate exercise, immune cells circulate through the body more quickly and are better able to kill bacteria and viruses. In other words, every time you do a H.E.A.R.T. workout session, your immune system receives a significant boost that increases your chances of fighting off cold viruses and more serious bacterial infections over the long term.

HIGH-INTENSITY EXERCISE IS A HORMONAL NIGHTMARE

Every time you exercise, you immediately change the hormonal environment inside your body and brain, an effect that can last up to 24 hours. Continuous high-intensity exercise accelerates aging by stimulating catabolic (negative) hormones and suppressing "good" hormones, such as growth hormone and testosterone. This is why people can exercise for months or even years without improvement in their bodies or fitness levels. One client, Muriel, exercised at high intensity for three years without losing a pound. In fact, she was still 20 pounds overweight when she sought help at the spa. Changing to the H.E.A.R.T. workout, which allowed her to stop punishing her body, she lost almost all her extra weight within twelve weeks —and had energy instead of feeling exhausted.

Sadly, high-intensity exercise may produce negative effects on aging, hormones, and the status of the immune system. I've had women come to the spa who ran marathons in their younger years, and the high-intensity running caused visible aging as some developed autoimmune diseases, such as asthma and arthritis, while others are now on heart rhythm medications for irregular heartbeats.

LOW-INTENSITY EXERCISE GIVES HEALTH BENEFITS

Because blood pressure often rises with age (and weight), exercise is of special importance as a natural therapy for keeping it in check. And consistent with the new theory of keeping exercise to a lower intensity, according to a report published in 1999 in the *Journal of Clinical Epidemiology*, low-intensity exercise results in greater blood pressure reduction than does high-intensity exercise. This report concluded that men and women with mild hypertension should get approximately 1 hour of low-intensity exercise four times a week to reduce their blood pressure. Your H.E.A.R.T. workout fits that prescription perfectly. Low- to moderate-intensity exercise also helps to reduce your lipid profile and improves glucose tolerance. In fact, if you had to choose between an after-dinner walk or a 5-mile race, you should choose the walk. You don't have to "go for the burn" to keep your blood glucose levels even. A study published in 1998 in the *Journal of the American Medical Association* found that increased participation in nonvigorous physical activity was as effective as vigorous physical activity in enhancing insulin sensitivity.

Low-intensity exercise is also beneficial for those with osteoarthritis (the "wear and tear" type of arthritis), improving physical function, aerobic capacity, and overall pain relief. And light to moderate activity is associated with lower coronary heart disease rates in women, according to a study published March 21, 2001, in the *Journal of the American Medical Association*. Stay tuned for more information on heart disease—the number one killer of women.

LOW-INTENSITY EXERCISE FEELS BETTER

Besides all the tremendous health benefits of low- to moderate-intensity exercise, it simply feels better. For too many years, exercise has been associated with pain, burn, and torment. But no more! Not only does moderate exercise burn more fat calories than heavy exercise, most people will engage in moderate exercise far longer than they would heavy exercise. For example, if you undertake power walking in your Zone One at a sustained, moderate clip, it will burn more calories than if you sprinted around the track and then had to spend several minutes recovering.

Dieting vs. Exercise:
Which Is Best for Weight Loss?

Clearly, a high-fat Western diet and inactivity are to blame for America's massive weight gain. And the hard-core truth is that your body is going to resist your efforts to change its weight—unless you let your metabolism know that this is the real thing. The most profound change to your metabolism will be the result of your H.E.A.R.T.

Your body wants to return to its *set point*, the weight you have been maintaining consistently. Heat production, muscle mass, blood sugar, mood, and fat-burning enzymes all affect your set point.

workout. When you're physically fit, the extra calories you consume are used for fitness activities rather than stored as fat, which causes you to gain weight. You may even need to consume more food. Let's compare the two methods of weight loss.

DIET FOR WEIGHT LOSS

When you go on a low-calorie or trendy diet but your muscles stay inactive, their protein is broken down for conversion into sugar, particularly with the popular high-protein diets. When you lose muscle, you lose calorie-burning ability, and your metabolism slows down. Also, when you skip meals and diet, your body goes into starvation mode and gets superefficient at storing the few calories you feed it. After a period of time, you regain the lost weight, along with a few more pounds, and it can be days, weeks, or even months before your metabolism recovers, because the body still thinks it's starving. This effect can happen as quickly as one skipped breakfast!

EXERCISE FOR WEIGHT LOSS

With exercise alone for weight loss, you will notice a significantly greater weight loss than with no activity at all. Exercise also improves fitness levels and overall body health. In a revealing study where two groups lost the same amount of weight on the scale—one through exercise alone and the other through a calorie-restricted diet—the exercisers lost a higher percentage of body fat. Remember, it's not just about lowering the number on the scale; it's about changing the shape of your body, and that happens when you reduce your percentage of body fat.

APPLE OR PEAR?

'm talking shape of your body, not what kind of fruit you like to eat. Apple body types are those that accumulate fat at the waistline (many men), and pears are those that carry more weight below the waist and around the thighs and upper legs. If you are an apple body type, you have a higher risk of developing heart disease, diabetes, high blood pressure, stroke, and even some cancers.

Here's a simple formula to tell if you are an apple or pear: break out your measuring tape, measure your waist in inches at its narrowest point, and then divide by your hip measurement in inches at the widest point. For women the score shouldn't exceed *0.80*. For men the score shouldn't exceed *0.95*.

For example, Carmen (a pear) has a waist measurement of 29 inches and a hip measurement of 41.

29 divided by 41 = .71 (acceptable—less than .80)

Gail's figure is definitely an apple with her waist at 38 and her hips at 37.

38 divided by 37 = 1.03 (too high—greater than .80)

Whether you are an apple or a pear with a growing waistline, it's time to start your H.E.A.R.T. workout to pare away (no pun intended) some of that visceral body fat, the type that hides close to organs deep within the recesses of the body and increases your risk of heart disease and diabetes. In fact, studies have shown that exercise reduces waistline fat more effectively than dieting.

DIET AND EXERCISE FOR WEIGHT LOSS:
THE FORMULA FOR SUCCESS

When you *combine* a proper daily diet and exercise, you will notice the greatest outcome. Not only will you lose more weight over the long term, you will have an easier time maintaining your weight loss. For example, burning 400 to 500 calories from exercise per day, along with consuming 400 to 500 fewer calories from eating the recommended whole foods on the Definition Diet per week, will result in a weight loss of *1½ to 2 pounds* per week—or *80 to 100 pounds* by the end of a year. Most important, the weight you lose will be pounds of fat—not precious water or your calorie-burning muscles.

Your H.E.A.R.T. Formula = Aerobic Training and Resistance Training

Both aerobic and resistance training appear to have positive effects on bone mineral density, glucose tolerance, insulin sensitivity, and weight control, and both are incorporated in your H.E.A.R.T. workout. For weight control, aerobic exercise is considered a significant calorie-burner, whereas resistance training assists the body in expending calories via an increase in lean body mass and basal metabolism. You always burn fat *after* aerobic and resistance exercise, but you only burn fat *during* aerobic exercise. Even though you don't burn fat when you weight-lift, you burn it afterward, when your muscles are recovering. Why don't you burn fat during the weight-lifting session? Because it's anaerobic (without oxygen).

In the past some women avoided resistance training because of the myth that women could not build strength—we were told that only men could have muscles. The truth is, the average woman can build strength at a slightly faster rate than the average man. Women also used to believe that they would get big and bulky if they trained with weights. We now know that women typically do not have the potential to develop large muscles because they do not have as much testosterone as men. And the biggest misconception is that when you stop working with weights, your muscle will "turn into fat." This is impossible! That's like saying an apple can turn into a banana—one cannot turn into the other. However, if you do stop working out, the muscle will atrophy (diminish), and your metabolism will slow down. When this happens, it is likely you will gain some fat.

AEROBIC TRAINING

When the body starts to use muscles to move, the demand for blood and oxygen at each muscle site goes up and the heart beats faster, giving the heart itself a workout. This demand for oxygen in the arm and leg muscles is where the term *aerobic* (with oxygen) comes from. We will use the term *aerobic* instead of *cardiovascular* (or *cardio*), because oxygen is going to be our friend in the H.E.A.R.T. workout. Aerobic exercise burns more calories than lifting weights during the actual exercise. But after an aerobic workout, the metabolism slows back down to normal in about half an hour to an hour, depending on the person. This time period of elevated fat- and calorie-burning is called the exercise "after burn."

RESISTANCE TRAINING

In resistance training, as long as the moving muscle has some type of resistance, it will respond by becoming stronger. The resistance can come from workout machines, free weights (dumbbells), cans of vegetables from the pantry, bands, iso-ropes, water, stairs, a step, an uphill climb, or even your own body weight. Your H.E.A.R.T. workout incorporates resistance training within each daily session. The body continues to burn calories at a higher rate for more than 1 hour after a resistance-training workout ends, and this calorie-burning can last as long as 2 hours. Your H.E.A.R.T. workout is designed to give you a maximum calorie- and fat-burning effect by combining aerobic exercise with resistance training.

Resistance training also increases muscle mass, which is lost during aging. In fact, studies indicate that women as young as twenty-four should add resistance training to their daily workouts. The American Heart Association also reports that regular resistance workouts benefit the cardiovascular system by lowering blood pressure and reducing cholesterol levels, which in turn reduce the risk of stroke and heart disease.

The H.E.A.R.T. workout adds muscle to your body without making you look like a bodybuilder. It firms and tones your body and reshapes and defines your muscles so that your body is actually smaller. That's because muscle weighs more than fat but takes up less room in your body. I am 5 feet 5 inches and weigh 135 pounds. But I also wear a size seven and can eat a lot of food without gaining weight.

Even though we know the value of combining aerobic and resistance training for an optimal workout, the fitness industry continues to separate the two programs, offering weight-lifting equipment in one room and aerobic classes or equipment in another. The traditional "bulky bodybuilder" way to exercise, with

LACTIC ACID

If you train hard enough to be out of breath, the fat-burning enzymes stop working because they are oxygen-dependent. If you're out of breath, you're burning just sugar and burning it only halfway. If you continue to exercise at that level, pyruvic acid accumulates in muscle and turns into lactic acid, which causes the "burning" pain we feel when we push ourselves too hard physically. We now know that "going for the burn"/"no gain without pain" actually accelerates the aging process, causing more harm than good.

sets and reps, continues to prevail, and using a personal trainer is considered the optimum way to work out effectively. (I personally think it's presumptuous for another person to tell you when you've done enough reps.) Listen to your body—it will tell you to do more or less. And remember, until you can motivate yourself to do that push-up, you're not an intrinsic exerciser and you don't "own" that workout—your trainer does. In the many years I have worked with women to reduce body fat, get in shape, and ward off chronic illness, nothing has been more effective than a combined hour of aerobic and oxygenated resistance training.

Your 24-Hour Turnaround

PREPARING TO WORK OUT

So there you have it. You know that the H.E.A.R.T. workout will put your Turnaround in fast motion, increasing your fat-burning potential within 24 hours. But dream with me for a minute. What if you continued the H.E.A.R.T. workout for one year—five years—a lifetime? Imagine the age-defying benefits you would experience in the way you look, feel, act, and react—each day of working out in your Zone One.

Determine your goals. As you prepare for your H.E.A.R.T. workout, it's important to establish goals. Setting goals will help turn your initial enthusiasm into a concrete and measurable reality. Without specific goals, you have no way to determine if the desired changes, particularly weight loss or a reduction in dress size, are taking place. Make sure to write these down in your Turnaround Journal to help you visualize the commitment. Make sure the goals are realistic—you should attempt something you can actually achieve. Don't set goals that will certainly lead to failure. Review small goals frequently and make changes as necessary. Some examples include:

1. I will *stay* with the workout for at least 30 minutes daily the first week.
2. I will *plan* to include this workout in my daily routine.
3. I will *think* positive thoughts about exercise before my workout.
4. I will *focus* on what I know is good for me instead of on how tired I might feel at the end of a workout.

If being skinny is your only motive for your Turnaround, and you haven't been skinny for twenty years, you'll probably fail. Yet if you focus on improving your overall health by incorporating the other TLCs with the H.E.A.R.T. workout, you will feel benefits immediately. Feeling good and feeling younger will keep you motivated to stick with the program, and before you know it, you will lose weight and reach that goal. While beauty is superficial and fleeting, optimal health is profound and lasting. Genuine beauty is the result of a larger commitment to all of your TLCs.

I usually have a knockdown, drag-out fight with my clients when we calculate how much weight they should lose each week. I'll admit that most of them are not thrilled by the idea of a reasonable weight loss of 1 to 2 pounds of fat each week. But the fact is, no matter how many calories you cut, 2 pounds of fat is the most that a human body can lose in a week. Any loss beyond that is muscle—and you do NOT want to lose your calorie-burning muscles!

BEFORE YOU BEGIN

Check with your doctor. If you are over forty years old and you haven't exercised for a while, it's a good idea to have a physical and talk with your doctor about appropriate exercise. Also check with your doctor if you have risk factors for cardiovascular disease, such as smoking, high blood pressure, high total cholesterol, diabetes, obesity, or a sedentary lifestyle. If you are experiencing occasional or frequent chest pains, feel faint or dizzy, or are taking prescription medication such as treatment for hypertension, make sure your doctor monitors your exercise and your progress.

Get a heart-rate monitor. It doesn't matter what age you are or how physically fit you are, it is very important that you have a heart-rate monitor and wear it when you do the H.E.A.R.T. workout, as your heart rate lets you know if you are exercising in Zone One. Look at competitive athletes, and you will see that almost all of them wear heart-rate monitors because it's the most efficient way to measure exercise and its results. As you see your heart rate go down during exercise and also at rest, you will know that your fitness program is working.

Log for success. Your Turnaround Journal is vital for charting your exercise progress. Get your journal out at the beginning of the week and pencil in your H.E.A.R.T. workout schedule for all 7 days. The H.E.A.R.T. workout can only become a habit if it's at the top of your priority list. If possible, try to schedule your workout in the morning—first thing on your agenda. As the day goes by you are more likely to find excuses to change your plan, such as unexpected events and errands.

TURNAROUND TIP

Try to avoid taking off two days in a row from your H.E.A.R.T. workout. Just forty-eight hours without exercise, and your metabolism slows down, your aerobic fitness begins to diminish, and your muscles start to atrophy. This holds true for everyone—no matter what shape you are in.

Zone One Training

Research has shown that your workouts will be more effective and efficient when you use your heart rate as a gauge for intensity. That's why I keep insisting that you rely on your heart-rate monitor at all times during exercise. A *zone* is a range of numbers that refers to the times your heart beats per minute. Your *Zone One* is the optimal personal training zone for you to achieve a young, lean, and healthy body. You calculate your Zone One with an equation that uses your resting heart rate and your maximum heart rate. The *resting heart rate* is measured when you first wake up in the morning before you get out of bed. The lower the number the better. You will see your resting heart rate go down as you become more fit. The *maximum heart rate* is the fastest your heart can beat for 1 minute. We use a standard measurement of 220 minus your age to get a predicted figure. A more accurate method is to have a treadmill test with your doctor. If you are on medication, which can increase or decrease your heart rate, or have any kind of heart abnormality, check with your doctor, as your Zone One may need to be adjusted.

CALCULATING YOUR ZONE ONE

Now let's calculate your Zone One, so you will know what the optimal workout intensity is when you get started with exercise. Get out your Turnaround Journal and find the resting heart rate that you recorded when you started reading this book. If you haven't taken your resting heart rate yet, read page 21 and get it tomorrow morning when you awaken. You will need it to calculate your zones.

ZONE ONE FORMULA

$$220 - age = a$$
$$a - \text{resting heart rate} = b$$
$$(b \times .55) + \text{resting heart rate} = \text{low end of Zone One}$$
$$(b \times .70) + \text{resting heart rate} = \text{high end of Zone One}$$

For example, if you are fifty years old and your resting heart rate is 60, then calculate:

$$220 - 50 \text{ (age)} = 170$$
$$170 - 60 \text{ (resting heart rate)} = 110$$
$$110 \times .55 = 60.5 \quad 60 + 60 = 120 \text{ (low end)}$$
$$110 \times .70 = 77 \quad 77 + 60 = 137 \text{ (high end)}$$

Your Zone One is 120 to 137.

Remember, the lower the heart rate (intensity), the more oxygen available, the higher the percentage of fat is burned. Training at 120 is just as good (if not better) than at 137. Studies have consistently shown that fatty acid oxidation (fat-burning) becomes approximately equal to the total amount of fatty acids available at 65 percent of your maximum heart rate—the middle of your Zone One.

YOUR INTERVAL ZONE

Your *Interval Zone* is a higher zone you will use once you've increased your fitness level and are able to sustain at least 30 minutes in your Zone One. In the Interval Zone, you improve your functional capacity. The number and size of your blood vessels actually increase, you step up your lung capacity and respiratory rate, and your heart increases in size and strength so that you can exercise longer before becoming fatigued. Staying in this zone for just 1-minute intervals produces incredible cardiovascular results. Fat-burning goes down in the Interval Zone, but if you return to Zone One after 1 minute or less, you will go back to optimal fat-burning. (Advanced workouts include 1-minute intervals for improved cardiovascular fitness.)

To calculate the high end of your Interval Zone, add 15 to the high end of your Zone One. For example: if your Zone One is 120 to 137, your Interval Zone would be 137 to 152 (137 plus 15).

EXERCISING IN ZONE ONE

Now that you've calculated your Zone One, use it to achieve a lean body!

low intensity + long duration = a lean body

Intensity is the level of exertion. Intensity (heart rate) refers to the level of exertion during exercise and is measured by your heart rate. To lose body fat, think *longer* (like long and lean muscles) workouts as opposed to harder when exercising. Hang out in your Zone One. If you can say to yourself at any time, "I could go at this pace for another hour," then you are at an appropriate intensity. If another hour is out of the question, then slow down and keep going at a lower heart rate.

Duration is how long you exercise. Duration (minutes) refers to how long you exercise. As you can see on the following time line, at 30 minutes you start burning significant amounts of fat. I always tell my clients that the most effective part of the workout is after 30 minutes. So consider that each 5 to 10 minutes you work out after the initial 30 minutes as icing on the cake for fat loss (or pounds off the hips). This is also when you start to increase the growth of fat-burning enzymes in your muscles. Don't worry about the distance you travel while exercising; the time you exercise is what's important.

If you look at world-class sprinters, you will notice that they are heavier than world-class marathon runners. That's because the marathon runner is a professional fat-burner, training at a lower heart rate for a longer time. To change your body and burn stored fat as fuel, you need to focus on long-duration exercise. Stored fat is used for fuel only after you first use the fat that you have eaten in the last 24-hour period, which has not entered your fat cells. This fat is far more available than the stored fat.

When you do your H.E.A.R.T. workout in Zone One, your muscles burn fuel from the following sources:

1. First the available sugar in your bloodstream for the first 8 to 12 minutes of your workout.
2. Next the available fat until you use it all up (this could be 30 minutes, or it could be 2 hours if you ate a lot of fat yesterday).
3. Last the stored fat. This is why you have to go for long duration. A 30-minute workout will not make your body lean. The bad news is: you start to use stored fat *only* after using up all the available fat. The good news is: if you follow the low-fat Definition Diet, you will start to burn stored fat sooner.

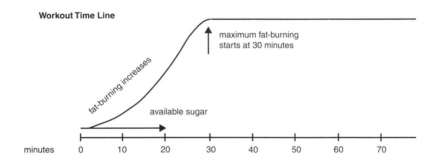

How often should you do your H.E.A.R.T. workout? For weight loss, my recommendation is at least five times a week for 60 minutes. While the exercise prescription for health is five times a week for 30 minutes, this will not produce weight loss. Again, longer-duration exercise is what burns stored fat. Some people routinely do aerobics three times a week and weight lifting three times a week. With the H.E.A.R.T. workout, the exercise is combined and extended to an optimal 60 minutes five times a week. I did this to help save time and to make both types of exercise more effective. Note: Never take two days off in a row!

Abdominal Alert: Three Effective Exercises

Always do your abdominal exercises *before* starting your H.E.A.R.T. aerobic and resistance workout. Eyebrows go up when I make this statement, and my clients invariably say, "But my trainer says . . ." Here are three reasons to do abdominal exercises first:

1. The ab muscles have a large blood supply before you start your workout, especially if you have been sitting around or you just woke up. When you start exercising, you send the blood to the muscles in the arms and legs and away from the abs. As you have learned, it's better to work a muscle that contains a good supply of blood and oxygen.

2. When your lower abs are contracted, your posture is better. Great posture keeps your back strong and protects it from injury.

3. I also think it's a good idea to do your abs in the morning before you go off for the day—just to make sure you get this exercise done before you start procrastinating.

"I do a hundred crunches a day—sometimes even more—but my belly sticks out worse than ever." I hear this all the time. How do I explain it? First of all, crunches (working your upper abs by lifting your shoulders off the floor) do *not* reduce the amount of fat around the middle of your body. Only Zone One exercise and the Definition Diet will get rid of this extra fat. Second, crunches work the upper part of the abdominal muscle and neglect the lower part that sticks out. If you watch people do crunches, every time they exert, their stomach protrudes slightly or greatly, making matters much worse.

The most effective way to work your abs is to engage them to move (functional abdominal effort) and to consciously contract them during the day—yes, even when you're seated at your desk. Ab exercises that are truly effective include the following.

Seated chair (beginner, also for those with back problems). Sit on the edge of a chair with only your toes touching the floor as far away from the chair as possible. Clasp your fingers behind your head and open your elbows until you feel your shoulder blades squeeze together. Do not pull on your head, and keep your neck relaxed. Gaze up at the ceiling with your eyes, and keep your chin slightly lifted.

Now lift one of your toes off the floor, bringing the knee toward the chest. Exhale as you lift the knee. Set the toe back down before you lift the other. Repeat until fatigued (not exhausted). I do these every hour that I'm seated at my desk (which was for many months while I wrote this book!).

Pelvic tuck (beginner, intermediate, advanced). Lie on your back with your heels resting on a chair or the bench at the gym. Make sure a 90-degree angle is formed by your heels, knees, and hip bones. Stretch one arm up and over your head on the floor while the other hand is resting on your lower stomach. Press your lower back into the floor (so you can feel the floor). This position reverses your pelvis, contracts your lower abs, and releases your lower back. Take a deep breath in, and on the exhale pull your belly button in as though it is trying to touch the floor as well. Do this mini pelvic tuck ten times. On the eleventh time, exhale and then tilt your pelvis even more so that your hips come slightly off the floor while you pull your belly button in. Don't be shy; you can't do too many of these; the more the better. They totally flattened my stomach just two weeks after my daughter, Riley, was born. If you can do this twice a day, that's great. It relieves lower back strain and pain and teaches you how to use your abdominal muscles with the breath.

Reverse curls (advanced). The pelvic tucks above will train your abs for this advanced level exercise. Lie flat on the floor, stretching your arms straight overhead and holding on to something heavy that will not move, such as the leg of your living room sofa or a piece of equipment at the gym. Crossing your feet at the ankles, lift them off the ground to the point where your knees create a 90-degree angle. Press your lower back to the floor as you contract your abdominal muscles. Making a pelvic tuck, reach your toes toward the ceiling, exhaling. Inhale as you return to the starting position, flattening your abs and your back on the way down. This movement is done slowly in both directions. Don't use your arms to pull and don't use momentum, but focus on your muscles. Once you can do 20 reps while holding on to something, try doing it with nothing to hold on to.

Warming Up: Mandatory for Burning Fat

I believe the warm-up is the most important part of a workout. Warming your muscles externally with saunas, heating pads, and massage is not effective for exercise and can actually decrease your level of performance. The important changes in chemical, neurological, and cellular muscle function all depend on warming the muscle from the inside out. Studies show that heart irregularities occur more often in people who don't warm up before exercise.

As you begin by slowly using your muscles, oxygen breaks away from the blood more rapidly and completely. In contrast, if you hop on a treadmill and begin running without warming up, your "cold" muscles will be oxygen-starved for the first few minutes, which means that right from the start you send the message to your body that there will be no oxygen available for fat-burning. Big mistake!

The rise in body temperature from your preworkout warm-up also accelerates the work of all those enzymes we've talked about. Fats and sugars are broken down quickly, and less lactic acid accumulates. Warm muscles are also more elastic, meaning that they are flexible (allowing for a greater range of motion) and are less susceptible to injury. Cold muscles don't absorb shock or impact as well making the workout more trumatic to your bones and joints. Another bonus of a preworkout warm-up is improved ability to send messages between the brain, spinal cord, and muscles. The end result is better reflexes and improved coordination.

During your warm-up, the capillaries that surround the muscles start to dilate, which brings more oxygen to the muscles and carries the waste products like carbon dioxide and lactic acid away.

The H.E.A.R.T. Workout Warm-up

Your warm-up can be a slow and carefully performed version of the upcoming H.E.A.R.T. workout. Here's a simple way to start:

- Move the blood and oxygen to all muscles of your body by deliberately walking with a large arm swing.

- If you have specific muscles that feel tight, start with small, slow movements, and gradually make them bigger and faster. For instance, for a tight Achilles tendon, start with small heel raises, and then make them larger as the Achilles tendons loosen up. (Stretching them first is a big mistake because a cold muscle is not flexible and does not want to be stretched.)

- During your warm-up, spend at least 5 to 8 minutes at a heart rate below your Zone One. This will ensure that all the necessary physiological processes are activated.

- Focus on your posture, abdominal control, and regular breathing during your warm-up.

- Replace any negative thoughts with positive affirmations (reread TLC 1). Pay attention to your self-talk. Replace thoughts such as "I don't feel like exercising" with "I will feel better after I warm up," or "I will feel great after I get moving." Imagine yourself strong and powerful. (Or as the Nike commercial says, "Just do it!")

The H.E.A.R.T. Workout Technique

Let's get started! Get on your shoes. Grab your heart-rate monitor and put it on. Drink another cup of water, and let's exercise.

aerobics + resistance = lean, healthy, and hormonally happy

You can take your current workout and modify it to include heart-rate specific exercise with aerobic resistance training (H.E.A.R.T.). For instance, you'll combine your aerobic workout (walking, biking) with a resistance workout (weights, isoropes) to increase the effectiveness of each one. Your goal with each session will be to use your muscles to elevate your heart rate. If you are not currently exercising, then use the chart to select your favorite type of aerobic and resistance exercise.

Here are some common combinations of aerobic exercise and resistance training that my clients use:

THE H.E.A.R.T. WORKOUT

AEROBIC EXERCISE	+	RESISTANCE TRAINING
Treadmill		Isometric rope or circuit resistance training[†]

Aerobic Exercise	+	Resistance Training
Stationary bike		Isometric rope or circuit resistance training[†]
Rowing machine		Slowly with medium resistance
Cross-trainer*		Slowly with medium resistance
Stair machine		Circuit resistance training[†]
Swimming		Swim gloves and kickboard
Walking (3 mph)		Isometric rope
Power walking		Hand iron gloves**
Biking		Circuit resistance training[†]

*This equipment provides both aerobic and resistance training.

[†]Circuit resistance training means integrating resistive sets of upper- or lower-body movements into your aerobic routine after you have reached "steady state," meaning that you are warmed up and your heart rate is stable. For most people this is between 15 and 18 minutes.

**Hand iron gloves are weighted gloves (1 to 3 pounds for each hand). These gloves are safer for the wrists and more convenient than holding dumbbells or any handheld weight while walking.

As you proceed with your workout, I want you to remember to:

- *Stop!* Stop running, hopping, and uncontrollably flinging your body parts around to elevate your heart rate. Stop using momentum! And stop working out at dangerously high heart rates; you now know the results. Your heart-rate monitor will tell you if you need to go harder or easier.

- *Go!* Instead, go with more muscle, awareness, and deliberate resistance. Judge the quality of your aerobic workout by how many muscles move you.

_____

Pulling (and Pushing) It All Together

Have I convinced you to use your muscles yet? There are several ways to accomplish this in your H.E.A.R.T. workout, and here are the general rules.

1. *Make your own resistance at the beginning of your workout by "recruiting" your muscles (that means keeping them tight and contracted), squeezing your buns, holding in your abs, and working out deliberately.* This deliberate resistance allows your muscles to warm up and have a blood and oxygen supply, and your coordination and balance will be better. Add resistance after you are 18 minutes into your workout (for intermediate and advanced workouts). Added resistance for your lower body could be an increase in elevation on your treadmill (slow the speed if needed) or an increase in difficulty on your elliptical cross-trainer, stair stepper, or stationary bike. If you are power walking, walk in the grass or sand, and if you are doing an exercise tape, add a step. Added upper-body resistance could be an isometric rope, hand irons, or free weights. If you are a new exerciser, do not add the extra resistance until you can sustain 40 minutes of aerobics. Continue to use your own muscle strength during this time.

2. *Use light to moderate resistance, allowing for constant and continued movement with your muscles.* At first this lighter resistance may seem easy, but as your muscles become fatigued, it takes more effort to complete the movement, so the muscles work harder and harder as the workout progresses, but without any pain or strain. Yes, the bodybuilder guy in the gym is correct: heavy lifting is required for *maximum strength*. But I want you to focus on your goals for a healthier, leaner body. There is rarely a time when you need to use the maximum effort of a bodybuilder, right? When you train for maximum strength, you create fatigue and trauma to the body. In many studies, people who completed a high number of repetitions with lighter weights had strength gains similar to those of people who completed a low number of repetitions with heavy weights. Study participants working out with lighter weights performed twice the number of repetitions at half the workload of the heavy-resistance group.

3. *Use handheld resistance instead of bars or machines for upper-body resistance.* Because there is a lack of "assisted" stability, more muscle fibers are needed to complete the movement.

4. *Use the abdominal structures (abs), the spine muscles, and the posture muscles (together these are called your core muscles) to "stabilize" all your movements.* Remember that the opposition muscles to your abs are your spine muscles, and it is important to keep them in balance by performing

movements that use both. When you're constantly being challenged to use multiple muscle groups ("moving with muscle"), including your arms, hips, legs, and back, you end up integrating, not isolating, muscle activity, and your core muscles are made stronger.

Walking uphill and doing reverse abdominal curls and yoga positions all help to keep abs and spine muscles in balance. A strong, stable core can make other sports, like hiking, power walking, and stepping, easier. For example, if your spine acts as a powerful base for your legs, you will be able to put more power behind each step and move with less effort. Core conditioning will also tone your torso and abs and keep your lower back healthy by improving your posture. If your core is strong, your lower ab muscles will be drawn in toward the spine and help you sit up straight.

Stop! Avoid machines that require no stabilizing or balancing, only pushing or pulling. They do not duplicate real life, in which balance and coordination help to produce movement.

Go! Choose handheld resistance that requires the use of the secondary and tertiary muscles for stability and balance in addition to the primary movement muscles.

5. *Use your own body weight to train the muscles in your lower body.* This rule always raises eyebrows when I inform a client that she won't be doing the 120-pound leg presses that her trainer previously prescribed, which she will admit actually made her thighs bigger instead of smaller. Your own body weight is adequate to train the muscles in your lower body. Use the elevation on the treadmill, increased intensity on the cross-trainer, a step video, or a power walk in the sand. The results will be lean and toned legs without the added size.

6. *Get down on the ground and do some good old-fashioned push-ups.* These are superfunctional and "real life" because you'll work out all your upper-body muscles at one time. Push-ups strengthen your chest and back muscles as well as your arms and abs. If you are a new exerciser, you can modify push-ups by putting your knees on the floor instead of just your feet while you do the exercise. Or you can do the push-ups by standing and facing a blank wall with your hands against the wall and your feet about 3 feet away from the wall. Aim for as many push-ups as you can do comfortably.

Dips are also great upper-body strengtheners. To do a dip, sit on the edge of a sturdy chair with your hands tucked under your hips, holding on to the chair. Slowly walk your feet about 3 feet away from the chair, sliding your bottom off the seat as you do. Keep your knees bent and your abs contracted. As you continue to hold on to the chair, slowly bend your elbows, lower your body toward the floor, and then push back up to the starting position as you exhale. Do as many dips as you can comfortably. You'll be able to do more as you build strength.

Beginner Level H.E.A.R.T. Workout

If you are new to exercise or haven't worked out in a while (or ever), I want you to start out with slow and easy workouts—and all in your Zone One. Aim for 30 minutes every day, and if you feel good when you get to 30, keep going—you'll get a greater fat and calorie burn. If you are more than fifty pounds overweight or if you have knee problems, get into a water aerobics class, start swimming laps, or slowly walk uphill on a treadmill to help boost weight loss safely.

Your goal is to build to 40 minutes or more *before* you add resistance to your H.E.A.R.T. workout. At this low level of effort, your body is learning to increase the rate of fat release from the cells and you are earning the enzymes the muscles need to burn the fat for fuel. Zone One is sometimes called the *fat-burning zone* because up to 85 percent of the total calories burned in this zone are fat calories.

Your Beginning H.E.A.R.T. workout could look like this:

- Choose a workout activity from this list:
  Walking/power walking
  Treadmill at a 2 to 4 percent grade going 3 mph or less
  Cross-trainer machine (preferably with arm workout)
  Swimming or pool class
  Low-impact aerobics or sculpting class
  Beginner aerobics tape

- Work out abs: Do the seated chair or pelvic tuck (or both).

- First 8 minutes: Using your selected aerobic activity, warm up with your heart rate below Zone One, using small, slow movements that are a "rehearsal" for your workout. For instance, if walking is your aerobic activity, start by walking slowly, making large but slow arm swings, and then build as you progress into your workout.

- Next 8 to 12 minutes: Stay at the low end of your Zone One. Make your own resistance, recruiting as many muscles as you can to make each movement. Remember to "move with muscle," making deliberate movements.

- Next 12 to 30 minutes (or longer, if you feel strong): Head toward the higher end of your Zone One if it is comfortable—but do not exceed the high-end heart rate. Remember, you burn more fat staying in your Zone One than you do with a higher heart rate.

- At 30 minutes: Cool down using stretches or yoga positions. Once you are able to go 40 minutes at the Beginner Level, you may move to Intermediate Level, in which you will add resistance training to your aerobic exercise.

Intermediate Level H.E.A.R.T. Workout

Your immediate exercising goal is to sustain longer training periods, which for most people means lowering your heart rate so that your body can carry more oxygen to your muscles and break into your fat storage cells. Soon you'll find yourself going the longer distances with a reduced heart rate—proof of your increasing level of fitness. At your Zone One intensity you should have no problem increasing your H.E.A.R.T. workout time to 1 hour.

Set 60 minutes as your exercise goal. But don't be shy—if you have more time, keep moving. All the great fat-burning benefits happen after 30 minutes, so if you have previously been exercising too vigorously but not losing weight, it's time to see results. Lower your heart rate to Zone One immediately, and exercise longer to burn more total calories from fat.

Once you can comfortably increase your Zone One workout to 1 hour (that may be today), I want you to add a resistance component at 18 minutes. You have two choices. You can either continue your lower-body workout and add an upper-body component (hand irons, isometric rope, or free weights), or you can choose a circuit routine. My favorite is on the Life Fitness treadmill or Cross Trainer elliptical machine. (Both interact with your heart-rate monitor to keep you in your Zone One.) After you have warmed up and are 18 minutes into your H.E.A.R.T. workout using either the treadmill or cross-trainer, press *pause,* step off the equipment, and stand in a semisquat position (knees bent, with your buns squeezed and your abs contracted). In this position, do one set of biceps curls at a weight that allows you to do at least 16 repetitions. Check your heart-rate monitor; your heart rate should stay in your Zone One. If it doesn't, use heavier weights next time. After completing the set, go back to your aerobic workout for 2 to 5 minutes, and then pause and work another muscle group with free weights. You can accomplish a complete upper-body workout within your 1-hour aerobic workout. Mix your circuit routine with your hand irons or isometric rope for a varied workout. Changing your workout around keeps the routine interesting and keeps your body from adapting to the same thing every day, which can cause a plateau effect.

A great H.E.A.R.T. workout for the Intermediate exerciser would look like this:

- Choose a workout activity from this list:
Outdoor power walking with hand irons or the isometric rope
Mountain hiking with two large water bottles
Inline skating with hand iron weighted gloves
Cross-country skiing
Treadmill training tape with hand iron weighted gloves
Treadmill training with isometric rope
Step class (Zone Training step tape) with weights or isometric rope (no dancing or bouncing)
H.E.A.R.T. workout exercise tape (order from my website)
Circuit training with free weights (dumbbells)

- Work out abs: Do pelvic tucks and/or reverse curls. Or if you are in the gym, try some hanging abs or the Roman chair—both are reverse curl methods. Ask the gym attendant to assist you with the equipment.

- First 5 to 8 minutes: Warm up at a heart rate anywhere below your Zone One (minimum of 5 minutes).

- Next 6 to 17 minutes: Pick up the pace and aim for the low or middle heart rate in your Zone One. Make your own resistance, recruiting as many muscles as you can. Remember to "move with muscle," as described in the Beginner section.

- At 18 minutes: Continue to do your aerobic exercise, and add upper-body resistance or start a circuit routine.

- At 55 minutes: Start to slow down, lower your heart rate, and stretch or do yoga poses. End at 60 minutes. On days when you have time, extend your workouts to burn extra calories from fat.

After 3 weeks of doing your H.E.A.R.T. workout at this level (five times a week or more), progress to the advanced workout.

Advanced Level H.E.A.R.T. Workout

No matter what your sport or fitness level, the H.E.A.R.T. workout will provide an excellent total body workout or cross-training for your specific sport. Engaging all the muscles of the body and moving in different directions will upgrade your current level of fitness and cross-train your body for any activity. A great H.E.A.R.T. workout could look like this:

- Choose your workout from the Intermediate Level list.

- Work out abs: Reverse curls.

- First 5 to 8 minutes: Warm up at a heart rate below your Zone One.

- Next 6 to 17 minutes: Pick up the pace. Make your own resistance by recruiting as many muscles as you can. Remember to "move with muscle."

- At 18 minutes: Continue to do the aerobic exercise and add upper-body resistance or start a circuit routine.

- At 22 minutes: Work out 1 minute at your Interval Zone heart rate (defined on page 100). Increase the intensity of the activity you are doing by adding extra weight or going faster or higher. Recover by lowering your heart rate back to Zone One immediately. Wait 5 minutes before doing another interval. Continue with upper-body resistance and intervals until 55 minutes.

- At 55 minutes: Cool down and stretch or do yoga poses.

Finish with Stretching: The Flexibllity Formula

As important as the H.E.A.R.T. workout is for keeping your lungs and heart fit, your body fat low, and your muscles strong, it also helps to keep your body flexible, by ending your workout with stretching. Even when we exercise regularly, we still spend time sitting at the computer, watching television, or working at a desk. During this sedentary time, our bodies get lazy, our muscles atrophy (shorten), and our joints lose their range of motion. Even if you're active, your body can lose its natural lubrication and stiffen with age. In fact, at adulthood the body's tissues have lost about 15 percent of their moisture content, becoming less supple and more prone to injury. If you are inactive, your muscle fibers start to adhere to each other, developing cellular cross-links that prevent parallel fibers from moving independently. Our once flexible muscles become shortened and unyielding. You can prevent or even reverse this effect of aging by stretching. Stretching slows muscle dehydration by stimulating the natural tissue lubricants. It pulls apart the cross-links and helps muscles reform and rebuild with healthy parallel fibers to keep us limber and injury-free.

Also be sure to stay hydrated during your H.E.A.R.T. workout. I give specific recommendations for increasing water before, during, and after your workout in the chapter on TLC 4.

It's not the actual muscle fibers that limit the range of motion. Rather, it's both the *connective tissue* and the involuntary action of our bodies called the *stretch reflex*. There are three types of connective tissue:

Tendons, which connect your bones to your muscles.
Ligaments, which bind bone to bone inside the joint capsules.
Muscle fascia, which makes up as much as 30 percent of a muscle's total mass and is responsible for about 41 percent of a muscle's total resistance to move-

ment. Many of the benefits derived from stretching—joint lubrication, improved healing, better circulation, and enhanced mobility—are related to the healthy stimulation of fascia. It is the only tissue that you can stretch safely.

When a muscle stretch goes too far or comes too fast, your muscles send out a neurological (subconscious) alarm, which triggers the *stretch reflex*—a protective contraction that limits the range of your movement or stretch. To gain flexibility, we need to move past this restrictive contraction. The opposite of *to contract* (or shorten) is *to stretch* (or lengthen).

So how do we keep ourselves young and flexible? Stretch at least once a day when your muscles are warm from the circulation of blood to the muscle. That happens at the end of your Zone One workout or after any physical activity.

The 30-Second Stretch

The end of your Zone One workout, while your muscles are still warm, is the optimal time to do a *passive* (relaxed) stretch. A passive stretch is good for cooling down and helps reduce postworkout fatigue. Research has confirmed that an effective stretch needs to be held for 30 seconds. In several studies, researchers found

that a stretch held for 30 seconds produced the same result as one held for 60
seconds. Take 5 minutes to relax and
stretch your hamstrings, quads, calf
muscles, Achilles tendons, and inner
thighs. Interestingly, the most important
(and neglected) upper-body stretch is the
front shoulder (anterior delt). All these
muscles and more can be stretched by
holding the postures in the yoga sun
salutation for 30 seconds or more (see
pages 116 to 118).

MIND OVER MUSCLE

According to science—and many ancient yogis—what limits your flexibility most isn't your body, it's your mind, or at least your nervous system. If you "relax into the stretch," you will gradually increase the length of the fibers.

In my decades of working with inflex-
ible people, I can promise you this: if you want to see increases in flexibility, commit to stretching twice a day (about 12 hours apart). I tell my clients that waiting
24 hours between stretch sessions allows your fibers to atrophy back to the same
length they were yesterday. They usually respond: "No wonder I still can't touch
my toes, even though I stretch every day!"

YOGA

The best type of flexibility combines improved range of motion with improved
strength, and no question, yoga provides both. In the practice of yoga you maintain the posture (a stretch position) long enough (90 to 120 seconds or longer) to
affect the connective tissues. Prolonged stretches like this can produce healthful,
permanent changes in the quality of the fascia that binds your muscles. If you
have never experienced yoga, take a beginner class (level one) or get private
instruction. Check my website for the latest in yoga tapes. The ashtanga yoga
practice, sometimes called "power yoga," produces both strength and flexibility.
At the end of my Zone One workout, I start with standing yoga postures (such as
the sun salutation) and transition to seated and lying down postures to stretch,
finishing with a 5-minute meditation.

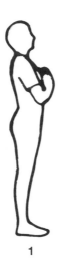

1

Stand erect with your feet together. As you exhale the breath, bring your hands together at heart level in prayer position (elbows out to the side). This is a mentally and physically powerful way to center the body.

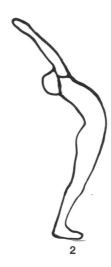

2

Inhale, stretching your arms up over your head alongside your ears, looking up, and arching your back from the waist, keeping your knees soft and your buttocks firm.

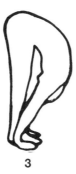

3

Exhale, stretching first forward and then downward in a smooth motion. Bring your hands to the floor beside your feet and your head to your knees. Your tips of toes and fingers should form a straight line. Bend your knees as much as you need to to accomplish this.

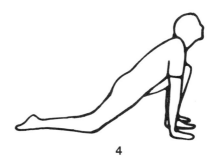

4

Inhale and hold your breath while reaching your right leg back to rest on the ball of your foot and tucking your left knee under your chest. If you're highly flexible, you can rest the top of your right foot on the floor.

YOGA SUN SALUTATION

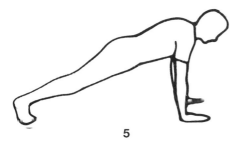

5

Still holding your breath, reach your left leg back, and with tight abdominals hold the push-up position on the balls of your feet.

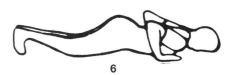

6

Exhale and bend the knees, placing the knees, chest, and forehead on the floor. Keep the hips lifted. If you're a beginner, you may place your chin on the floor.

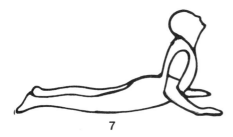

7

Inhale as you slide your body forward, lowering your hips, pointing your toes, and lifting your chest and chin toward the sky, with elbows slightly bent and pressed into your ribs. The front of your legs and top of your toes are touching the floor. Shoulders are down so there is no tension in your neck.

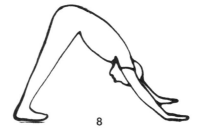

8

Exhale as you tuck your toes under, lifting your buttocks and bringing your body into an inverted V, without moving the hands or feet. Press your heels toward the floor and drop your chest in toward your legs. Bend your knees as needed.

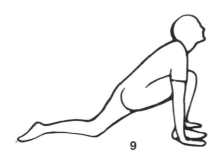

9

Inhale as you bring your right foot forward between your hands. Keep your fingers and toes in a straight line.

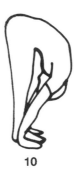

10

Exhale and bend forward, bringing your left leg up to meet the right and dropping your head to your knees. Straighten your legs as much as possible.

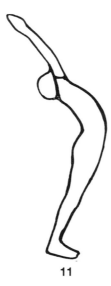

11

Inhale as you bring your arms forward and up above your head alongside your ears. Look up and arch your back, keeping your knees soft and your buttocks firm.

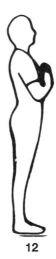

12

Exhale, returning your hands to the prayer pose. Repeat the entire sequence, this time stepping back with the left leg first.

YOGA SUN SALUTATION

FLEXIBILITY—FAST!

Proprioceptive Neuromuscular Facilitation (PNF) is a neurological technique that kind of tricks the stretch reflex and gets you fast gains in flexibility. If you are injured or have back problems, I advise working with a professional to learn this technique.

If you have tight hamstrings, try this PNF experiment: While bending forward, just short of your maximum stretch, lift your toes off the floor (heels feel as if they are pressing into the floor) and hold for 5 to 10 seconds. Then drop your toes and see if you can relax a little deeper into the forward bend. The PNF stretch alters the stretch reflex by having you contract a muscle at near-maximum length, easing the pressure on your muscle spindles and sending signals that it's safe for the muscle to release further.

Multitasking Can Keep You Committed

Multitasking can help you to stick with your Turnaround goals by saving valuable time and creating less guilt over time "selfishly spent." While it's *not* selfish to spend time on oneself, most women have been taught to constantly think of others and ignore their own needs.

Some ways to multitask with the H.E.A.R.T. workout include using your treadmill while you're catching up on the latest novel, returning phone calls, talking to your kids about school, chatting with a friend, or even having a conference call with business associates. If you are training in your Zone One, talking will be effortless. I frequently use my treadmill training time to return client phone calls, make appointments, and dictate charts. Sometimes I talk to clients while they, too, are on their treadmills, burning fat and getting in shape hundreds of miles away.

MAKE CHANGES, IF NECESSARY

I know life can get crazy sometimes with kids, commitments, and chaos. As a parent and a professional, I know that all the Turnaround planning in the world is futile when you are hit with life's interruptions. Many things can interfere with the best-laid plans for exercise—the weather can change, the kids can get sick and have to stay home from school, you may have to travel on business, or Mom could stop by for a long visit.

It's always important to have Plan B available in case your original workout plans are foiled. I don't want to hear any excuses for stopping your workouts for a week or two! Especially when interruptions occur and your stress level gets unusually high, the best way to calm down and regain a sense of control is to exercise. If your regular workout does not fit into your interrupted schedule, you could also try something new. The main thing is that you stick with your commitment to exercise and move around more. Here are two suggestions:

1. *Schedule a personal trainer, and do not cancel.* Make sure the trainer follows the H.E.A.R.T. method of working out. If you have a tight budget, share the cost of the trainer with a few friends—just ask the trainer for a semiprivate session. Don't worry, it's done all the time!

2. *If your work hours change or the kids' schedules have thrown your daily routine out of whack, use it to your advantage.* Try a new workout class (at your YWCA or a local health club) during the off time, or seek out a walking trail in a city park. Walk around the soccer field while the kids are at practice, or walk at a local mall when you have to wait to pick them up from an after-school activity. Check my website for a new H.E.A.R.T. aerobics tape, or trade exercise equipment with a friend so you can try something new. Don't let change throw you off—work with it to your advantage!

Intrinsic Exercise = Loving Your Exercise

In TLC 1, I gave you the right tools to use to begin loving yourself *and* your exercise. I want you to conceptualize, visualize, emotionalize, and—most important—actualize your workout right now. Here are some hints for loving your workout, alone or with social contact:

- Try a H.E.A.R.T. treadmill workout or exercise tape in the privacy of your own home. If you are a beginner or lack the inner confidence to exercise with a group, having your "home gym" makes sense and allows you to exercise whenever you want to. My recommendation for the most effective workout is the Life Fitness treadmill or Cross Trainer. The interactive Zone Training programs automatically adjust resistance to keep you in your target heart-rate zone for optimal fat-burning or cardiovascular conditioning. Add an assisted pull-up and dip station, and you have a complete H.E.A.R.T. workout. Check www.24hourturnaround.com for contact information.

- If exercise bores you no matter what you do, use distraction to stay with the program. Listen to music or books on tape while walking out-of-doors or on your indoor treadmill. Once you get into the exercise habit, take a tip from new research which claims that if you become involved with the act of exercising (mind to muscle), the workout will produce a better result. That means really focusing on the moment—how the exercise feels.

- Exercise while you watch television. Many of my busiest clients find that the evening news is a good time to get in an extra 30 minutes of their H.E.A.R.T. workout. Or you can wait for Oprah to come on in the afternoon, and get inspiration and exercise—two for the price of one.

GRAB A PARTNER

Many people find that exercising with others keeps them motivated and excited about their workouts. Here are some fun tips for extending your exercise network:

- Organize a couples' get-together for a hike and healthy lunch rather than cocktails and a heavy dinner.

- Invite some neighbors to go bowling for activity (and a few laughs) instead of grabbing a late movie and pizza.

- Exercise with your partner. Research shows that exercising with your partner increases your odds of sticking with it. Enjoy the way your healthy, sexy bodies move while you exercise together.

- Walk with friends or colleagues at lunchtime, or invite them to work out to an exercise tape with you on the weekend.

- Start an early morning power-walking club in your neighborhood or office complex. All it takes is getting up an hour earlier—and the motivation of friends and the exercise "date" can keep you committed.

- Take your kids to the park and do a H.E.A.R.T. power walk around the perimeter while they play on the swings.

Uh-Oh! The Weight-Loss Plateau

So you've finally hit that plateau? Don't worry. This is common after doing the same exercise every day. Your body simply gets used to the level of exertion or the routine you are asking it to perform. In return, it maintains your weight and fitness level at that point. What's more, since you have put on a few pounds of muscle, the weight on the scale seems to be staying the same. Or, perhaps more realistically, maybe you're eating more calories than you think you are or not burning as many calories as you expected. No matter what causes you to hit the proverbial weight-loss plateau, here are some ways to move forward once again:

- Try a new workout. Change your equipment or make the weights heavier. Rotate your equipment. Take a power yoga class.

- Upgrade your fitness program. When you stop losing weight, it's time to up the ante. Add some extra activity to burn more calories, such as taking an evening walk or joining a sports team (volleyball, softball, bowling, tennis, baseball). Just make sure you don't sabotage your new activity by going out for a beer after the game! Opt for the stairs instead of the elevator, and park farther away from the mall to force yourself to walk more.

- Go for a goal. There's nothing like a challenging goal to give your workouts new meaning. Track your resting heart rate and set a goal of a 5-point reduction.

- Check your measurements at the end of twenty-one days. Commit to raising your fitness level and the elevation on your treadmill.

- Plan a spa vacation in Hawaii that includes workout activities and hikes. Take the family on a bike trip to visit country inns. Go canoeing. Participate in a race or a walk for charity in some scenic spot you've always wanted to visit. Take a walking tour of your favorite city.

Spirituality and Exercise

While it may seem odd to link spirituality with exercise, more than 800 published journal studies show that spirituality is related to improved physical and mental health. Here are some ways to increase your spiritual strength while you also strengthen your body:

- Listen to spiritual or motivational tapes.

- Use your CD or tape player and headphones to listen to sacred music, religious songs, or New Age music that soothes the soul.

- Use "prayer walking," a concept developed by Janet McHenry. When you go outside for a H.E.A.R.T. power walk, say a prayer for your family members, your neighbors, leaders in your community, passersby, and more. The

Huichol Indians of Mexico did thirty-day walks to pray to the maize gods; monks still stroll in groups while reciting psalms; and Buddhists practice mindful walking as they pray. Prayer walking is a similar concept.

Turnaround Essentials

FOR YOUR FAMILY

Research suggests that too much television viewing may lead to a higher body mass index (BMI). In a recent study, people who watched just 2 extra hours of TV per day had higher BMIs than people who watched less TV, even though both groups exercised the same amount. Watching television for 3 hours a day between the ages of two and seventeen equals two years of television watching. Choosing more active leisure-time activities may help keep the pounds off.

It may become tempting to skip your regular workouts once you reach a desired weight. But before you do, I want you to know that thin people need regular exercise, too. You can be a "skinny fat person" and your clothes fit well, but you may still have too much body fat compared with your amount of muscle.

Studies show that even if you are not overweight, a sedentary lifestyle can increase your risk for heart disease. To keep your heart healthy and strong, do your H.E.A.R.T. workout for at least 30 minutes on most days of the week. (This 30-minute prescription is *not* intended for weight loss.) With additional exercise, thin people will see benefits including lowered blood pressure, controlled stress, prevention of blood clots, balanced hormones, and controlled cholesterol. Many people also experience an improvement in mood, self-esteem, and confidence from regular exercise.

Remember, your H.E.A.R.T. workout is essential for your Turnaround. No matter how religiously you follow the Definition Diet or how strictly you adhere to the hydration plan or eliminate alcohol from your diet, without the H.E.A.R.T. workout you will not get the amazing 24-hour results that I guarantee. Start your H.E.A.R.T. workout today.

TOTAL LIFE CHANGE 3

The ABC's
of the Definition Diet

F YOU LOVE to eat as much as I do, then you need to get the facts straight about food. In this Total Life Change, I'm going to teach you how to eat a lot of the right foods—whole, natural foods.

"How can you eat a lot of food and still lose weight and keep it off? That makes no sense at all." Marla, a seminar attendee with a lengthy history of eating disorders, didn't buy my theory of the Definition Diet—and even openly challenged what I was saying. So I asked Marla to define the basis of her latest weight-loss program. Her response was typical: "First you eliminate all food containing carbohydrates, and then you deprive yourself of the food you crave to avoid overeating and weight gain." Now admittedly, this unhealthy practice of food denial and elimination is the basis for most diet books, but as I firmly told Marla, this form of deprivation dieting is an unhealthy, obsolete philosophy and will *not* result in permanent weight loss. And even worse, many of these diets have harmful side effects.

What if the goal of your diet were discovering fabulous whole foods and adding them to your daily meal plan? What if I said that deprivation was *out* and satiety (being satisfied and full) was *in*? Well, that's exactly what I will teach you with the Definition Diet. This antiaging diet is based on whole, natural, low-fat foods that are high in fiber, which promotes efficient fat-burning during exercise and every other hour of the day. With the Definition Diet, you follow a regular 3/500 eating plan, which means eating 500 calories or less of the whole food choices every 3 hours to fill you up, boost metabolism and mood, balance hormones, supply energy to the brain and the body, and promote healing sleep. Because of the high nutritional content of the Definition Diet, your health and the way you look will improve immediately.

This new way of eating is not complicated or mysterious. It is not designed to "trick" the fat cell. It's not about "fighting" your fat after forty or even "attacking" your fat. The Definition Diet is not about "false fat" or low- and high-fat lies. (Trust me. Your fat cells are way too smart for any of that.)

The Definition Diet is about becoming leaner, healthier, and younger—but it's not just about food. Losing weight and keeping it off for a lifetime both involve all your Total Life Changes, from your H.E.A.R.T. workout to increased hydration to destressing and healing sleep, each supporting the others to help you stay slim.

Note: weight loss isn't as tricky as weight maintenance, for three obvious reasons:

1. Weight loss usually happens in a reasonable period of time, anywhere from four to thirty weeks. Weight maintenance is forever, and that's a long time.

2. During the period of weight loss, you get attention and support from the people around you. This attention goes away after everyone gets tired of telling you how good you now look.

3. The weight-loss process in itself is highly rewarding, giving you an improved sense of well-being, great looks, and even new clothes. During weight maintenance, it's the same old you—only smaller.

This is where the ABC's of the Definition Diet come into play. In a nutshell, they give you specific guidance in how to quickly and safely lose weight, and then the answers on how to maintain a normal weight for the rest of your life. They include:

- *A for Attitude.* You will learn the facts you need to formulate a healthy attitude toward food.
- *B for Best Choices, Bad Choices, and Better-Informed Choices.* You will learn which food choices will help you stay healthy, lose weight, and halt or even reverse aging.

- *C for Cleansing and Cleaning.* You will learn safe and easy ways to purify your body, cleanse your palate, and clean out the pantry so you are not tempted by unhealthy foods.
- *D for the Definition Diet.* You will learn about specific foods and eating schedules for a personal dietary plan, why these foods increase your body's metabolism and burn calories, and the best way to eat these foods for weight loss and super energy.

Now let's examine the ABC's in detail to begin your attitude check—and body, mind, and mood transformation.

A Is for Attitude

For 99 percent of the time humans have lived on earth, our diets have consisted mainly of plants and some very lean wild game. Only over the last few thousand years have we changed from hunter-gatherers to farmers, and finally to automobile drivers headed for the drive-thru lane at fast-food restaurants. While we are genetically programmed to thrive on a diet of nuts, seeds, plants, honey, wild game, and water, we are gorging instead on greasy fries, doughnuts, potato chips, fatty beef, and sugary colas. As you start your attitude change, let's look at some of the foods our ancestors originally ate and see how dramatically our diets have changed. I'm then going to give you the skinny (literally) on why the foods you eat may be adding inches to your waistline and hips and how you can easily *turn around* your attitude—and size—by making better food choices.

BACK TO OUR ROOTS

	ANCIENT MAN	MODERN MAN
FRUITS AND VEGETABLES	Ate three times the variety of fruits and vegetables that we do, which along with legumes and nuts provided 65 percent of daily calories and 100 to 150 grams of fiber.	Eats 9 to 17 grams of fiber daily. Takes vitamin and mineral supplements to get the nutrients our ancestors got with whole food.

	ANCIENT MAN	MODERN MAN
LEGUMES AND NUTS	Ate nuts and legumes in their natural state, which provided healthful fats, fiber, protein, and other nutrients; no added salt or flavorings.	Eats nuts that are highly salted and limited legumes, usually packaged in cans.
GRAINS, PLANTS, AND SEEDS	Ate plants "as is" with no milling, refining, enriching, or processing.	Eats plants that are highly processed, reduced in fiber and nutrients, and filled with added preservatives.
MEAT	Ate lean wild game (3 to 12 percent fat) and fish, particularly fish, such as salmon, sardines, mackerel, and herring, which contain high levels of omega-3 fatty acids (lacking in modern diets).	Eats "factory grown" animals that are filled with saturated fats (25 to 40 percent fat), hormones, and antibiotics, known to increase the risk of cardiovascular disease, obesity, and a host of other chronic illnesses.
DAIRY PRODUCTS	Did *not* eat dairy products, because animals were not yet domesticated.	Eats many dairy products that are high in saturated fats, man-made hormones, and antibiotics.
REFINED SUGAR AND OILS	Ate fruits and honey for natural sugars; did not eat oils.	Eats more than 120 pounds of refined sugar a year—per person; consumes many types of oils that are known to lead to heart disease and some cancers.

Beware of any book that claims you can lose weight simply by slashing calories—for that's a very small part of the antiaging, weight-loss picture. Also watch out for diets that encourage "restricted" calories or skipped meals in favor of a drink or bar. In some cases these diets call for total fasts for rapid weight loss in which fewer than 200 calories are consumed in a day. This type of program guarantees loss of your lean body mass (muscles) and slowed metabolism. Your muscles are your natural calorie-burners and will help you become lean and defined fast if you follow the Definition Diet.

Turn Around Your Attitude:
Seven Changes You Should Make

ATTITUDE CHANGE 1:
REALIZE THAT CALORIES DO COUNT

While many popular diet plans claim that a high-fat or high-carb diet is the trigger for weight gain, that's not the whole story. Whether the food is fat, carbohydrate, or protein, *all calories count,* and a high-calorie diet without an equal increase in activity will certainly boost the number on your bathroom scale.

Now when you compare calories to get the most food and nutrition for your allotment, you need to know that there are 9 calories per gram of fat and 4 calories per gram of both carbohydrate and protein. It makes sense that low-fat choices will let you eat *more* food. Eating excess fat calories can indeed make you fatter than if you ate excess carbohydrate and protein calories. This is because the body expends energy (burns calories) to convert excess carbohydrates and proteins to stored fat. Fat, on the other hand, is ready to roll right into that fat cell with very little effort (fewer calories burned). So if you are inclined to overeat, select your weapon carefully: stay within your allocated calorie range and choose from no-fat or low-fat carbohydrate or protein foods for high energy and greater satiety. The Definition Diet provides food choices that are high in fiber and low in fat, so that counting calories is not necessary, even though calories still count.

ATTITUDE CHANGE 2:
EAT FOOD IN ITS NATURAL STATE

We now realize that eating food in its natural form (raw) is better for us in many ways. Not only are raw foods excellent sources of vitamins, minerals, antioxidants, enzymes, phytonutrients, and fiber, but the body actually uses extra calories just to process or break down the food to absorb the nutrients (sort of like aerobics for the gastrointestinal system). In contrast, cooked foods are rapidly digested and easily assimilated with *no* energy required to break them down, so you wind up with more net calories.

To see how this works, let's look at an apple. An apple contains roughly 75 calories and a host of disease-fighting nutrients, plus fiber to end constipation and suppress appetite. When an apple is baked, the calories stay the same, but the vitamins, minerals, and enzymes are destroyed by the heat. On the other hand, if you eat the apple raw, your body must warm it to prepare to digest it, a process called the thermic effect, which requires 7 calories. The end result? Your body ends up with only 68 calories, along with all those great nutrients. I realize that 7 calories may not seem like a lot, but when you run the total for all the raw food you can eat in a week, this number could jump to as many as 700 calories. No wonder ancient man was so lean!

REALITY CHECK

- *20 minutes* = the average amount of time it takes to work off the calories consumed in 1 minute, even if those calories come from healthy foods
- *9 calories* = the number of calories per gram of fat
- *4 calories* = the number of calories per gram of carbohydrate or protein

DID YOU KNOW THAT . . .

- If you eat an extra 100 calories of fat, you only burn 3 calories to process this food for storage as fat?
- If you eat an extra 100 calories of carbs or protein, you burn 25 calories to convert them for storage as fat?

Beware of diet books that analyze different metabolic syndromes (Syndrome X, Y, or Z), trying to convince you that Americans do not have the ability to eat healthy unprocessed (raw) carbs and to exercise. These syndromes disappear once you become active and eliminate processed food. Also beware of books that put you in the "average American" category to determine a food plan. We're each unique, which is why the Definition Diet works so well. You pick and choose your favorite whole foods, eat them at your convenience, and get the results necessary for your body's health.

A salad is another great example of how raw foods can boost calories burned for weight loss. Not only does a salad contain a high percentage of fiber, it also requires a lot of calories for the body to digest it. This means that a fresh, colorful salad gives you fewer net calories—the perfect choice for weight loss and weight control. You might try my favorite dinner salad, lovingly referred to as "the trough" by my husband. (I describe this in detail in the chapter on recipes, page 372.)

ATTITUDE CHANGE 3:
EAT PROTEIN TO REBUILD AND REPAIR THE BODY

With all the low-carb, high-protein diets around, protein is of special interest these days. Yet before I give my clients the Definition Diet, I always ask them what they think protein is used for in the body.

Some clients answer that protein increases energy levels. The truth is that your body first uses the glucose from fruits, vegetables, and sprouts for energy. Then it uses starch and fat. The last thing the body uses for energy is protein.

Some clients say they need protein to help boost endurance. Yet excess protein provides your body with an overload of nitrogen, which can actually cause fatigue. People pumped up with protein (bodybuilders) are not known for their marathon-running abilities. True?

And then there are clients who think they need added protein for strong bones.

Wrong again. Too much protein has been linked to osteoporosis, the weakening of bones that leads to painful fractures. It might surprise you to know that the strongest bones on the planet belong to vegetarians.

We know that protein is most important when you are a rapidly developing infant, and Mother Nature calculated out the protein thing for us. Mother's milk is 2.38 percent protein at birth and drops to 1.2 to 1.6 percent protein in six months. (Not exactly a 40/30/30 plan.) But why is protein important for adults? We use protein for rebuilding and repair. Protein helps to *rebuild cells* (the billions that we lose every day) and *repair cells* when we are injured or sick.

To figure how much protein you need each day, the U.S. government Food and Nutrition Board has calculated an easy formula: *0.36 grams for every pound of body weight in healthy men and women.* For example, if you're 140 pounds, you need *50 grams of protein* (.36 × 140) per day; at 175 pounds, you need *63 grams.* Keep in mind that these recommendations are approximate, as each of us is different.

You may not realize that protein is available in foods low in saturated fats, such as fish, nuts, legumes, soy products, and vegetables. Use this chart as a guide in adding plant-based protein to your daily menu.

HOW TO GET A DAY'S WORTH OF PROTEIN

	GRAMS OF PROTEIN
½ cup soybeans	12.5
3 egg whites	10
½ cup brown rice	2.5
3 ounces salmon	24
8-ounce smoothie with soy milk	4
1 slice sprouted-wheat bread with almond butter	15

ATTITUDE CHANGE 4:
AVOID TRENDY HIGH-PROTEIN DIETS

Contrary to what you may have read in the latest diet book, high-protein diets are downright dangerous. Not only does this lopsided eating style promote unhealthy habits, it may increase your disease risk over the long term.

With a high-protein diet, you often limit the intake of fruits, vegetables, whole grains, and, shockingly, sometimes all of the above. Yet these are the foods that contain the vitamins, minerals, fiber, antioxidants, and phytochemicals necessary for halting and even reversing aging and for treating and preventing diseases. These diets are generally associated with higher intakes of total fat, saturated fat, and cholesterol compared with the average diet. Overconsumption of meat is associated with heart disease and cancer (not to mention the threat of deadly mad cow disease). A high-protein diet is especially risky for those who have diabetes, as it may speed the progression of the eye disease diabetic retinopathy, a common complication of diabetes, which is often heralded by hypertension and traces of protein in the urine (proteinuria). And excess protein leaches calcium out of your system, putting you at higher risk for early osteoporosis and painful, debilitating fractures.

After two or three days on a no- or low-carb diet, pyruvic acid from faulty fat metabolism builds up very slowly in your muscles. Without sugar (carbs), muscle turns fatty acids into ketones, which spill into your blood, creating a dangerous condition called ketoacidosis or ketosis. While the authors of high-protein diet books claim that ketosis indicates that the muscles are burning lots of fat, they are dead wrong. All ketosis shows is that the muscles are burning fat *halfway*. You're not burning lots of fat, you're burning a little fat incompletely.

When weight loss is achieved on high-protein diets, it happens through two mechanisms:

1. Ketosis induces diuresis, which results in a loss of fluid weight. For every gram of protein metabolized for weight loss, 3 grams of water are excreted from the body. Dehydration promotes aging and disease conditions.

BOOK REVIEW

You'll learn a lot from books that detail the Japanese diet. This Asian eating style is high in plant and soy proteins that give us much-needed protection from aging and disease. The Japanese diet also includes plenty of heart-healthy fish and plants from the sea (like seaweed) that contain amazing minerals.

COMPLETE PROTEIN?

One of the biggest fallacies ever perpetuated is that there is a need for so-called complete protein. Protein is composed of amino acids, the building blocks of the human body. Twenty-three amino acids are needed by the body, and fifteen of these are manufactured in the liver. The other eight must come from food, so the body can build a complete protein. These amino acids are found amply in fresh fruits, vegetables, and legumes. Just eat a varied plant-based diet, and you will get all the amino acids you need without eating meat. Don't kid yourself—you do not feel better eating meat. Your body hates to digest that type of protein because it is a lot of work—8 to 15 hours of work, as a matter of fact. To digest fruits, vegetables, and grains, your digestive system works 20 to 90 minutes.

2. The low calorie count of high-protein diets results in the weight loss, *not* the low carbohydrate intake. But this weight loss occurs at a tremendous price for the human body because of the risk of losing muscle and the injurious effect on the body's organs.

ATTITUDE CHANGE 5: CHANGE YOUR METABOLISM

"I'm fat because I have a slow metabolism and I'm over forty." If I've heard that statement once, I've heard it a thousand times. Basically, metabolism is *all* the chemical reactions that occur in your body, including the reactions that take place in your brain, liver, digestive tract, muscles, heart, lungs, and every other tissue or organ. The bad news? Your metabolism is programmed to sustain a set weight, which could be higher than your ideal weight. So what does that mean when you want to reduce your weight? The minute you start to eat fewer calories, your metabolism asks your body to get by on fewer calories, and your body complies by holding on to every calorie it can. Just think of how many friends you have who have lost weight quickly on a popular new diet only to gain it back. No matter how you do it, quick weight loss is *guaranteed* to *slow* your metabolism. And as you just learned in TLC 2, exercise is the key.

TRUE OR FALSE?

- *When we eat carbs, they are turned into fat and we gain weight.* **False.** Carbs not used immediately by the body are stored as glycogen in the liver and muscles. The muscles use this as energy. (Unless you lie on the couch all day, in which case you deserve to be fat!) The liver sends the stored glycogen back to the bloodstream to supply energy to the brain as needed.

- *The brain functions exclusively on glycogen (carbs).* **True.** The liver has the capacity to store carbs for about 10 to 12 hours. Carbs need to be constantly replenished, or the brain will die. That's why we naturally crave carbs. When I tell this to clients they are relieved because the popular press has led many to believe something is very wrong with them if they crave carbs.

- *When you eat too many carbs throughout the day, they will be converted to fat.* **True.** But keep reading: if you eat too much of anything—protein, carbs, or fat—it will be converted to fat. Let's quit blaming carbs, especially the healthy ones.

- *Eating fewer carbohydrates will deplete your stores of glycogen and then burn more fat.* **False, false, false!** Fat is only broken down by combining with glucose and oxygen to yield energy. You cannot burn fat without glucose or carbs! I honestly think these self-proclaimed experts on nutrition promote half-truths like "carbs are fattening" because they think we can't understand the real, somewhat more complex message.

In study after study comparing groups of people who dieted with and without exercise, the nonexercisers invariably regained more than 90 percent of their weight, while the exercisers on average kept off every pound. Exercise helps the adrenal glands to function properly—another weight-loss boost. When the adrenal glands release their hormones, your energy and resistance to fatigue are improved, which contributes to calorie-burning.

BOOK REVIEW

n a 2001 review in *Circulation,* the American Heart Association took a strong stand against high-protein diets. In the study, the AHA evaluated the Atkins, Zone, Protein Power, Sugar Busters, and Stillman diets. They found that weight loss from high-protein diets usually results from the diuretic effect of restricting or eliminating carbohydrates, reducing caloric intake, and ketosis-induced appetite suppression. The AHA was particularly critical of popular diets that promised quick results by eating steak, bacon, fried eggs, and other high-protein foods while cutting back on carbohydrates such as potatoes, pasta, vegetables, and fruit. High-protein diets can lead to short-term weight loss through loss of body fluid because carbohydrates attract water. And in the long run, high-protein diets can lead to ketosis, the body's natural response to starvation.

The American Medical Association recommends that those individuals who want to lose weight and keep it off consume the bulk of their daily calories from carbohydrate-rich foods such as whole-grain cereals, fiber-rich fruits and vegetables, and nonfat dairy products. About 15 percent of calories should come from lean protein sources such as fish and soy, and no more than 20 percent of calories should come from fat. The AHA notes that this healthier diet may also help lower blood pressure and reduce the risk of osteoporosis, liver failure, gout, and some forms of cancer.

ATTITUDE CHANGE 6: EAT HALF YOUR DAILY CALORIES FROM WHOLE CARBOHYDRATES

Carbohydrates contain simple and complex sugars along with fiber and provide your body with the energy it needs to function and be productive. Whole carbs are found almost exclusively in plant foods, including fruits, vegetables, peas, beans, and grains. (The only animal-derived foods that contain a significant amount of carbohydrates are dairy products.)

Carbohydrates are also the main source of blood glucose, which is a major fuel for all the body's cells and the only source of energy for the brain and red blood cells. I know I've said it before, but your brain will die without carbs! The good news is that the carbs you do not immediately use are held in reserve (in the muscles and liver) for later that day.

The foods that have given carbs a bad name—manufactured cookies and chips, processed snacks, white bread, and white pasta—are not to be confused with healthy, whole carbs from nature. They're two completely different things.

ATTITUDE CHANGE 7: REDUCE TOTAL FAT TO 20 PERCENT OF DAILY CALORIES

While some fat is necessary to feel full and for the body to function normally, you can get all of this fat from whole food sources, such as seeds, nuts, plants, and fish. As you decrease total fat in your Definition Diet, you will get the following health benefits:

- Decreased levels of dangerous blood lipids (LDL or "bad" cholesterol and triglycerides); increased levels of HDL or "good" cholesterol, all important for reducing the risk of heart disease
- Improved immune response, helping you ward off diseases from the common cold to cancer
- Improved memory and mood
- Reduced effects of aging
- Reduced body fat

While you're cutting total fat, do not go off the deep end and eliminate it from your diet. I find it amazing how Americans still religiously follow low-fat diets yet continue to get even fatter. More than 60 percent of American adults are overweight or obese. Could it be that the low-fat diet you tried was loaded with extra calories from manufactured "fat-free" foods? Try nature's low-fat foods instead!

Your Turnaround Formula for Weight Loss

Some people use a low-fat diet as an excuse to binge on fat-free cookies, chips, or bagels. Others think eating a huge plate of pasta with a bowl of potatoes is following a low-fat diet (at a total of 900 calories). While both foods are low in fat, the formula for weight loss is simple:

- When you eat *fewer* calories than you use, your body metabolizes the stored calories (fat) and you lose weight.

- When you eat the *same* amount of calories your body uses, your weight stays the same.
- When you eat *more* calories than you use, you gain weight.

Some new research by the U.S. Department of Agriculture confirms the truth: the only diets that keep weight off in the long term are those that advocate low fat intake and foods high in complex carbohydrates. And that's the Turnaround bottom line—no pun intended!

So how much fat should you consume in order to lose weight or maintain a normal weight? The American Heart Association and the National Cancer Institute take the easy way out with their 30 percent recommendation. This figure was based on what researchers believed would be a reasonable level of compliance by Americans—meaning that they allowed a higher percentage because they assumed Americans could not stick with anything lower. Don't be an average American.

To lose weight and keep it off, you have to keep your fat intake to about *20 percent* of your daily calories. If you are over thirty-five, or if you're headed in that direction, you will *not* lower your body fat and stay there if you get *more* than 20 percent of your calories from fat. How do I know this? From personal experience

KNOW YOUR FATS

Monounsaturated fat comes from oils that are liquid at room temperature, or better still, plant foods (olives, flaxseed, nuts, and avocados). Monounsaturated fat is actually good for you. New research suggests that these fats may reduce your LDL ("bad") cholesterol level without lowering the good (HDL) cholesterol, helping to reduce your risk of cardiovascular disease.

Omega-3 fats are highly polyunsaturated fats found in fatty fish (anchovies, sardines, shad, mackerel, tuna, and salmon), flaxseed, and nuts. Studies show that the heart benefits of these omega-3 fats extend beyond the effect on cholesterol to possibly reducing the tendency to form blood clots, resulting in protection against heart attacks. Omega-3s are hormone-friendly and great for the skin, and they help to protect the brain.

Polyunsaturated fat comes from oils that are liquid or soft at room temperature, including corn, soybean, sunflower, safflower, and sesame oils. While polyunsaturated fat lowers LDL or "bad" cholesterol, it also lowers your HDL or "good" cholesterol, which you want to increase. There are some very preliminary studies questioning whether polyunsaturated fats might be linked to the onset of certain cancers. Other studies link these oils to reduced aging of the immune system. These oils are *not* on your Definition Diet.

Cholesterol is found in meat, dairy, and egg yolks. Food cholesterol increases blood cholesterol, adding to your risk of heart disease.

Saturated fat comes from animal sources, whole milk dairy products, and some oils. Saturated fat is found in red meat, butter, cheeses, luncheon meats, cocoa butter, coconut oil, palm oil, and cream. It is wise to avoid foods that contain saturated fats.

Hydrogenated fat is made during a chemical process called hydrogenation, in which naturally unsaturated liquid oil changes into a solid and more saturated form. The greater the amount of hydrogenation, the more saturated the fat has become, which can raise your blood cholesterol levels. To keep your heart healthy, avoid foods with hydrogenated oils on the ingredients list, such as snack foods and commercially baked products.

Trans fats are formed during the process of hydrogenation and are found naturally in certain foods, including stick margarine, fried foods, snack and fast-food products, commercial breads, crackers, pastries, and many processed foods. A word of warning for margarine lovers: the food chemists achieved more than they expected when they created margarine—it is just as unhealthful as butter, if not more so.

(being a woman over fifty) and from professional consulting, having worked with tens of thousands of women on a weight-loss regimen.

B Is for Best Choices, Bad Choices, and Better-Informed Choices

Every day you make choices about the food you eat—the types of food, the times you eat them, and the quantity. But are the choices you make really working for you, helping you to stay lean, healthy, and young? Research shows that more than 70 percent of premature aging and disease is the result of the food choices we make, *not* the result of genetics. The truth is, while you cannot change your family genes, you can take control of the food you eat, and making just a few small changes in your diet can make you both look and feel younger. The following represent the best and worst food choices you can make.

BEST CHOICE: FIBER UP

Fiber plays an important role in the Definition Diet. This calorie-free substance, found mainly in low-fat plant foods, is mostly indigestible and passes through the body intact. Fiber also fills us up. I don't know about you, but the very fact that I have something available to eat that will fill me up and is low in calories puts this

WHOLE FOOD FAT (REAL FAT) VS. PROCESSED FAT

When you eat olive oil your body says, "Hey! This looks familiar, but where's the rest of the olive?" Sorry, but olive oil is a processed food. But when you eat an olive, your body recognizes the olive as a whole food from nature and knows what to do with each part of the food—the fat, the fiber, and the nutrients. The key? To get the healthiest daily allotment of fat in your diet, eat whole foods—nuts, avocados, olives, fish, and seeds.

valuable whole food source at the top of my list. We know that foods high in fiber speed up digestive processes, helping the body rid itself of waste products more quickly. Yet even though fiber gets a good rap, the average American eats only 9 to 17 grams of fiber a day (our Stone Age ancestors ate 100 to 150). Your goal? To eat 50 grams of fiber daily on the Definition Diet.

There are numerous reasons for striving to get 50 grams of fiber each day, all scientifically substantiated. For instance, we know that a low-fat, high-fiber diet reduces blood estrogen levels in women, helping to balance hormones. We also know that women on high-fiber diets have a lower incidence of breast cancer. And studies show that a high-fiber diet keeps blood sugar levels balanced, resulting in less hunger and more weight loss. In one study published in May 2001 in the *New England Journal of Medicine,* researchers compared the results from eating 24 grams of fiber each day with those from eating 50 grams of fiber. They reported that the daily calories of the participants did not vary between the diets, but the high-fiber diet led to a significant reduction in blood sugar levels. On average, blood sugar levels were 8.9 percent lower on the high-fiber diet. And as expected, the high-fiber diet reduced concentrations of cholesterol and triglycerides, important factors in cardiovascular disease. In fact, a study from the Harvard School of Public Health revealed that with every 10 grams of fiber eaten, the risk of heart disease drops 20 percent. Now that's worth another helping of whole-grain cereal, broccoli, or kidney beans, isn't it?

Other studies confirm the same—that a high-fiber diet benefits overall health, prevents disease, and helps to maintain a normal weight. For example, a 1999 study at Northwestern University published in the *Journal of the American Medical*

Association showed that a 10-gram increase in the daily intake specifically of cereal fiber decreased the risk of heart attack by 29 percent. Studies in Hawaii have suggested that plant-based diets low in calories from fat, high in fiber, and rich in legumes (especially soybeans), whole-grain foods, vegetables, and fruits reduce the risk of endometrial cancer—a definite plus for women.

And finally, studies show that people who eat a high-fiber breakfast are not as hungry in the late afternoon as those who don't eat fiber in the morning. Soluble fiber, found in foods like oatmeal, barley, beans, and rye, slows the emptying of your stomach and your intestine. Your goal? Start your day with at least 6 or more grams of fiber for breakfast.

THE FATS-ALZHEIMER'S CONNECTION

In his new book, *The Memory Bible: An Innovative Strategy for Keeping Your Brain Young*, Dr. Gary Small, director of the UCLA Center on Aging, tells us that eliminating most fats from our diets lowers our risk for Alzheimer's disease. However, eating omega-3 fats (from fish, nuts, and avocados) helps to keep brain cell membranes soft and flexible, decreasing the risk for cognitive decline and benefiting the memory.

Fiber content of food (listed from highest to lowest)
1. Whole grains, including cooked cereals and breads made from barley, oats, buckwheat, rice, rye, quinoa, spelt, wheat, and corn. (Processed cereals, grains, and bread made with flour don't count.)
2. Legumes, including lentils, peas, and beans (including nonfat refried beans, nonfat garbanzos on salad, and soybeans).
3. Nuts, seeds, and dried fruits. High in calories—eat in moderation.
4. Root vegetables, including yams, carrots, beets, and potatoes.
5. Other vegetables, including broccoli, green beans, and leafy greens.
6. Fruit, including berries, pears, apples, and prunes. (Juice has *no* fiber.)
7. Lettuce, cabbage, celery.
8. Meat, chicken, milk, cheese, eggs (contain no fiber).

"Nothing will benefit human health and increase chances for survival of life on Earth as much as the evolution to a vegetarian diet."

—Albert Einstein

THIS IS A TEST!

re you a sinker or a floater? You can find the answer to that question in your toilet. Sinkers need a lot more fiber in their diet. Fill your diet with stone-ground grains, nuts, fresh and dried fruits, vegetables, and legumes to try to get your 50 fiber grams daily.

What is your transit time? This test is not optional. At your next dinner, eat a large spoonful of corn kernels (frozen or fresh) and do not chew them. Or eat some fresh or canned beets. Then watch for whole corn or deep red (from the beets) in your stool. The most accurate method of determining your transit time is with charcoal tablets. Your local pharmacy or supermarket carries these for the treatment of gas. Immediately after a bowel movement, take 20 grains (5 to 10 tablets) with water. Watch for the charcoal-colored bowel movement and determine your transit time.

- 10 to 18 hours: you have a healthy digestive system.

- 18 to 24 hours: you need more water and fiber in your daily diet.

- More than 24 hours: waste matter is sitting too long in your colon. Toxic substances that were supposed to be eliminated may be irritating your colon and getting absorbed back into your bloodstream. Once in the bloodstream, they are sent to all parts of your body and brain. You need increased fiber and water. If you are a carnivore, consider going without for a while and increasing your fresh vegetables, fruits, seeds, grains, and legumes.

BETTER-INFORMED CHOICE: VEGETARIANISM

Vegetarianism has existed for centuries. Today millions of people are vegetarians, and the numbers are growing as more doctors and wellness practitioners talk about the deleterious effects of animal products on the body. Likewise, environmentalists reject meat because of the resources wasted in producing animal products for consumption.

While there are different types of vegetarians (see What's in a Word), I urge you to consider this healthy eating style as part of your Turnaround. Not only will you look younger and feel more energetic, but the internal you will benefit as well. Vegetarians, in general, have lower serum lipids, lean physiques, later puberty, and reduced disease. Low-fat vegetarian diets may be especially protective in regard to some cancers including breast, colon, and prostate cancer.

The low-fat, high-fiber vegetarian diet helps to lower high blood pressure and your weight, among other health benefits. In a revealing study of 428 college students published in March 2000 in *Obesity Research,* researchers compared adherence to a vegetarian diet vs. a weight-loss diet. They found that there was a stronger commitment to the vegetarian diet in that 62 percent of vegetarians remained on their diet for more than a year, whereas 61 percent of weight-loss participants followed their diet for only one to three months.

In case you're worried about getting adequate protein on a vegetarian diet, most vegetarian diets meet or exceed the Recommended Dietary Allowances (RDA) for protein consumption.

WHAT'S IN A WORD?

Vegetarian: eats exclusively plant foods.

Lacto-vegetarian: eats dairy products along with plant foods.

Lacto-ovo vegetarian: eats eggs and dairy products along with plant foods.

Fishetarian: eats a vegetarian diet with the addition of fish.

Vegan: eats plant foods, vegetable oils, and seeds only. The strict vegan excludes all animals (beef, poultry, and fish), animal products (eggs, dairy, and honey), and the wearing and use of animal products (silk, wool, leather, lanolin, gelatin).

BAD CHOICE: MEAT

What do we really know about red meat? The facts may turn your stomach!

- People who eat red meat five or more times a week are three times as likely to suffer from heart disease and breast cancer, and four times as likely to develop colon cancer as people who eat no meat or eat red meat less than once a month.

RED ALERT!

Many people aren't aware that their gastrointestinal flu symptoms could be the result of something they ate. The culprit is often food-borne microbes that breed in undercooked ground beef or poultry, eggs, mishandled dairy products, or fresh produce tainted by animal waste. In a survey conducted by the nonprofit Center for Science in the Public Interest, researchers concluded that 75 percent of food-borne illness came from animal sources.

- Meat overtaxes the digestive system, stresses the liver and kidneys, and depletes calcium from the bones.

- Red meat increases the uric acid level in the body, which is a risk factor for gout, a form of arthritis that causes excruciating pain in your toes and other joints. The average piece of red meat produces more uric acid than your body can eliminate in a day.

- Cows in the United States are given antibiotics to keep them disease-free. These drugs are passed on to humans who consume animal food.

- More than 90 percent of U.S. beef cattle today receive hormone implants, including zeranol, trenbolone acetate, progesterone, testosterone, and/or estradiol. These hormones are used to make the cattle gain more weight (bigger cows = more money).

- Of the pesticides Americans consume, 90 percent do not come from vegetables and fruit, as most people assume, but from meat and dairy products.

According to *National Geographic,* the three most consistently disease-free and long-lived people on earth are the Abkhazians of Russia, the Vilacabambans of Ecuador, and the Hunzas of Pakistan. These populations have no obesity, cancer, or heart disease, and many live to be more than a hundred years old. The men are physically active and still fathering children at a hundred years of age. By the way, these people are incredibly lean. The diet of all of these people consists of 70 to 80 percent high-water-content foods such as raw, uncooked fruits and vegetables. And then there are the Americans. *The average American carnivore devours 100 pounds of animal fat every year.*

BETTER-INFORMED CHOICE: DAIRY

I hope you will agree with me when I say that cow's milk is designed for baby cows. The human is the only mammal on earth that drinks milk after weaning. The cow on the range will kick the calf away when it is time for weaning. In fact, all animals have a natural instinct that tells them milk is not a proper food after weaning time.

There are numerous reasons to avoid dairy. Here are just a few you should consider:

- A high percentage of cow's milk contains bovine growth hormones that are unnatural and unhealthy for humans. (Bovine growth hormones stimulate growth in immature cattle and increase milk yield in lactating cows.)

- What the dairy industry calls "nature's perfect food" turns a 50-pound baby calf into a 450-pound cow in one year. If you want to put on a few pounds, go for it—because high-fat dairy will do the trick.

- Whole-fat dairy products are linked to heart disease, autoimmune diseases such as arthritis, childhood diabetes, kidney stones, allergies, nasal congestion, depression and mood swings, respiratory problems, canker sores, and mad cow disease.

- In the Nurses' Health Study, a study of 120,000 female nurses who have shared their lifestyle and medical data with Harvard University researchers

FEED THE PEOPLE, NOT THE COWS!
(FACTS FROM *THE FOOD REVOLUTION*)

The fact is, there is enough food in the world for everyone. But tragically, much of the world's food and land resources are tied up in producing beef and other livestock, while millions of children and adults suffer from malnutrition and starvation.

What we know

- Number of underfed and malnourished people in the world: 1.2 billion
- Number of overfed and malnourished people in the world: 1.2 billion
- Experiences shared by both the hungry and the overweight: high levels of sickness and disability, shortened life expectancies, lower levels of productivity
- Children in Bangladesh who are so underfed and underweight that their health is diminished: 56 percent
- Adults in the United States who are so overfed and overweight that their health is diminished: 55 percent

What we know

- U.S. corn eaten by people: 2 percent
- U.S. corn eaten by livestock: 77 percent
- U.S. farmland producing vegetables: 4 million acres
- U.S. farmland producing hay for livestock: 56 million acres
- The National Dairy Council funded a study in which postmenopausal women drank three additional 8-ounce glasses of skim milk (to provide a total of 1,500 milligrams of calcium daily) compared to the control group of postmenopausal women. The council was not thrilled when the results, published in the *American Journal of Clinical Nutrition,* found that women who drank the extra milk actually lost more calcium from their bones than the control group of women who did not drink it.

What we know

- Countries with the highest consumption of dairy products: Finland, Sweden, United States, England
- Countries with the highest rates of osteoporosis: Finland, Sweden, United States, England
- Calcium intake in rural China: one-half that of people in the United States
- Bone-fracture rate in rural China: one-fifth that of people in the United States
- Foods that when eaten produce calcium loss through urinary excretion: animal protein, salt, and coffee
- Amount of calcium lost in the urine of a woman after eating a hamburger: 28 milligrams
- Cow's milk provides more than nine times as much saturated fat as soy beverages.
- Soy beverages provide more than one hundred times as much essential fatty acids as cow's milk, so provide a far healthier quality of fat.
- Soy beverages, unlike cow's milk, provide substantial amounts of substances known as *phytoestrogens* (genestein, daidzen, and so on), which lower both heart disease and cancer risk.

since 1976, researchers found no evidence at all that higher intakes of milk reduced osteoporosis or bone-fracture incidence. In fact, the study found that the relative risk of hip fracture for women who drank 2 glasses or more of milk per day was 1.45 times higher than for those who drank 1 glass or less per week.

- In the Physicians Health Study, researchers at Harvard University and Brigham and Women's Hospital in Boston tracked 20,885 men for eleven years and confirmed a link between higher consumption of dairy products and prostate cancer.

CALCIUM ABSORPTION RATES

Not all calcium is equal when it comes to being absorbed and utilized by the body. A comparison of some common foods shows that calcium from vegetables is better absorbed than calcium from dairy.

FOOD SOURCE	ABSORPTION RATE (%)
Brussels sprouts	63.8
Mustard greens	57.8
Broccoli	52.6
Turnip greens	51.6
Kale	50.0
Cow's milk	32.0

BAD CHOICE: SUGAR

When you start eating a diet higher in plant foods, your body will have all the natural sugar (glucose) that it needs for energy, and your sugar cravings will diminish. I have watched this happen with my clients for twenty-six years. Not only does sugar give you a lot of wasted calories and increased body fat, it actually depletes your body's store of necessary B vitamins. And that's not all. Sugar has been proved to do even more damage, including the following:

- Leaches calcium from hair, blood, bones, and teeth
- Interferes with the absorption of calcium, protein, and other minerals
- Retards the growth of valuable intestinal bacteria
- Causes unnatural imbalances in blood sugar levels
- Is associated with diabetes, obesity, rheumatism, gout, hypoglycemia, acne, indigestion, arteriosclerosis, and even mental illness
- Ferments in the stomach, stops the secretion of gastric juices, and inhibits the stomach's ability to digest
- Accelerates aging, ill health, and weight gain

BETTER-INFORMED CHOICE: CAFFEINE

This central nervous system stimulant, used by more than eighty million Americans, is the only food ingredient that actually mimics the stress response, giving you an increase in heart rate, blood pressure, and glucose availability to the brain that increases alertness. But caffeine can create problems when overused or if you are sensitive to its effects, leading to nervousness, heart palpitations, restlessness, anxiety, and insomnia (definitely a no-no if you need to increase healing sleep and destress using mind-body innercise).

Eating the foods recommended in the Definition Diet will keep your blood sugar levels balanced, helping to reduce the craving you have for caffeine. If you find it difficult to cut out caffeine altogether, limit your intake to morning only and

VANILLA LOW-FAT LATTE

Try low-fat vanilla soy milk in your coffee. You can even get a latté with vanilla soy milk at many restaurants and coffee specialty shops. Studies linking caffeine and osteoporosis found that women who drank 2 cups of coffee but no milk daily over a lifetime had weaker bones than coffee drinkers who also drank a glass of milk each day. We know that soy milk works better than cow's milk for prevention of osteoporosis, so go for the latte—a little coffee with a lot of soy milk!

opt for organic products. The pesticides used on coffee bean plants are very toxic. My secret? I pour one cup of organic coffee with added low-fat vanilla soy milk when I crave caffeine. After drinking half of it, I wait awhile and get involved in something else. Most of the time I don't even want the other half-cup. (Of course, you could be amazingly disciplined and just pour a half-cup to start!)

BAD CHOICE: FAST FOOD

Fast food is a $115 billion industry, and there are no signs that it's going to slow down anytime soon, especially with all the advertising that lures us into believing there is an effort to make it more healthful.

Even if you stay away from fast-food burgers or other meat products, the other foods on the flashy menus are high in calories and saturated fats—guaranteed to pack on pounds and clog your arteries. In fact, did you know that fast food is your principal source of trans fats—one of the emerging risk factors for heart disease? (Trans fats have that special taste that stays in your mouth, making you crave even more of those unhealthy french fries.)

"Americans now spend more money on fast food than on higher education, personal computers, computer software, or new cars."
—Eric Schlosser in *Fast Food Nation*

BAD CHOICE: PROCESSED FOOD

Processed foods are no longer in the original state as provided to us by nature; they are the opposite of a whole or natural food. Most processed foods come in a bag, bottle, box, can, or wrapper and can exist without refrigeration. Not only are vitamins and minerals reduced in most processed foods, but these altered foods are usually high in calories and contain sugar, white flour, and trans fats. (Go ahead and check the labels if you don't believe me!)

C Is for Cleansing and Cleaning

Just as we take our cars in for an oil change and tune-up to keep the engine running at an optimal level, we must periodically cleanse our bodies so that they will be efficient and productive. To prepare your body for the Definition Diet, I urge you to first consider a detox cleansing. Detoxification will help keep your bodily systems running smoothly and will give you increased energy and peak performance in all you do. If your colon is not fully releasing the waste that accumulates after each meal, that waste turns toxic. The toxic waste leaks back through the wall of your colon and goes straight into the bloodstream, creating an unhealthy body—one of the major obstacles to losing weight. When your body is not up to par, what's the first thing it seeks? Nourishment, which translates into an uncontrollable desire for more food.

TIME FOR A COLON CLEANSE

When your body is toxic, you have less energy for exercise, adding to your weight-control problem. You are more susceptible to viruses, bacterial infections, and chronic illness, and aging is accelerated. Cleansing the systems of the body frees up more energy for cellular regeneration (antiaging) and weight management.

To get started with your detox program, I want you to head to the health-food store and ask the staff to recommend a "colon cleanse," a natural product that gently stimulates the colon to eliminate bodily waste. These products typically come in a powdered form and can be stirred into water or a glass of juice. After drinking, you should notice a difference in bowel elimination within 24 hours. And while you are at the health-food store, order a freshly squeezed apple-carrot juice to begin your detox juicing program.

DETOX WITH JUICE FASTING

BENEFITS OF JUICING

- Slows the aging process
- Eliminates or modifies smoking, drug, and drinking addictions
- Rids the body of toxins
- Motivates you to stay on your Definition Diet because you feel cleaner, healthier, and have more energy
- Provides the best multivitamin/mineral supplement money can buy

Fasting is the best detoxifying method known to health and wellness experts, and a 24-hour juice fast once a month hereafter will accelerate the elimination of toxins from your liver, kidneys, lungs, bloodstream, and skin. Do not fast for more than this 24-hour period, especially when you are trying to lose weight. When you restrict calories on a lengthy fast, your metabolism will decrease, making weight loss virtually impossible.

When you do a juice fast, make sure you use at least 80 percent vegetables, with apple as the only allowed fruit. This is the only day of the month that juice is allowed on the Definition Diet. Make sure your juicer uses the whole vegetable, including the fiber, if possible. I use the K-Tec Champ HP 3 to make whole, raw vegetable juices and soups. I also use it to make fresh peanut butter and homemade healthy ice cream. For more information on the Champ, call 800-748-5400 or visit www.K-TecUSA.com. If your only option is to buy prepared juices, stick with the health-food store variety or a food outlet that juices on demand. Try to avoid commercially produced juices as they are pasteurized and devoid of important nutrients.

THE SEVEN KEYS TO A SUCCESSFUL JUICE FAST

1. Limit your fast to one 24-hour period each month.
2. Use 80 percent vegetables, and dilute the juice 25 to 50 percent with filtered water.
3. Drink freshly made juice every 3 hours.
4. Make sure you get adequate calories in your juice (no fewer than 1,200 for the day).
5. Use a variety of vegetables for the best result.
6. Drink the juice alone, not with solid food.
7. Drink slowly to allow for better assimilation.

NOW CLEANSE THE PALATE

Your sense of taste is crucial in learning to love new and healthy foods. (If they don't taste good, we end up going back to our less healthy favorites.) Taste receptors have specialized surface proteins that detect different molecules dissolved in saliva. New taste receptors are regenerated approximately every eight days, and these taste receptor cells collect together in bunches of forty to fifty cells to form your taste buds. This is exciting and encouraging news because it means we can acquire a taste for new and different foods.

An important study published in June 2000 in *Appetite* concluded that with repeated exposure, the desire to eat, degree of fullness, and intake of a less-preferred food can actually increase over time. This study confirms the fact that if you at least try new foods that are good for you, in time you may actually love them. Try a new food such as soy in different recipes, and your new taste buds will learn

REALITY CHECK

The following lists foods from the highest to lowest in nutrients. See how processing zaps the nutrient value?

- Fresh raw fruits and vegetables
- Juiced veggies consumed immediately
- Dehydrated or dried foods (lose 2 to 5 percent of nutrient value)
- Fruits and vegetables that are freshly picked and frozen (immediately lose 5 to 30 percent of nutrient value)
- Lightly steamed vegetables (lose 15 percent of nutrient value, more if not crispy)
- Cooked foods—baked, broiled, boiled, grilled, steamed too long (lose 40 to 100 percent of nutrient value)
- Cooked leftovers reheated in the microwave (lose 90 to 99 percent of nutrient value)
- Canned foods, deep-fried foods, and foods with additives (lose 100 percent of their nutrient value and have toxins added to them)

to love this healthy addition. Make a commitment to stick with the new food for eight days. I also suggest sticking with "real food," which is edible whole food in its natural state. Real food is not processed, has no chemical additives, and comes to us from Nature as a "complete package," meaning that it contains everything necessary for your body to process and assimilate that food.

DO A DIET UPGRADE

Good Choice	Bad Choice
Sprouted-grain bagel	Grocery store egg bagel
Organic corn tortilla	White flour tortilla
Fresh orange	Orange juice
Brown rice	White rice
Whole, natural food	Processed food

FRESH VS. FROZEN

Typically, fresh produce that is ripe has higher amounts of vitamins and minerals than frozen produce. But there are some exceptions. For instance, frozen produce that was picked at the peak of ripeness may be more nutritious than fresh produce that was picked before it was ripe and then stored for a long time. Ask the produce manager about the selection at your grocery to see how long it was stored before appearing in the bins. If you can't find out by asking, learn how to assess produce for freshness. If it is mushy, bruised, moldy, limp, or brown instead of green, yellow, or orange, don't buy it!

EAT CLEANSING FOODS: BUY ORGANIC

I find it encouraging that organic foods are no longer considered "fringe" choices and are widely available in most grocery stores. Studies have shown that organically grown foods have an even higher vitamin and mineral content than commercially farmed produce, partly because of the quality of the soil in which they are grown. The benefits add up to improved health and longevity for those who choose organic. Here are some other reasons to buy organic.

1. Pesticides have been linked to cancer, birth defects, nerve damage, and genetic mutations.

2. Pesticides are contaminating water and killing sea life and other important organisms and are not in the best interest of our planet's health and well-being.

3. The negative effects of pesticides on children are four times greater than on adults, and eating organically will positively affect their health in the future.

4. Organic foods aren't really more expensive in the end. It may appear that carrot for carrot you are spending more at the health-food store, but the money you are giving the government for pesticide regulation and testing, hazardous waste disposal and cleanup, and damage to the environment

makes that nonorganic carrot more expensive—not to mention your eventual medical costs.

5. Organic produce is usually locally grown, so fruits and vegetables can be picked riper. The taste is much better, and they contain more vitamins. Foods grown close to home and in the proper season will have the best flavor because they're less packaged and refrigerated.

6. Federal rules require organic products to be free of genetically modified (GM) ingredients. Safety testing is inadequate and government rules too lax to protect us from the potential risks of GM food.

CLEAN OUT THE REFRIGERATOR AND PANTRY

As you prepare now to begin the Definition Diet, I want you to remove everything from your refrigerator and pantry (a good time to clean both), and then only put back the very healthy foods. Take stock of what foods you have, and read the labels on dressings, condiments, and sauces. If they have sugar, hydrogenated oil, additives, food coloring, or preservatives, toss them now. I want you to replace them with healthier foods. Give away any cans, jars, and boxes of processed foods that are not on your Definition Diet. (The Salvation Army will take them for their food drive.)

D Is for the Definition Diet

You are what you eat. Nutrition _defines_ your age. Every night when you go to bed and make those billions of brand-new cells for your young and healthy body, you make them from what you eat and drink. If you want to take advantage of this antiaging miracle, eat great food. Research now shows that more than 70 percent of premature aging is not the result of genetics but of the lifestyle choices you make, including diet. A few small changes can be helpful, but a commitment to the Definition Diet will have a definite effect on how you age.

You are what you eat. Nutrition _defines_ your health. If there is any doubt in your mind about diet and good health, bookmark this page and spend a few minutes reading about antiaging and disease, starting on page 328. Forget genetics, forget what happens on the SAD (standard American diet), and stop being an average American. Your diet defines your health—the health of your heart, your skin, your mind, and the planet!

You are what you eat. Nutrition *defines* your body. There is a huge misunderstanding that's perpetuated by the bodybuilding community that you have to lift heavy weights on a regular basis to have muscle definition. I am here to tell you otherwise. Having a defined body is the result of (1) eating a diet low in fat and high in nutrients and (2) working out in your Zone One. Nothing more, nothing less. Being "defined" does not mean you have to have large, masculine muscles, either. If your muscles are small but toned and your body fat percentage is low, you will see those beautiful, long muscles you were born with, and you will look defined and fit.

DEFINITION DIET PYRAMID

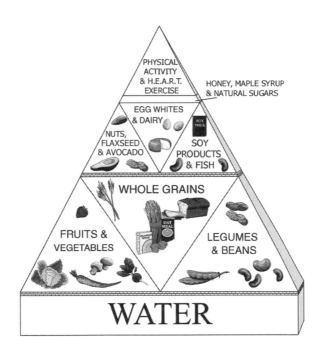

The Definition Diet focuses on nutrition and health but will help you lose and maintain your weight for life. You can't maintain weight loss if you are unhealthy. Unhealthy people gain back the weight they lose on fad diets. Let's start today, knowing that you can eat more food because it contains fewer calories. You will never be hungry, because you will eat every three hours. You will lose weight and keep it off, because you will increase your metabolism. Your sex life can be better. You will have better focus and memory throughout life.

As you plan your Definition Diet, there are foods that you must eat every day. These whole and natural foods are high in fiber, hormone-friendly compounds, and antiaging phytonutrients and have the right amount of protein, fat, and carbohydrate to guarantee weight loss.

EVERYDAY FOODS ON THE DEFINITION DIET

- 4 to 7 servings of vegetables with a minimum of 2 servings raw
- 2 to 4 servings of fruit
- 4 to 8 servings of cooked whole grains, sprouted bread, whole-grain cereal (for weight loss, choose 4 servings); whole-grain pasta can be added after three weeks on your Turnaround.
- 2 servings fish, dried beans, egg whites
- 1 to 2 servings of soy (beans, tofu, soy milk, tempeh)
- 1 ounce (½ ounce for weight loss) nuts and seeds (flaxseed is a superstar)

DEFINITION DIET SAMPLE DAILY MENU

7:00 A.M. BREAKFAST
5-egg-white omelet with green onions, red bell pepper, and fresh basil
2 ounces cooked oatmeal with ½ cup raspberries and cinnamon
Optional: latte (organic coffee) with ½ cup low-fat vanilla soy milk or ½ cup iced vanilla soy milk

10 A.M. SNACK

Ezekiel cinnamon-raisin bread (made by the Food for Life Company and available at health-food stores) topped with 1 teaspoon almond butter (or peanut butter)

1 P.M. LUNCH

Salad bowl (Jay's Trough) with 1 cup spinach, ½ cup each raw red cabbage and orange bell pepper, tomato slices, red onion, 1 ounce California avocado, ½ cup cooked soybeans, and nonfat organic salad dressing from health-food store

1 cup tomato-vegetable soup

3 P.M. SNACK

Smoothie (½ banana, ½ cup strawberries, ½ cup low-fat vanilla soy milk, and ice, blended)

6 P.M. DINNER

3 ounces broiled salmon on top of ½ cup spicy black beans

½ cup brown rice

½ cup crisp steamed broccoli

½ cup crisp steamed green beans

8 P.M. DESSERT

Raw apple, sliced

TOTAL CALORIES   1,410

ANALYSIS OF DEFINITION DIET SAMPLE DAILY MENU

Nutrient	Grams	Percentage of Daily Caloric Total
Protein	90	26
Carbs	188	55
Fat	28	19
Fiber	49	

MAKE A TRADE-OFF

Trade salt and butter for fresh herbs and spices; they possess antioxidant properties that can help guard against cellular injury and aging. Try the following vinegars, herbs, and spices to add more flavor to your whole foods:

Basil	Curry	Parsley
Bell pepper (freeze-dried green, red, yellow, mixed)	Garlic powder	Pepper
	Marjoram	Peppers (dried, from mild to hot)
Celery flakes	Mint	Rosemary
Chives (dried)	Mustard	Thyme
Cilantro	Onion powder	Turmeric
Cinnamon	Oregano	Vinegars (balsamic, flavored, wine)
Coriander	Paprika	

START WITH VEGETABLE SUPERSTARS
(4 to 7 servings)

Cruciferous vegetables. Cruciferous vegetables play a starring role in your Definition Diet. These nutrient-packed vegetables include arugula, broccoli, broccoflower (a combination of broccoli and cauliflower), brussels sprouts, cabbage, cauliflower, kohlrabi, radishes, rutabagas, and turnips. As members of the cabbage family, cruciferous vegetables are extremely low in calories, high in fiber, and have high levels of antioxidants. Some new findings show that substances found in cruciferous vegetables dramatically decrease the amount of DNA damage that occurs when cells are exposed to carcinogens. These veggies are also believed to have the greatest benefit in lowering the risk of ischemic stroke.

TURNAROUND TIP

Eat cruciferous vegetables soon after you buy them, whether you eat them raw or cooked. Cook only until tender-crisp. If you have leftovers, don't keep them for

THE FEELING

Where did the word *hungry* come from anyway? *Hunger,* an Old English derivative meaning a desire or need for food, is what I tag "the feeling." When your body feels hungry, it's actually seeking nutrition. When you eat food that has no or low nutritional value, it won't be long before your body gets the feeling again, because it didn't get what it needs. If you eat nutrient-dense foods, you simply won't be hungry as often—therefore, you won't eat as much. So what should we eat when we get "the feeling"? I always tell my clients to picture themselves as the first women on earth and then ask, "What's available to eat?" There are three words that best describe that picture: *whole, natural,* and *low-fat.* I encourage you to choose foods that fit the following descriptions when you get "the feeling."

1. *Whole foods:* foods picked directly from nature and eaten, whether off a tree, bush, plant, or dug up out of the ground
2. *Natural foods:* whole foods prepared without preservatives, colorings, flavorings, processing, or canning
3. *Low-fat foods:* whole and natural foods are typically low-fat, except nuts, seeds, and avocados, which have healthful fats

more than a day. For kids, use a low-fat cheese sauce to tempt finicky eaters, and make a nonfat yogurt dip to dress up raw veggies.

Leafy green vegetables. Leafy green vegetables, also low in calories and high in nutrients, are another plus for your Definition Diet. You can choose from beet greens, bok choy (Chinese cabbage), chard, collards, dandelion greens, kale, mustard greens, and spinach, among others. A half-cup of cooked kale, collard greens, or spinach delivers at least 13 milligrams of the carotenoid called lutein, which is shown to help prevent narrowing or hardening of the arteries.

TURNAROUND TIP

Try adding bok choy to your diet for a healthy dose of indoles. These compounds may inhibit cancer, particularly breast cancer. Bok choy is also high in calcium. Chop the bok choy and use raw in your veggie bowl, or sauté it in a stir-fry with other vegetables. If you aren't used to the stronger-flavored greens, use your favorite romaine lettuce for the base of your veggie bowl and add small amounts of the other greens to establish a taste for them.

Roots and tubers. Other choices for your Definition Diet include vegetables that grow below the ground. These fiber-rich and nutrient-dense vegetables include beets, carrots, celery root, daikon, fennel, jicama, kohlrabi, parsnips, potatoes, sunchokes (Jerusalem artichokes), sweet potatoes and yams, radishes, rutabagas, and turnips.

FOCUS ON FRUIT
(2 to 4 servings)

Fruits, two to four each day, are a delicious part of the Definition Diet. You can choose an apple, banana, berries, carambola, cherries, citrus, kiwi, mango, melon, peach, pineapple, pomegranate, tomato, or an array of dried fruits (raisins, cranberries, peaches, figs, plums), among others. Don't forget prunes, which are a top antiaging food and, as we all know, great for digestion. Eat whole fruits with the peel, as they are highest in fiber; avoid fruit juices, which are high in calories and sugar. (One medium fruit equals one serving; ½ cup berries equals one serving.)

SPROUTS

There isn't a better source of nutrients (and certainly nothing fresher) than sprouts. I tell my kids that sprouts are "living food" for growth. And I tell my big kids (my clients) that sprouts are full of enzymes for optimal antiaging and rejuvenation. Low in calories, sprouts take up a lot of room on your plate and make a salad or sandwich interesting. Many beans are also sprouted and available for salads. My favorites are the little green and brown pea, lentil, and adzuki sprouts. (Because of the risk of food-borne bacteria with sprouts, make sure to wash them thoroughly upon purchase and store them safely in the refrigerator.)

TURNAROUND TIP

Despite the fact that trendy diets have banned the banana, I am here to tell you it's an amazing and very filling food. A regular-sized banana contains only about 100 calories and less than 1 gram of fat. Bananas contain about 10 percent of your recommended daily allowance of potassium, a necessary mineral for normal blood pressure. Frozen organic berries are a "must-have" staple for the freezer to use for instant smoothies, and dried fruit is easily stored in purses and briefcases for snacks.

ADD WHOLE GRAINS
(4 to 8 servings of cooked whole grains, sprouted bread, and whole-grain cereal—4 servings for weight loss; you may add whole-grain pasta after three weeks on the Definition Diet)

While refined grain products do not support good health, whole grains—brown rice, millet, oats, barley, and others—are very low in fat and reduce the risk of heart disease and some cancers, not to mention that they are mandatory to keep your skin from aging. Because whole-grain foods influence carbohydrate metabolism, some recent studies suggest that these foods may reduce the risk for developing type 2 diabetes.

DEFINITION DIET VEGGIE BOWLS
(JAY'S TROUGH—FORMALLY KNOWN AS SALAD)

A veggie bowl will be your new friend for life. Side effects? It will give you a healthy, lean, and long life, and for practical purposes it's a simple way to make a quick meal. Put at least two chopped raw vegetables into your veggie bowl (tomatoes, carrots, peppers, purple cabbage, cauliflower, celery, onions, and more), and then add some favorite toppings for flavor. (Optional: one crisp-steamed veggie per bowl.) Unlike salads, lettuce is not the main ingredient in a veggie bowl. In fact, I don't put any lettuce in my bowl. Instead, I use arugula, kale greens, and sprouts as the base. From there, the sky's the limit!

TURNAROUND TIP

Add any of the following toppings to your base:

- Three sliced Greek olives (67 calories) for taste and oil
- ¼ to ½ cup edamame (soybeans), garbanzos, kidney beans, or black beans
- A dozen almonds (about 80 calories) for taste, fiber, calories, and protein
- A spoonful of grated strong-flavored cheese, an entire mandarin orange, a few raisins, or some soy nuts. Get creative!
- Nonfat organic salad dressing from the health-food store
- Any of the free herbs, spices, and vinegars previously listed

Whole grains include all three parts of a grain kernel: the bran, germ, and endosperm. Sprouted-wheat bread, some whole-grain breakfast cereals, brown rice, barley, and oatmeal are all super whole-grain choices on your Definition Diet. (One slice sprouted-wheat bread, ½ cup cooked brown rice, 2 ounces cooked oatmeal, ½ cup dry cereal, or 1 cup cooked whole-grain pasta equals one serving.)

TURNAROUND TIP

You have many options for including whole grains in your daily diet. Combine canned red beans with rice, salsa, and fresh tomatoes, and roll it in a corn tortilla. Or add rice or exotic grains to your veggie bowl for an extra filler. (Cooked orzo is amazing in spinach salads!)

Sprouted-grain bread vs. your current favorite. Why is bread considered a no-no on most diets? Because it is made from flour—a highly processed product from a wonderful plant. Your body sees flour much the same way it sees sugar—both are highly refined and low in nutrients and fiber. If your family insists on eating bread made from flour, your best choice is bread with whole-wheat flour listed as the first ingredient. (Don't be fooled by bread that lists the first ingredient as "wheat flour.")

The Definition Diet's answer to eating bread is "sprouted-grain" bread, which is the actual wheat, rye, or oat plant sprouted (just like sprouts) and made into bread. You are in for a treat when you taste it. To make sure you get the correct type, look for the word *flourless* on the label. My favorite is Food for Life's Ezekiel Bread, which comes in sesame, cinnamon raisin, and other varieties. Alvarado St. Bakery also makes sprouted-grain tortillas, burger buns, and bagels, which are found in most health-food stores. Yes, we can safely eat bread again and stay lean and healthy!

Cereal grains vs. processed cereal. I can promise you there is nothing that comes in a box at the grocery store that is whole. When you look at cereal, you want to recognize something that looks as if it came from a plant. An orange Fruit Loop doesn't vaguely resemble anything from nature, nor do flakes, puffs, squares, alphabet letters, stars, or O's. On the Definition Diet, go for the *real* thing. Here are some suggestions:

- Angelika's Skin Antiaging Cereal. Angelika, our skin specialist, created this recipe to be filling, antiaging, and healing for most skin problems: I eat this

FRUIT OR VEGETABLE?

While most of us use tomatoes, avocados, and cucumbers as vegetables in salads, sandwiches, and sauces, they are really considered part of the fruit family of foods. This special grouping also includes eggplant, okra, peppers, plantain, and squash.

EAT YOUR ENZYMES

After the age of thirty-five, we are all headed for aging trouble. This may start with laugh lines or crow's feet on the face, but it ends with a saggy butt and wrinkled knees. Help! Enzymes are the magic ingredient to combat aging and promote weight loss. Not only do enzymes aid in food digestion and nutrient assimilation but they stimulate brain cells and help to repair tissue, skin, organs, and cells.

The big contributor to enzyme deficiency is a poor diet. Raw whole organic foods contain powerful enzymes, while foods that have been cooked, processed, and refined are virtually "enzyme dead." Make sure your diet contains some of the following sources of enzymes: avocados, papayas, pineapples, bananas, mangos, and the richest source of all—sprouts. Superoxide dismutase (SOD), the antioxidant enzyme that counteracts free radical damage, is found in barley grass, broccoli, brussels sprouts, cabbage, wheat grass, and most green plants.

three times a week, and my fifty-plus skin looks twenty years younger. You can find the recipe on page 371.

- Kashi (from the health-food store) is another delicious whole-grain cereal that is great. It is high in protein and fiber. Avoid kashi with added oil and sugar.

- Granola should be purchased at the health-food store. Buy the low-fat variety (read the label and watch out for added sugar and oil), and make sure it has no more than 3 grams of fat per serving.

You will see faster weight-loss results if you make pasta your second choice after whole grains—and hold off on the white-flour or egg noodle variety. Check the shopping list in the recipe chapter for Definition Diet pastas that will fill you up and boost good health.

TURNAROUND TIP

Go for a small serving of the noodles and a big helping of veggies on top. Slather freshly chopped tomatoes (or use fat-free organic tomato sauce in a jar) and your favorite herbs all over a serving of pasta. You can add soy crumbles (frozen) to the sauce or have a veggie burger diced on top for added protein. A great product is Soy Protein Pasta, with 13 grams of soy protein per serving, made by Crum Creek Mills (888-607-3500 or www.crumcreek.com).

INCLUDE FISH, DRIED BEANS, AND EGG WHITES
(2 servings)

Heart-healthy fish, dried beans, and egg whites are excellent sources of protein yet are very low in fat and calories. For instance, you can choose from an array of dried beans such as black beans, garbanzos, split peas, red lentils, baby limas, and pinto beans, among many others. Try fat-free refried beans for dips, wraps, or Mexican dishes. (½ cup cooked beans equals one serving.)

PORTION CONTROL

The Definition Diet does not generally focus on portion control. I've yet to find many clients who are still hungry for more after eating the required high-fiber, low-fat foods. Still, portion control will become important if you ever get sidetracked on your diet. (I don't like to use the words *slip* or *cheat*.) Especially when you have company, go out to dinner with friends, or get caught up with holiday festivities (and high-fat or rich foods), portion control allows you to enjoy the moment while sticking to the Definition Diet. I find that most of my clients feel less guilt using portion control as they plan and allow for a small sliver of pumpkin pie at Thanksgiving (instead of a large slice with whipped cream) or one or two Hershey's Kisses after dinner instead of the usual handful. Remember, sidetrack with control—portion control.

Egg whites are high in protein (about 4 to 5 grams per egg white), low in sodium, fat-free, and about 16 calories each. This versatile food can be scrambled, made into an omelet with low-fat or soy cheese, used with a slice of sprouted-grain bread for French toast, or boiled and chopped up to toss on salads or vegetables. (Five egg whites equals one serving.)

For those who enjoy fish, you can choose from many different types for your Definition Diet, including tuna, mackerel, sardines, salmon, herring, and white fish. While no fish is off-limits, allowing you to enjoy shrimp, lobster, crab, and scallops, I still encourage fish high in omega-3 fatty acids. Sardines are the richest source of the omega-3 fatty acids eicosapentaenoic acid (EPA) and docosahexaenoic acid (DHA). Sardines are also the richest source of the heart- and energy-friendly antioxidant co-enzyme Q10. And they are extremely high in energy-rich DNA and RNA, the amino acid protein-building blocks of life—not to mention the calcium boost they give your bones. The top estheticians and skin care experts in the world will tell you that the omega-3 fat in sardines and salmon is essential for young and healthy skin. Check with our experts when you come to Hawaii. (3½ ounces of fish equals one serving.)

TURNAROUND TIP

EPA and DHA are omega-3 fatty acids found in cold-water fish (salmon and sardines). But many vegan diets are devoid of EPA and DHA, while vegetarian diets provide small amounts if dairy products are eaten. If you are vegetarian or vegan, the EPA and DHA can be synthesized by the body given sufficient dietary intake of linolenic acid from soybeans, walnuts, Brazil nuts, wheat germ, and flaxseed.

GO SOY!
(1 to 2 servings of soy—beans, tofu, soy milk, tempeh)

Of all legumes, soybeans have the highest concentration of protein. Most beans contain 20 percent protein by volume, while soybeans have more than 40 percent. Soy products are cholesterol-free and high in calcium, phosphorus, and fiber. Soy protein has been shown to be nutritionally better than animal protein and can be used as your sole source of daily protein.

As Barry Sears, Ph.D., writes in *The Soy Zone*, "Besides being rich in protein, soy has unique properties that help your body maintain steady insulin levels even better than other protein-rich foods, such as meat or chicken." Soy is also high in an amino acid that helps the body use the carbs stored in the liver to keep your body supplied with energy, which helps to eliminate hunger, and it's high in fiber.

Soy has the extra benefit of isoflavones, which are disease-fighting phytochemicals. As I explain in TLC 7, these substances, found only in plants, mimic the female hormone estrogen and have been proved to help ward off heart disease and cancer. Soy also contains choline, a proven memory booster that also helps maintain the structural integrity of membranes surrounding every cell in the body. Choline plays a role in nerve signaling, cholesterol transport, and energy metabolism. In fact, the American Heart Association (AHA) recently added soy protein to the limited list of foods they suggest should be eaten every day.

So how much soy should you eat each day? The AHA states that you can benefit greatly with 25 to 50 grams per day of soy protein. For instance, ¼ cup of roasted soy nuts has 62 milligrams of isoflavones; ½ cup of tempeh or tofu has 35 milligrams, and 1 cup of enriched low-fat soy milk has 32 milligrams.

THE SOY CURE

When philanthropist Michael Milken was diagnosed with advanced prostate cancer in 1993, he wasted no time in switching from his daily egg-and-bacon-sandwich breakfasts to a low-fat vegetarian diet. He also founded CaP CURE, the Association for the Cure of Cancer of the Prostate. Through research supported by CaP CURE, Milken learned that cutting down on fat was not enough—that soy protein could be an important missing ingredient in his diet. So he incorporated soy and other cancer-fighting ingredients into his diet, along with other Total Life Changes in *The 24-Hour Turnaround.*

Michael took his commitment to researching and fighting prostate cancer to the next level. He created a couple of cookbooks with all our favorite dishes modified to include soy. In the beautifully photographed *The Taste for Living Cookbook,* Beth Ginsberg collected more than seventy-five of Milken's favorite dishes, from Greek Spinach Pie in a Phyllo Nest to Devil's "Fool" Cake with Cocoa Frosting. (Substitutions can be made, such as having low-fat turkey in place of tempeh in a sandwich.) Proceeds from the sales of *The Taste for Living Cookbook* go to further CaP CURE's research.

Of course, soy protein is not just limited to the bean or white tofu. I want you to try the following soy products for added taste, texture, and healing isoflavones:

- To satisfy a craving for a salty, crunchy snack, try roasted soy nuts.
- Use edamame (the Japanese name for the beans in the pod) on salads, in soups, and as a topping for pasta.
- Add vanilla soy milk to your morning oatmeal, fruit smoothies, or cappuccino.
- Substitute soy yogurt, cream cheese, or milk for dairy products in your favorite recipes.
- Soy crumbles, available in your grocer's freezer, take on the flavor of other foods, so use these in chili, tacos, and soy loaf.

NUTS AND SEEDS
(½ to 1 ounce—½ ounce for weight loss)

While nutritionists used to warn that nuts were the dieter's downfall, we now know a whole lot more about these heart-healthy fats. Nuts are full of arginine, the amino acid that helps your body make nitric oxide, which helps blood vessels dilate and thus lowers blood pressure. Nuts are high in vitamin E and other cancer-fighting antioxidants, which prevent damage to DNA and cells from chemicals called free radicals. Walnuts, peanuts, almonds, and Brazil nuts, among others, are known to help reduce high cholesterol levels, particularly the LDL ("bad") cholesterol that increases your risk of heart disease. And get this: a 1-ounce serving of your favorite nuts is a great source of protein, potassium, magnesium, iron, phosphorus, zinc, and thiamin. Nuts are also high in phytochemicals and phytosterols.

Peanuts are technically categorized as legumes, but we'll call them nuts in the Definition Diet. Peanuts are high in monounsaturated fats and also contain resveratrol, the same antioxidant found in grapes and wine. This substance has an anticlotting effect similar to aspirin's and may result in reducing tumor growth. Organic nut spreads, such as almond or peanut butter, have no trans fatty acids and are an excellent source of omega-3 fatty acids and your R&R protein. In a recent study published in the *Tufts Nutrition Review,* researchers found that people may lower their risk for heart disease by 25 to 39 percent if they eat a serving of nuts five or more times a week.

Flaxseed is vital to your 24-Hour Turnaround, and I eat it daily. Flaxseed is heart-healthy because it contains alpha-linolenic acid, an essential fatty acid that we need yet our bodies cannot manufacture. Essential fatty acids are needed to regulate blood pressure, manufacture cells, and more. (Alpha-linolenic is an omega-3 fatty acid similar to the ones found in fatty fish.) These tiny black seeds, which can be used ground or

---

WHAT'S IN A DEFINITION DIET SERVING OF NUTS?

14 peanuts

11 almonds

10 pecan halves

9 cashews

8 walnut halves

4 Brazil nuts

10 hazelnuts

2 tablespoons flaxseed

HOW TO USE CHEESE AS A CONDIMENT

- Order your sandwiches without cheese. Or use no-fat, low-fat, light, or reduced-fat cheese or soy-cheese slices on your sandwich.
- Use low-fat mozzarella in your homemade dishes like lasagna or ravioli or opt for a nutritious soy cheese.
- Have an ounce of real cheese occasionally so you do not feel deprived, but save it for special occasions.
- Use freshly grated Parmesan and Romano cheeses for flavor; a little goes a long way.
- Make homemade pizza with lots of sauce, garlic, veggies, and olives, then add a sprinkling of your favorite cheese.

whole, also contain lignans, which have antioxidant actions and help protect against certain cancers.

Flaxseed has become the nutrient superstar lately; a new Canadian study found that ground flaxseed could help women with breast cancer. Scientists with the University Health Network in Toronto report that flaxseed used in muffins was able to slow down tumor growth in breast cancer patients. Fifty women who had been recently diagnosed with breast cancer were divided into two groups. One group ate a daily muffin containing 2 tablespoons of ground flaxseed. The other group ate ordinary muffins. After forty days, the flaxseed muffin group had slower-growing tumors. At this point it's not known whether the benefits are the same from flaxseed oil.

TURNAROUND TIP

Use nuts daily, but use them sparingly. While they are a nutrient-dense food, they are also high in calories. If you are seeking weight loss, keep your intake of nuts to ½ ounce each day. At the spa we use nut butters as toppings (hold the butter) and as part of snack time. Almonds are a great source of vitamin E. Peanuts and peanut butter have anticancer properties and make a great topping on toast or a slice of banana or piece of celery. Walnuts are also a great snack and can add something special to a muffin or be tossed in your whole-grain cereal for extra crunch and protein. (I love walnuts in my "trough.")

Add flaxseed to your casseroles, as sprinkles in your veggie bowl and whole-grain cereal, and in baking wholesome breads and muffins.

Fine-Tuning the Definition Diet

STRATEGY 1: COUNT FATS TO CONTROL CALORIES

Rather than counting calories, I want you to choose one of the fat-gram categories listed below, depending on your activity level. If you are sedentary or moderately active, try to keep your total daily calories to 1,500, with 20 percent from fat, or 33 grams of fat. If you are active and exercise regularly, you can boost this daily amount to 1,800 calories, so your 20 percent from fat will equal 40 grams. The lower the amount of fat you eat today the more of your own body fat you will burn in the next 24 hours while you exercise, during your daily activities, and even while you sleep.

calories × 20 percent = total fat calories ÷ 9 (9 calories in a gram of fat)
estimate fat grams

Sedentary/moderately active:
1,500 calories × 20 percent = 300 calories ÷ 9 = 33 grams of fat

Active/exercise regularly:
1,800 calories × 20 percent = 360 calories ÷ 9 = 40 grams of fat

---

ALL FATS ARE NOT EQUAL

Fats	Calories	Fat Grams	Fiber Grams	Protein Grams	Other
1 tbs peanut butter	90	8.0	1.29	4.0	Calcium, potassium, vitamin E
1 tbs almond butter	95	9.0	2.00	4.0	Calcium, potassium, vitamin E
⅓ avocado	100	9.8	1.21	1.0	Folic acid, potassium

FATS	CALORIES	FAT GRAMS	FIBER GRAMS	PROTEIN GRAMS	OTHER
1 tbs butter	100	12.0	0	1.0	None
1 tbs mayonnaise	100	11.0	0	0.2	Vitamin E
5 medium Greek olives	111	11.0	1.30	1.0	Calcium, potassium, iron
1 tbs olive oil	135	14.0	0	0	Vitamin E
3 ounces salmon	130	5.0	0	23.0	Omega-3, potassium, vitamins A and E
3 ounces sardines	152	9.0	0	20.0	Omega-3, potassium, vitamins A and E

As you can see from the chart, a tablespoon of olive oil has almost the same calories as a serving of salmon. Yet the salmon has 23 grams of protein and is filled with omega-3 fats for your skin. Consider that most recipes call for 2 to 4 tablespoons of olive oil just to sauté the garlic and onions! Then add the oil that goes all over your fresh salad (say another 4 tablespoons, or more than 500 calories and 56 grams of fat). If you find that hard to believe, measure your salad dressing at dinner tonight. A great alternative is one of the organic fat-free dressings. Then you can save your calories and fat grams for some real food. Or put your favorite vinaigrettes with the smallest amount of extra-virgin olive oil in a spray bottle, and spritz a small amount over your salad for flavor only.

STRATEGY 2: COUNT FIBER GRAMS AT EACH MEAL

Use the following fiber gram counter to choose some of the foods for your minimeals and consume the total of 50 grams of fiber daily. Be sure to have at least 10 grams of fiber or more for each meal; for snacks, include foods that will provide 2 grams or more. Also refer to other food lists, including Corrine Netzer's *The Complete Book of Food Counts* and Annette B. Natow and Jo-Ann Heslin's *The Most Complete Food Counter*, for more extensive selections and fiber counts.

FIBER, FAT, AND CALORIE CONTENT OF SELECTED FOODS ON THE DEFINITION DIET

	PORTION	CALORIES	FAT GRAMS	FIBER GRAMS
BREADS				
Bagel, sprouted-wheat	1	140	0.5	2.0
Corn tortilla, stone-ground	1	58	0.5	1.5
Ezekiel Bread	1 slice	80	0.5	3.0
Sprouted-wheat tortilla	1	110	2.0	4.0
CEREALS/GRAINS				
Angelika's Cereal	½ cup	140	2.0	6.0
Barley	½ cup	90	0	5.0
Brown rice	½ cup	110	0	2.0
Buckwheat/Kasha	1 cup	154	1.0	4.5
Low-fat granola	½ cup	150	3.0	4.0
Oat bran	1 ounce	87	1.8	5.7
Oats, uncooked	½ cup	145	2.0	4.5
Quinoa	½ cup	159	2.0	3.0
DRIED FRUITS				
Apricots	¼ cup	77	0	3.0
Dates	2 medium	45	0	1.5
Figs	2 medium	40	0	2.0
Prunes	3 medium	50	0	4.0
Raisins	1 ounce	80	0	1.2
FRUITS (RAW)				
Apple (with skin)	1 large	75	0	4.0
Avocado, California	½ cup	177	17	4.9
Avocado, Florida	½ cup	112	8	5.3
Banana	1 medium	90	0.5	3.0
Blueberries	1 cup	81	0.5	4.0
Cantaloupe, cubes	1 cup	56	0.4	2.0

	Portion	Calories	Fat Grams	Fiber Grams
Fruits (Raw)				
Grapefruit	½ medium	40	0.1	2.0
Orange	1 medium	64	0.1	3.3
Papaya	½ medium	80	0.2	2.9
Peach	1 medium	42	0	2.0
Pear	1 medium	90	0.6	4.0
Plum	1 small	35	0.4	1.0
Raspberries	1 cup	60	0.5	8.5
Strawberries	1 cup	50	0.6	4.0
Tangerine	1 medium	37	0.1	2.0
Vegetables (Raw)				
Artichoke	1 medium	60	1	4.5
Bean sprouts	½ cup	18	0	1.8
Beans, green	1 cup	44	0	4.0
Beets	1 cup	54	0.1	3.5
Broccoli	1 cup	40	0	4.5
Brussels sprouts	1 cup	62	0.4	4.0
Cabbage	1 cup	22	0	2.0
Carrot	1 medium	35	0	2.0
Carrots, cooked	1 cup	70	1	3.8
Cauliflower	1 cup	28	0	1.8
Corn, kernel	½ cup	89	1	3.2
Kale, cooked	1 cup	36	0	5.0
Lettuce, romaine	1 cup	12	0	1.0
Peas, green	½ cup	59	0	4.0
Peas, sugar snap	½ cup	57	0	3.5
Potato	1 medium	136	0	4.0
Spinach	1 cup	9	0	1.0
Spinach, cooked	1 cup	52	0.2	5.8
Squash, zucchini	1 cup	22	0	1.0
Yam	½ cup	78	0	2.7

	PORTION	CALORIES	FAT GRAMS	FIBER GRAMS
LEGUMES				
Beans, garbanzo	½ cup	130	1.3	5.5
Beans, lima, kidney, baked	½ cup	120	1	10.0
Beans, refried	½ cup	100	.5	6.0
Lentils	1 cup	190	1.0	8.0
Soybeans	½ cup	127	5.8	4.0
Soy milk, light	1 cup	90	2.0	2.0
Tofu, light	½ cup	87	5.0	1.0
Split pea soup (approx.)	1 cup	190	0.5	16.0
SNACKS				
Popcorn (air popped)	3.5 cups	90	1	4.5
Sunflower seeds	½ ounce	82	7	1.6
Almonds	½ ounce	80	7	1.8
Almond butter	1 tablespoon	90	8	0.7
Walnuts	½ ounce	75	6	1.1

STRATEGY 3: DEFINE YOUR EATING SCHEDULE: THE 3/500 RULE

Every time you eat, you boost your metabolism from the thermic effect of digestion. Many dieters make the mistake of spacing their meals too far apart, which can slow your metabolism and lower your blood sugar, forcing you to binge or overeat at your next meal and the next day. Just 16 hours without food, and your metabolic rate drops to a protective "starvation" level. Your body starts to panic, fearing that it may not get food for a long time, and works to preserve every calorie it gets by decreasing your metabolic rate. If you go without eating, you will store fat.

Enter the storage zone. Let's think about what this means in terms of sleeping and breakfast. If you eat dinner at 6 P.M. and do not eat breakfast until after 10 A.M. the next morning, your body will be in the "storage zone." This is a dangerous zone to be in if weight loss is your goal. Because the body is fearful that food is not going to be available, it tries to store every calorie that comes its way. So skipping

3/500 ON THE GO

Because high-calorie meals stimulate extra insulin, the fat storage hormone, here's a suggestion if you go out for lunch: order your favorite salad with your favorite side of grains for a total of about 600 calories. Take half of it home or back to the office and eat it around 3 P.M. for your midafternoon snack. It's easy to stop at 300 calories when you know you can have the rest in a couple of hours. Restaurant portions are often twice what you should be eating anyway, especially the places that "super size" the menu selections.

breakfast and opting for an apple at 11 A.M. turns that innocent apple into a source of fat on your thighs. This storage effect can hang around for days and even weeks. To keep this from happening, always eat breakfast, and then stay with your 3-hour eating schedule.

Frequent eating keeps you energized and zaps hunger. Frequent eating maintains your blood sugar level, which keeps your energy level up and your appetite down. In a study published in 1999 in the *International Journal of Obesity and Related Metabolic Disorders,* researchers reported that test subjects had less perceived hunger and ate 27 percent fewer calories when the food for the day was broken into a "multimeal plan." In another study published in December 1999 in *Appetite,* researchers discovered that smaller, multiple meals spread evenly through the day enhanced the control of appetite. The researchers felt that a reduced insulin response and the release of gastric hormones accounted for the reduction in appetite.

The 3/500 rule. The Definition Diet rule is to take in *500 calories* or less every 3 hours. The sample menu on pages 160 to 161 gives you an example, in that some of the meals are close to 500 and the snacks are 200 or less. These minimeals don't have to be labeled breakfast, lunch, or dinner. I want you to redefine your thinking about food intake so that having the "big three" is not always necessary. Plan special and convenient times to have a pleasurable eating experience. I like to take a 10 A.M. break and sit in a hammock on the beach with a big smoothie. My sister picks up her kids at school and brings them home for an egg-white omelet at 11 A.M. After a nutritious high-protein lunch, they head back to school with sharper minds and a greater attention span. Always keep a handy zip-lock snack in your bag, backpack, or car so when 3 hours have passed, you can easily eat your snack— and avoid sending your body into the storage zone.

STRATEGY 4: EAT SNACKS

I want you to eat two or three snacks each day on the Definition Diet. Studies have shown that the size of the snack is what fills you up, rather than the amount of calories. In other words, go for volume. Have a giant smoothie made with nonfat yogurt instead of ice cream. Have a few nuts with a large ripe apple instead of lots of nuts. Both the amount of snacks per day and the volume of low-fat food per snack contribute to your feeling of satisfaction—not just for then but for the whole day.

Code your snack food. Coding is a technique for food education that I have been using with families for over twenty years. If you have children ages two to six, coding is a great tool for teaching good eating habits. After implementing this program in several homes, I realized the psychological value for adults as well. Here's how to code: make small servings of snacks using the ideas below, and store them in

ARE YOU OVER FIFTY?

As I approached fifty I became increasingly interested in how metabolism could be stimulated to stay lean. I found that the thermic effect of food was incredible! Studies confirm that it becomes even more important to use the 500-calorie mini-meal rule to stay lean after fifty (no meal should total more than 500 calories). For instance, in a study done at Tufts University, metabolism was compared in two groups of women, one in their twenties and the other fifty and older. While both groups used calories efficiently after consuming meals of 500 calories or less, the frightening effects of more than 500 calories explained the weight gain in the fifty-plus crowd. It seems that the older women burned 30 percent fewer fat calories than the younger women.

I have tested this theory on my clients and on myself and found that when we combine the 3-hour cycle with the 500-calorie limit and begin the eating cycle upon arising, the results are astonishing. The 3/500 philosophy is an important part of the Definition Diet and should be used, in my opinion, by all women. After all, we will all be fifty someday.

Note: Raw food can boost this effect even more!

MY FAVORITE A SNACKS

- Frozen fruit, such as bananas, grapes, and berries
- Ezekiel cinnamon-raisin bread with almond or peanut butter
- Cut-up raw veggies with a creamy nonfat dip
- Hummus with carrot sticks
- Bean dip with cucumber slices
- Almonds and prunes
- Edamame beans, lightly salted

MY KIDS' FAVORITE B SNACKS

(Hint: Eat these with an A snack to upgrade their nutritional content to a B+.)

- Rice crackers
- Baked tortilla chips
- Whole-wheat pretzels
- Healthy low-fat muffins
- Imagine Food's puddings and nondairy frozen desserts
- Popcorn (without added salt or butter—use a sprinkling of Parmesan or Romano cheese for flavor)

SOME OCCASIONAL C SNACKS

(These snacks will help with the transition from junk snacks to A snacks. Use as needed, but try to limit to twice a week.)

- Frozen juice bars
- Frookwich sandwich cookies (fruit-juice sweetened)
- Healthy hot chocolate made with soy milk (available at health-food stores)
- Healthy low-fat muffins

zipper-sealed sandwich bags or small plastic containers. Code the treats with colored stars, dots, numbers, or my A, B, C system.

Always have a variety of the A snacks available. Because the letter *A* comes first in the alphabet (and signifies the best grade!), kids understand how this stands for the best snacks they can eat. B snacks are acceptable, but explain to your child why they are not as healthful, and that they should always opt for an A snack before choosing a B snack. The C stands for *caution,* meaning you should eat them less frequently—because they have less nutrition. Limit C snacks to just a few times each week.

Know When to Supplement

There is no one vitamin and mineral pill that can give you the full range of phytonutrients (beneficial chemical compounds naturally found in plant foods) that you get by eating whole food. That's why eating a variety of fruits, vegetables, grains, nuts, seeds, and beans is so important. The word *supplement* means "in addition to," and that's exactly how I want you to use your vitamins and mineral supplements. Eat whole food, and then supplement with a high-quality and well-balanced vitamin-mineral formula.

I have spent years researching supplements and have come to this conclusion: the main goal of the vitamin industry is for us to buy many bottles of their products. Surprise—their priority is profit! If you get a good multiple vitamin complete with enzymes (check my website for recommendations), you will have ample protection unless you have a true vitamin deficiency, in which case check with an osteopathic or naturopathic doctor for herb and therapeutic nutrient recommendations. Don't self-prescribe high-potency nutrients, as studies are now confirming that some may do more harm than good.

WHY BREAKFAST?

Eating breakfast is essential to help control eating *after* dinner. When you eat fiber in the morning, it affects how full you feel at the end of the day. Many people skip breakfast almost as a way to test their willpower. They figure that if they go as long as possible without eating, they'll be better off. What happens when you finally start eating? Most times you lose control and consume enormous amounts of food.

EIGHT TIPS FOR CHOOSING A MULTIVITAMIN

1. *Make sure the supplement is produced in a reputable lab.* There are many choices for multivitamin and mineral supplements in stores and on-line.

Because the Food and Drug Administration (FDA) does not regulate the manufacturing and packaging of vitamins and minerals or the claims made on their package labels, look for a supplement that is produced in an FDA lab. This will ensure that ingredients need to be documented going into and out of the lab. (Check my website for some names of labs that are highly regarded.)

2. *Find a multivitamin that divides the daily dose into three pills.* For some vitamins and minerals, such as water-soluble vitamin C and calcium, it's better to divide the daily dose and take 3 tabs at least 3 hours apart. This increases absorption and lets more of the supplement influence your body's chemistry. Bottom line? A one-a-day is not effective!

3. *Make sure the pill dissolves.* Drop a pill into warm water. If it does not dissolve in between 14 and 21 minutes, the chances are great that it won't dissolve in your stomach, making the nutrients unavailable to your body.

4. *Purchase a multivitamin-mineral formula that includes enzymes.* My favorite enzymes are papain (from papaya) and bromelain. Take the vitamin with your meals, and you will digest your food (and extract the nutrients) more efficiently. The enzymes will also help boost the effectiveness of the supplement in the body.

5. *Make sure the vitamin agrees with you.* Drink half a glass of warm water before taking it and half a glass afterward. The water will help the vitamin dissolve. If, after a few days, the multivitamin seems to be causing stomach upset, switch to another brand.

6. *Read the label.* Check the list of ingredients to make sure you are not allergic to any of the products. For instance, some people have allergies to wheat, which could be used in the supplement.

CHOOSING BEVERAGES

I t won't surprise you if I say opt for water first on the Definition Diet. It is the healthiest beverage you can drink. If you need more variety, choose herbal tea, which is calorie-free and delicious, and even has health benefits. Black tea consumption has been shown to affect blood vessel function. Studies show an association between consumption of green tea and reduction in the risk for cancer and heart disease. Green tea contains a family of naturally occurring chemical compounds called polyphenols, which have an antioxidant effect in the body. Some interesting studies indicate that green tea increases fat oxidation for reasons other than the caffeine. There are a variety of green teas available at most health-food and grocery stores. Your family may enjoy them as well.

7. *Remember that* expensive *doesn't mean "better."* Save your pennies and skip the specialty versions, such as "women's vitamins," that add cost but not value. These "special formulas" have increased certain nutrients based on claims that a nutrient can alter a physiological condition. A problem occurs because, in real life, one nutrient helps your body absorb others. If you megadose on one, you can throw off that perfect system devised by nature. The basic Turnaround rule: your body will use what it can from a supplement and excrete the rest (but see below). *Balance* is the key word. Better to take a low- or moderate-dose formula that works synergistically with your food than pay big bucks for excess you'll never use.

8. *Get supplements that are in a whole food base rather than synthetic fillers.* The vitamin label will list this information. The whole food ingredients supply the missing components that are nature's top-secret ingredients.

WHEN MORE IS LESS

Taking large doses of certain vitamins can be dangerous. The fat-soluble vitamins (vitamins A, D, E, and K) pose a particular threat, as they are stored in body fat and

MEALTIME TIPS

Eat slowly. Did you know that eating fast can inhibit fat loss? I knew that'd slow you down some! It takes 15 to 20 minutes for your body to let your brain know that you are finally full. If you eat a bunch of calories (even nutritious calories) in a hurry, you can still feel hungry even though you've eaten more than you need. To speed fat loss, eat slowly and deliberately, and carefully chew each morsel. Don't pick up your fork until you've finished the bite in your mouth. Use a slow-down strategy like starting with a raw veggie salad (major chewing involved) or a hot soup. Eating quickly and mindlessly means you lose the pleasure of eating. Maybe that's why you're still unsatisfied when you've finished an adequate meal.

Eat intentionally. Studies have revealed that watching TV while eating may cause you to consume more calories, so make sure your eating environment is conducive to pleasurable dining—not listening to the late-breaking news. Unfortunately, the same applies to radio listening and my favorite routine, talking on the phone. I'm happy to report that eating with other people seems to slow us down in the calorie department. Perhaps it's because of the "conversation factor."

are not easily eliminated from your body. Nutrients stored in body fat can reach toxic levels over time, so you must be knowledgeable about vitamins and use caution.

Taking a separate high-dose mineral supplement can be a problem because minerals also remain in the body for a long period of time. If you get most of your nutrition from whole foods and complement this with a balanced multiple vitamin and mineral supplement with enzymes (not a megadose) that you take three times a day, you won't need to worry about vitamin or mineral toxicity.

CALCIUM AND YOUR BONES

There is some evidence that increased calcium intake does *not* prevent early postmenopausal bone loss. In fact, some studies confirm that in addition to adequate calcium intake, more effective therapy appears to be required when the goal is to

FOR THE TOUGH BIRDS

While I do not include poultry (or red meat and pork) on the Definition Diet, if you want to include birds in the diet, please read *Prisoned Chickens, Poisoned Eggs* by Karen Davis and be aware of the following:

- Free range is most likely the safest.
- Hormone-free is important to your health and your 24-Hour Turnaround.
- Cook and eat the bird without skin or added fat.

increase or maintain bone-mineral density. That therapy is your H.E.A.R.T. work-out, in which you combine weight-bearing, bone-building exercise with heart-strengthening aerobics and muscle-building resistance training. I'll talk more about ways to keep bones strong in TLC 7. For now, if you are taking a good multivitamin-mineral supplement, chances are good that your calcium supplementation is adequate.

IF YOU MUST HAVE DAIRY, READ THIS

Organic (hormone-free), nonfat dairy products—including skim milk, nonfat yogurt, and cottage cheese—are relatively low in calories and contain protein and calcium (but are not the best sources of either). If you are not allergic to dairy and choose organic products, dairy can supplement your diet in many ways. I am adamantly opposed to cruelty to animals and ask that you please buy free-range and organic if you choose to add dairy.

- Cottage cheese is a good snack when combined with fruit.
- Yogurt and fruit can be a snack or dessert.
- Nonfat milk is a good substitute for full-fat in coffee or cereal.

EATING OUT WITHOUT PIGGING OUT

Think about it. Restaurants are in the business of pleasing the customer. Almost all restaurants offer healthy food choices or will accommodate your requests. Dining out gives you the opportunity to try new foods that you may not be including at home.

Restaurant rules:
- Have a huge glass of water first.
- If you are familiar with the restaurant's menu, mentally commit to your order ahead of time.
- Don't be shy about asking how certain dishes are prepared. Most chefs are more than happy to modify dishes.
- Choose an appetizer, a side of veggies from one menu item, and another veggie off a different item to make your own meal.
- Ask the waiter if he can check with the chef for a low-fat, vegetarian suggestion. Often they will make you something special.
- Call the restaurant 4 to 6 hours ahead of time and plan your dish with the chef. I do this when I'm having dinner with people I've never met.
- I always call the restaurant ahead and ask the hostess to instruct the waiter to hold the bread basket and instead serve a platter of crudités with nonfat dressing. Bread can be brought in single servings instead of basket style, at which time you will pass. Restaurant bread is off limits. Sorry.
- Request all entrées grilled, broiled, or baked dry with sauces on the side so that you can dip sparingly.
- No salad dressing. That's where the fat grams and calories will drown you. I've been taking my own nonfat dressing to restaurants for twenty years. It never fails—everyone wants to use my dressing!

Bon appétit!

UNDERSTANDING RDAs

The Recommended Dietary Allowance (RDA) and the Percent Daily Values are general guidelines. You may need more than these numbers, especially if you are dieting, under stress, or have had an illness. You can input the foods you eat using a nutritional software program (check my website) and get running totals of your nutrient intake compared with the RDAs. Nutri-Counter makes a pocket nutrition calculator that also gives you calorie, fat gram, and fiber information on the foods you choose for your daily menu (a great way to log your food for weight loss). An intake of nutrients that is below the RDA does not necessarily mean that a medical problem exists. Then again, an intake at the RDA level or slightly above may not be enough for your situation. We all have our very own need for nutrients based on age, activity level, and health. Once again, if you eat the Definition Diet, nature will nurture you.

MUSCLE MYTHOLOGY

Protein, creatine, and amino acid supplements for bigger and stronger muscles? Forget it! Protein supplements are expensive, they don't work, and excessive amounts of protein could even be harmful. I have owned three fitness clubs and a couple of aerobics studios, and I have a client list of thousands. I could make a lot of money selling protein supplements, trust me. But I also have to sleep at night. Protein supplements do not work and can upset the natural balance of your health, at the very least. Containing 4 calories per gram, excess protein is stored in the body as fat, not muscle, and large amounts of protein can exacerbate kidney problems.

In many studies, people who lifted weights achieved no greater strength gains when taking a protein supplement than they did when working out without taking the supplement. So why do people claim to see a result when starting a protein-replacement product?

- They usually start a workout program at the same time.
- Taking replacement products is a regimen. When humans commit to a regimen, they typically follow changes in more than one area, meaning that

GET HEART SMART

The B vitamins (B6, B12, and folic acid) have gotten some recent press in the healthy heart category. In scientific research, folic acid has prevented neural-tube defects in babies and also lowered blood levels of homocysteine, an amino acid that irritates blood vessels and is linked to heart disease. Scientists now realize that B vitamins play a role in the blood's clotting factor, making your body more likely to form blood clots and obstruct blood vessels if you are deficient. There are some studies linking a deficiency in vitamin B6 with increased homocysteine levels and thus increased risk of heart disease.

Recently the FDA approved limited health claims for these supplements, and because the FDA is typically very conservative in allowing claims, we can assume there is a legitimate association between these nutrients and heart disease. You get vitamin B through whole-grain products, lentils, chickpeas, spinach, black beans, kidney beans, oranges, and broccoli.

they eat healthier, drink more water, avoid drinking alcohol and smoking cigarettes, and get more sleep.

- The placebo effect: if you believe it to be true, it often has just that result (discussed further in TLC 8).

BLENDER DRINKS

Once again I repeat, *eat whole foods* first. In all my searching for nutrient-dense foods, I have found one blender drink, called the Ultimate Meal, that is superb. This complete and nutritious blender meal is made by Sam Gerard, a gentleman from Santa Barbara, California, who dedicates his time to finding the highest quality of nutrition from whole organic foods. You can find out more about the Ultimate Meal by going to his website at www.UltimatLife.com. (My favorite Ultimate Meal recipe is on my website under "Favorites.")

FOR THE KIDS

Approximately 30 percent of American children are overweight, with an alarming 13 percent classified as obese, according to the latest studies released by the Surgeon General. It breaks my heart when a mother comes to me looking for an answer to her child's increasing weight. Exercise and activity play a key role in maintaining a normal weight for a child or adult.

To lose weight or maintain a healthy weight, make sure your children have limited television and computer time. Instead, provide opportunities for them to be involved in outdoor activities and recreational sports. Help kids learn how to pack their own lunches and snacks so the choices are up-front and available. Keep all junk food off the premises so they're not tempted to binge on high-fat, high-sugar foods. Also, talk to your children about the reasons for the Definition Diet. Preface your statements with "because I love you" to help them understand that some food restrictions do not mean that "Mommy is punishing me."

And most important, learn to say no. Being a mom, I realize the easiest thing a parent can say is yes, and the hardest is no. Saying no to junk food teaches your children self-control. It teaches them to respect their bodies by eating healthy food, giving them the intrinsic skills to say no later on to smoking, drinking, and drugs.

FOR YOUR HUSBAND

Colon and rectal cancer are the third most common causes of cancer deaths in American men. Eating red meat and drinking

STAY MENTALLY SHARP

A recent study revealed that low blood levels of vitamin B12 and folic acid might be related to the development of Alzheimer's disease. Dr. Gary Small reminds us in *The Memory Bible* that tuna and salmon are excellent sources of B12. If you're a vegetarian, be sure to take a multiple vitamin that includes all the B vitamins.

RED ALERT!

While adequate, safe amounts of amino acids are found in food, self-dosing on amino acid supplements should be avoided. The delicate balance of amino acids in food is not present in these supplements. Ingesting the supplements and upsetting the balance can be risky.

FAT-BURNING ENZYMES

Don't let anyone fool you into buying bottled fat-burning enzymes. Enzymes are just proteins, nothing more. So how can someone make claims about enzymes burning fat? Because while they are in the bottle they are, in fact, enzymes that *could* burn fat *if* they made it to your muscles. But the catch is this: the minute those so-called fat-burning enzymes hit your stomach, your stomach acids attack and destroy them. They become ordinary proteins again. Save your money, okay? Make your own fat-burning enzymes by doing your H.E.A.R.T. workout in your Zone One.

alcohol (specifically beer) are strongly linked (a quadrupled risk) to these deaths. While men who exercise have a lower risk of colon cancer, this may be because exercise stimulates regular bowel movements. Urge your husband to stick to the high-fiber plan to increase regularity and give added protection against colon cancer. Then calculate his Zone One and loan him your heart-rate monitor. Encourage him to start an exercise program to decrease his risk of all diseases.

Consumption of fatty fish and soy reduces the risk of prostate cancer for men. A study of 6,272 Swedish men with a thirty-year follow-up showed that men who ate no fish had twice to three times the frequency of prostate cancer of those who ate moderate or high amounts. Learn to prepare salmon using herbs and low-fat sauces to increase flavor, and your husband will stop asking "Where's the beef?" at suppertime.

Final Thoughts

As you start the Definition Diet, take one day at a time. You surely didn't gain your weight or get out of shape in one week—or month! Each and every 24 hours can be a nutrition turnaround, creating a leaner, younger, and healthier body.

The good news is that food can be a positive force in your life, giving you more strength and energy, making you look and feel great and actually grow younger every day. I believe there is within all of us an innate desire to make food choices that create a healthier life for ourselves, our children, and our planet.

TOTAL LIFE CHANGE 4

Healing Hydration

HAVE A love affair with water. I love to be in it; I live next to it; and drinking more than 10 glasses of it each day has kept me lean, young looking, and healthy.

I guess that's why it's hard for me to understand why so many women ignore their daily water requirements. Clients from around the world come to the spa in Hawaii for information on weight loss, antiaging, and wellness. Yet when I tell them to start a hydration program, they give the same response: "Yes, I know I'm supposed to drink more water to stay healthy, but I'm really here for the latest anti-aging and weight-loss information."

I'll never forget Kristin, a thirty-four-year-old dancer from Los Angeles, who said she avoided drinking water because it made her "look fat and feel bloated." Kristin, a tall, striking blond with a great figure, looked at me like I was crazy when I told her the best way to stop water retention was to give her body what it needs—even more water!

I know both professionally and personally that water is a main factor in looking younger, staying healthy, and—the biggest bonus of all—losing weight. Yet I also realize that many people don't understand what this "silent nutrient" actually does in the body and how we must continually replenish it to stay well. Before I explain why water is the antiaging "cure," go pour yourself a tall glass of water and start to enjoy the amazing health benefits as you read.

Water, Water, Everywhere

Because more than two-thirds of your body weight is water, this liquid is just as important as oxygen for keeping you alive. Imagine every cell, tissue, and organ—all depending on water to function. Water keeps your body alive by stabilizing its temperature, eliminating toxins and waste products, carrying nutrients, and maintaining blood volume. Water is also the medium in which cell chemical reactions take place. You could go for weeks without food, but you will live only a few days with no water.

WATER IN . . .

Once the water you drink enters your body by absorption through the mouth, esophagus, and gastrointestinal tract, it starts to saturate all the body's thirsty cells. If you weigh 150 pounds, you have about 10 gallons of water in your body. Of this amount, approximately 6 to 7 gallons are inside your cells, 2 gallons are in the space surrounding the cells, and slightly less than a gallon is in your bloodstream. Did you know that blood plasma is 90 percent water?

The amount of water in your body right now is closely related to the amount of electrolytes (sodium, potassium, calcium, and magnesium), and your body works 24-7 to keep the total water and blood sodium level constant. If you eat salty foods, possibly boosting the sodium level in the body too high, your body will retain water to dilute the excess sodium. (Many women experience this during the premenstrual phase of their monthly cycle—and yes, drinking more water, not less, is the cure.) Your body's natural response to water retention is supposed to be an increase in thirst, but for unknown reasons, many of us have lost our thirst indicators, especially if we're over forty.

TOXINS AND WASTE OUT

On a normal day, your body uses water to metabolize food, remove waste, regulate temperature, and more. Water then leaves the body primarily as urine excreted from the kidneys. The average water loss is about 2½ quarts of water through different means such as urine, bowel movements, perspiration, and evaporation by the lungs when you exhale (about 3 cups of water). You don't need your calculator to figure out how much water should be coming in!

The minimum amount of water just to replace the normal 2½-quart fluid loss could be 10 glasses a day. However, for a 24-Hour Turnaround, just consuming the amount your body loses is not enough. If you want weight loss and antiaging results, it's time to *up* the ante!

THE DANGER ZONE

What happens when you become ill with a gastrointestinal flu and more water is going out than coming in? Or when you get overheated and don't take in enough liquids to keep the body balanced? Consider what ensues when you're faced with chronic stress, and even more fluids are required. Most people are oblivious to the onset of dehydration, due in part to the lack of thirst. By the time your thirst indicator kicks in, you are already 1 to 2 percent dehydrated, at which time with luck the body will rush to the rescue and trigger behaviors that cause you to drink more water or lie down until the body cools off. Finally, when dehydration becomes severe and you lose too much water, your life can be threatened. The amount of blood in the body is diminished, and all the organs are affected, especially your heart, which goes into overload trying to pump blood to the major organs. You may feel symptoms of headache, dry mouth, flushed skin, and fatigue. If dehydration worsens, you may get low blood pressure, dizziness, rapid heart rate, and kidney failure, or even death.

There is a serious need to replenish this water supply constantly if you want to stay young, vital, and healthy. Even minor dehydration can trigger devastating internal reactions, such as:

- Dehydrated body cells that age faster
- Water retention because of high sodium levels (influences blood pressure)
- Increased risk of bladder infections that could harm the kidneys
- Increased constipation
- Decreased fat-burning
- Diminished fuel to the brain

24-Hour Turnaround Solution

Unfortunately, the statement "drink more water" has never been convincing enough for my clients to make this Total Life Change. That's why I have to present the correct information—facts, data, studies, and successful strategies from professionals (my "water lecture") to convince my clients (that's you) to start this important TLC immediately. Before I give you some surefire ways to hydrate your body, take the following quiz to help determine your 24-Hour Turnaround Solution.

True or false? Everyone needs only 8 glasses of water each day.

False. If we all drank 8 glasses of water each day, we'd be a much healthier world. But the truth is that our water needs vary, depending on our age, health status, activity level, and climate. For example, during exercise you can lose up to 3 pints of water an hour from sweating. Yet if you jog on a hot day, that number can jump to 3 *quarts* of water an hour. People rarely drink enough water to replace what they've lost during exercise. Loss of fluid limits the amount of blood the heart can pump with each stroke. Eventually the amount of blood delivered to the working muscles becomes inadequate, causing the heart rate to go up.

A small child may not require 8 glasses of water each day, while someone who weighs 190 pounds and exercises may need at least a gallon (16 glasses). If you have cardiovascular disease, check with your doctor, who may want to monitor your intake of fluids.

True or false? It's best not to drink before you exercise in order to avoid nausea and cramping.

False. Exercise or vigorous activity elevates the temperature of the body. If adequate water is not taken in before and during exercise, the body loses its ability to cool itself properly. Fatigue can set in

RED FLAG SYMPTOMS OF DEHYDRATION

Headache
Dry mouth
Flushed skin
Dry or flaky skin
Fatigue
Irritability/bad mood
Low blood pressure
Dizziness
Rapid heart rate
Kidney failure

ARE YOU RETAINING WATER?

Press the thumb of one hand into your shinbone (about midway between your ankle and your knee). Hold the pressure for 30 seconds. When you lift your thumb off, can you still feel or see a dent in your leg where you were pressing? If the answer is yes, keep reading. What you just did was press the extracellular water out of that spot, and it will take a little time for it to go back to being smooth. This simple 30-second test shows that you are holding water in places you shouldn't, and the first line of defense is to drink more water. Let your body know that you're not in a drought, so it can stop hoarding!

and, in some cases, dangerous dehydration. The American College of Sports Medicine recommends drinking a minimum of 6 ounces of water every 15 minutes during training. The most important time to drink water for fat loss is 1 to 2 hours prior to exercise. Consume 8 to 16 ounces if possible. If you exercise right after you awaken, go to bed hydrated and start with your water ASAP.

True or false? A little water is necessary for survival. But 8 to 10 glasses would cause you to feel bloated and retain water, with swollen hands, ankles, and feet.

False. Drinking enough—or better yet, extra—water is the best treatment for fluid retention. While diuretics offer a temporary solution by forcing out stored water, along with some essential nutrients, the body perceives the water loss as a threat and will store the lost water at the first opportunity. Within a day or two, the fluid retention quickly returns. When you are dehydrated, your body starts hoarding water and packs it in between the cells (extracellular water), which is commonly known as bloating. In a study published in 1998 in the *American Journal of Physiology,* researchers concluded that postmenopausal women who took estrogen replacement therapy actually retained more water than those women who did not.

True or false? The sports drinks that athletes use are the best for hydrating during the hot summer months or during exercise.

False. Not necessarily. Sports drinks contain fruit juice or are high in sugar and electrolytes (potassium and sodium). These drinks add unnecessary calories,

HOT FLASH!
HYDRATE YOUR LEAN, SEXY MACHINE

Metabolically active tissue (lean body mass) has the highest percentage of water (75 percent). Keep that lean body mass hydrated, and let it work for you! Lean muscle is your calorie-burning equipment. Water also helps to maintain muscle tone. A hydrated muscle can grow, speeding up your metabolism. A dehydrated muscle can only catabolize (tear down). See TLC 2 for more information on speeding up your metabolism.

The bottom line (and you know which bottom I'm talking about) is that if you want your muscles to burn fat, you'd better give them water—and plenty of it.

and unless you are doing extremely strenuous exercise for more than 90 minutes, pure water is actually far better. Because the body must digest the calories in the drink, the sugar or juice content slows the emptying of the water and increases the amount of time until the water reaches the cells.

True or false? Soft water is easier to drink and is tolerated better than hard water.
False. Soft water may taste better, but it is also high in sodium; hard water is high in calcium and magnesium. There is no reason to substitute soft water for hard, and chances are you don't need the extra sodium, which can cause water retention and even increase your blood pressure.

Three Reasons to Hydrate—Right Now!

I often consult with clients who have a host of medical problems, some quite serious. On the initial client questionnaire, I ask them to tell me about their health, medications they are taking, past illnesses, and daily habits—including how much water they drink. I never cease to be amazed at how many of these clients could resolve their illnesses if the health-care provider had educated them about diet and hydration. I have spoken with doctors across the country, and most tell me that

H₂O STATS FOR EXERCISERS

- Electrolytes (sodium, potassium, calcium, and magnesium) are all lost in sweat in varying amounts. Electrolyte losses are less in conditioned individuals.

- A 1.9 percent decrease in body weight because of dehydration results in a 10 percent decrease in ability to deliver oxygen to the cells and a 22 percent decrease in physical performance. Reduced oxygen to the muscle cells equals reduced fat-burning.

- If you're 3 to 4 percent dehydrated, your heart rate and body temperature increase significantly.

- The substances in concentrated fluids (juices, sports drinks, sodas) delay emptying from the stomach and availability to the body.

- Cold fluids leave the stomach most quickly. It's recommended that water consumed during exercise be cold but not iced, but it's fine to follow your preference.

- Weigh yourself before and after a workout as an experiment. Every 2-pound weight loss during an exercise session equals 1 quart (4 cups) of water loss. This shows how important it is to stay hydrated. This water weight loss from exercise can result in feelings of weakness and nausea.

- If you're 2 percent dehydrated, it will take you 24 to 36 hours to rehydrate at the cellular level. Physical ability is reduced during this time.

- During exercise, blood flow to the skin is increased, and our three million sweat glands allow us to release heat and cool down.

DID YOU KNOW THAT . . .

- The kidneys can't function properly without enough water. When they don't work to capacity, some of their load is dumped onto the liver. The liver's primary function is to turn stored fat into energy for the body. If the liver is doing the kidneys' work, it metabolizes less fat, and weight loss stops!

- The National Cancer Institute says that the drinking of chlorinated water (tap water) increases one's risks of developing bladder cancer by 80 percent.

- Unintentional chronic dehydration is associated with serious diseases, including asthma, renal dysfunction, endocrine system and adrenal fatigue, high blood pressure and other cardiovascular problems, arthritis, ulcers, pancreatitis, digestive difficulties, and lower back pain.

- While this may be radical reporting, some scientists believe that brain cell dehydration is the primary cause of Alzheimer's disease. With prolonged dehydration, brain cells begin to shrink, and many of their functions begin to be lost, such as the transport system that delivers neurotransmitters to nerve endings.

- Drinking more water and liquids can benefit those with asthma. Water helps to liquefy the thick mucus, making it easier to expel.

- The mucous membrane that lines the stomach to protect it from hydrochloric acid is 98 percent water.

- Dehydration stresses the body; chronic stress can lead to further dehydration.

- An effective way to prevent migraines is the regular intake of water.

- Common colds and the flu frequently lead to dehydration.

medical school students are not given information about the role of water in the human body—and how we can affect our health positively by drinking more.

Because a shortage of water in the body could result in symptoms and signs that are similar to disease symptoms, conventional medical doctors may overlook hydration as a natural way to resolve the patient's problems. On page 200 I've listed just a few of the many health conditions that can be influenced by hydration of the body. Perhaps the greatest health discovery of the twenty-first century will be that natural medicine—water—can halt or even reverse a variety of health conditions.

1. HYDRATE TO LOSE WEIGHT

If you want to lose weight, there is *no* question that you must drink plenty of water. We know that water helps the body metabolize stored fat. Medical studies have shown that a decrease in water intake will cause fat deposits to increase, while an increase in water intake can actually reduce fat deposits. If that doesn't make you start drinking, read this: mild dehydration will *slow your metabolism* by as much as *3 percent*. That statistic alone sends most of my clients to the water cooler in the middle of a consult. When you reduce calories and increase exercise, you need more water to get rid of waste products from the fat that is being burned.

If you've been depriving your body of water and start drinking 10 glasses of water each day, you might see the number on the scale go up. This gain is not fat and will not change the size of your body. The water-weight gain is a good thing, as this extra water will help you lose the fat pounds.

Other weight-loss benefits with increased hydration include the following:

- Proteins and enzymes of the body function more efficiently in solutions that are water-dense. In a nutshell, this means that your rate of burning old fat is going to go up.

- Liver function is boosted to its fat-burning max.

- Water provides a no-calorie energizer during times of great stress. Think about it. The reason we tend to gain weight when we're under chronic stress boils down to one simple fact: we eat. We eat to feed our troubles, to console our spirit, and most important, to meet the brain's added need for energy to sustain the round-the-clock "fight or flight" activity. However, only about 20 percent of these calories reach the brain. The rest head for our hips (unless our activity level goes up). With water as a source of energy instead of food, this storage does not happen. Brain cells are 80 to 85 percent water. Supply your brain with the nutrient it *really* wants when you are stressed: good old H_2O.

● Water fills you up so that you eat less.

2. HYDRATE TO END CONSTIPATION

Water helps rid the body of waste, which includes both urine and feces. The formula I give my clients is simple: *10 glasses of water equals softer stools and less constipation.* When the body gets too little water, it siphons what it needs from internal sources, mainly from the colon. But when you drink at least 10 glasses of water each day, normal bowel function usually returns.

3. HYDRATE TO REJUVENATE AGING SKIN

Water is also important for skin texture and tightness. Your skin tone is a very important indicator of ample water intake. When enough water is present in the cells, the skin has more elasticity and better color, and it ages much more slowly. Water also helps to prevent the sagging skin that usually follows weight loss. Shrinking cells are buoyed by water, which plumps the skin and leaves it clear, healthy, and resilient. Any insult (sunburn, the wrong skin products) or injury (cuts, wounds, abrasions) to the skin will lower its ability to act as a barrier against foreign substances. Water helps to heal this protective organ.

Filtered, Bottled, or Tap?

So what type of water should you choose? Is the tap water in your kitchen sink safe to drink? Or should you purchase expensive bottled water? What about filtered water—not as expensive, but is it safe? The U.S. Environmental Protection Agency mandates that all public water supplies be filtered, treated with chlorine, and tested regularly for the presence of fecal coliform bacteria, such as *E. coli,* found in the intestines and fecal material of humans and animals. Bottled water is usually tested regularly for the same reasons.

The use of chlorine to disinfect our drinking water became standard practice in the early 1900s. Shockingly, we don't use chlorine because it's the safest or even the most effective means of disinfection; we use it because it's the cheapest. In spite of all our technological advances, we still essentially pour bleach in our water before we drink it. The long-term effects of chlorinated drinking water have just recently been recognized. According to the U.S. Council on Environmental Quality, the cancer risk among people drinking chlorinated water is 93 percent higher than among those whose water does not contain chlorine, such as bottled or filtered water. On a personal note, while I'm against fluoridation because of proven harmful effects to humans, many dentists lavishly use it on patients' teeth—and it's still commonly found in drinking water.

Years ago Dr. Joseph Price did a landmark study on chickens and wrote a highly controversial book entitled *Coronaries/Cholesterol/Chlorine.* In the study, hundreds of birds were divided into groups. One group was given water with chlorine and the other water without chlorine. When the group raised with chlorine underwent autopsies, every chicken showed some level of heart or circulatory disease; the group without chlorinated water had no incidence of disease. The group with chlorine had poor health and a reduced level of activity; the group without chlorine grew faster, larger, and displayed vigorous health. The poultry industry took the study seriously, and as a result, most large poultry producers use dechlorinated water. I'm not an expert in this field, but it seems like common sense that if regular chlorinated tap water is not good enough for chickens, it probably is not good enough for us!

When chlorine is added to our water, it combines with other natural compounds to form trihalomethanes (THMs). These chlorine by-products are highly carcinogenic and trigger the production of free radicals in the body, which cause cell damage. Although concentrations of these THMs are low, it is precisely these low levels that cancer scientists believe are responsible for the majority of human cancers in the United States.

Breast cancer, which now affects one of every eight women in North America and is on the rise, has been connected to the accumulation of chlorine compounds in the breast tissue. A 1993 study carried out in Hartford, Connecticut, by Dr. Mary Wolff, an epidemiologist from Mount Sinai School of Medicine, revealed that women with breast cancer have higher levels of chlorination by-products in their breast tissue than women without breast cancer. Experts say these chemicals are attracted to fatty tissue. Wolff's study was the first of its kind in North America.

If that doesn't make you leery of what you've been told about "safe water," keep reading: up to two-thirds of our harmful exposure to chlorine comes from breathing the steam during that hot shower or bath and the absorption of chlorine compounds through the skin. A warm shower opens up the pores of the skin and allows for accelerated absorption of chlorine and other chemicals in water. The steam our kids inhale while soaking in the tub can contain up to fifty times the level of chemicals in the tap water they drink due to the fact that chlorine starts to vaporize almost immediately. Inhalation is a much more harmful means of exposure since the chlorine gas (chloroform) we inhale goes directly into our bloodstream. When we drink chlorinated water, the toxins are partially filtered out by our kidneys and digestive system (although I'm not recommending that you ask your kidneys to do this). The chlorine vapors are a strong irritant to the sensitive tissue and bronchial passages inside our lungs—so much so that chlorine was used as a chemical weapon in World War II. The inhalation of chlorine is a suspected cause of asthma and bronchitis, especially in children.

Chlorine in shower water also has a very negative effect on our skin and hair, depleting them of moisture and elasticity and leaving them with a dull, dry appearance. Take a closer look at your kids when they come out of the swimming pool and have discolored hair, red eyes, and flaky skin. Now here's the really bad news: we usually have higher levels of chlorine in our tap water than the recommended safe level for swimming pools. Unreal? If you don't smell the chlorine when you pour a glass of water, that's because your glass of chlorinated water is minuscule compared with the pool you swim in. Nonetheless, chlorine is in the tap water and is toxic to your system.

There are organizations that are fighting for the elimination of chlorine from our water supply, but unfortunately, we know the consequences could be devastating to our health because of the resulting harmful bacteria and water-borne diseases. So how do we protect ourselves? We can remove the chlorine from the water we drink, shower, and bathe in using one of the inexpensive home water filters that are made for this purpose. Check my website for the best brands; I'm always updating information on products to keep you well. Until your filter comes, drink bottled water, or to lessen the effects of the drinking water, fill an open-top jug with water and let it stand in the refrigerator or on the kitchen counter. The chlorine that is dissolved in the water will evaporate, and the smell will go away too.

Water Alternatives Are No Substitute for H$_2$O

Let's look at some common "water alternatives" to see why you cannot substitute them for fresh, natural water.

Fruit juices. While fruit juices have some nutritional value, they are not a good Definition Diet choice because they are very calorie-dense, meaning that there are many calories in a small serving. Did you know that 8 ounces of juice typically contain 120 calories? Not to mention that the fiber has been taken out, which puts that glass of juice in the sugar category. Also, if you substitute fruit juice for water, it may take the place of other nutritious whole foods—a very good reason to eliminate juice from a child's diet. My clients have immediate results when they eliminate juice from their daily diets and stay with whole fruit, which also gives them the added benefit of high fiber. Water plus fiber is a guaranteed cure for constipation, and it fills you up too.

If you're dying of thirst on a hot day or after strenuous exercise, don't reach for that carton of OJ; juice doesn't do the trick. The nutrients in the juice will slow down the absorption of the water by your dehydrated system. And don't forget, by the time you are thirsty, you have passed the level of mild dehydration and are headed into the danger zone.

Caffeinated drinks. Human beings are the only animal whose thirst mechanism is not in sync with the need for water. Maybe it's the common practice of overindulging in water-depleting fluids that creates this alarming out-of-sync thirst regulator. Caffeine, one of the main components of most sodas, is a drug. Caffeine has strong addictive properties because of its direct action on the brain, and it works as a diuretic. For those cola, coffee, or tea addicts, caffeine is one of the main reasons you crave these drinks every day and are never satisfied with just one. Quality food, moderate exercise, and extra sleep will all increase your energy and decrease your need for caffeine.

Artificially sweetened diet drinks. Remember Kristin, the young dancer who avoided drinking water for fear of being bloated? After adopting the 24-Hour Turnaround, she called me one evening before a show to say that increased liquid consumption had made her bloated, and she had gained—not lost—4 pounds. When I asked her what she had been eating and drinking, she said she was living off artificially sweetened diet drinks—not pure water. Kristin said the more she drank, the hungrier she became.

I explained to her that when you eat or drink a fake sweetener, the sweet taste stimulates your tongue, and the brain programs the liver to prepare for acceptance of new energy (calories). However, if this sweet taste is not followed by calories (food), you will feel a sudden urge to *eat*—and chances are great that you will not be craving a fresh garden salad! The more sweet taste without accompanying calories, the greater the urge to eat—and that can turn into overeating or binge eating, so the "bloat" you feel may be just plain added fat. That information alone changed Kristin's beverage consumption from diet drinks to water immediately.

Carbonated water. Although carbonated or soda water is rich in minerals, unfortunately these minerals are not present in a form that our bodies are able to use easily. Unlike the minerals in fresh fruits and vegetables, those in mineral water are easily deposited in our joints, muscles, and tissues. Excess amounts of mineral water can cause stiffness, gall or kidney stones, and premature aging of the skin. Stick to the plain old version. Some of us these days seem to be addicted to bubbles. Could it be because those sodas tasted so good? The bubbles in mineral

WHERE'S OUR WATER GOING, ANYWAY?

According to John Robbins, author of *The Food Revolution,* Americans know that their water is not pure. This is evidenced by the fact that each year they spend more than $2 billion for bottled water and home tap-water treatments.

In 1997 the U.S. Senate Agricultural Committee issued a lengthy report on livestock waste in this country, stating, "untreated and unsanitary, bubbling with chemicals and disease-bearing organisms . . . [the livestock waste] goes onto the soil and into the water that many people will bathe in and wash their clothes with and even drink . . . [and] it's poisoning rivers and killing fish and sickening people."

What do we really know about the water that is approved to drink? The facts are a bit startling, I must warn you:

- To produce 1 pound of California beef requires 2,464 gallons of water, according to the Water Education Foundation.
- Nearly half the water consumed in this country is used for livestock, mostly cattle.
- The amount of water that goes to produce a 1,000-pound steer would float a naval destroyer.

Must we live with such blatant abuse of our earth's perfect natural resource? No, there are answers! Perhaps a cultural shift toward a plant-based diet would help plug the drain through which much of our water is being lost. There is no other single action that is as effective for saving water as eating a plant-based diet.

water are formed by carbon dioxide, a waste product that the body tries to eliminate. It doesn't make sense to force carbon dioxide into the body when it has gone to so much trouble to get rid of it in the first place. Limit your intake of mineral water and bubbles to social occasions, when they are a far better choice than an alcoholic beverage or a can of soda.

Alcohol. After a night on the town (or that innocent glass of wine with dinner), we cannot process food properly, expel wastes efficiently, repair damaged muscle

WATER DEFINED

The Food and Drug Administration regulates the bottled water we purchase. Here are some FDA definitions:

- *Artesian water* is water drawn from a permeable stratum of rock overlaid by impermeable rock in which the water level is above the natural water table.

- *Purified water* is demineralized water (also called distilled water) that is produced by ion exchange or by reverse osmosis (passing it through filters to remove dissolved solids).

- *Mineral water* contains large quantities of minerals collected as it passes through layers of rock and earth to the well or spring.

- *Spring water* flows naturally from an underground formation without the use of drills or pumps.

- *Sparkling water* contains carbon dioxide gas, either from nature or from science.

- *Soda water* is carbonated water that contains sodium bicarbonate.

tissue as quickly, or keep vital organs functioning well. Have you ever noticed that if you have numerous glasses of wine with dinner, your workout suffers the next morning? Should you go to the gym anyway, thinking the best thing to do is sweat it out? *No.* You're dehydrated, and the best choice for you is to stay home and drink water. What about that "can't seem to get it going today" feeling that you associate with laziness? Having a bottle of water will help remedy this and give you a boost of energy; having a beer in the afternoon or wine with dinner will add to these lethargic feelings.

Janis loved wine. It didn't matter what kind—every day at 4 P.M., this forty-five-year-old mother of two teenagers poured herself a wine spritzer. At 6 P.M.

she had two glasses of wine with dinner. No wonder she had a sluggish feeling, a slow metabolism, and difficulty concentrating each morning. Janis thought it was her hormones—we blame everything on hormones these days—but it was the wine. I gave Janis the facts about her evening wine habit: that it takes up to 48 hours for the body to expel all traces of alcohol (yes, wine) from our bodies. One night of drinking can cost you a couple of days of efficient workouts, effective weight loss, and cellular repair, not to mention the damaging effect on your skin, the organ that everyone sees! You'll learn more about the effects of alcohol in TLC 5.

RED FLAG

In terms of cumulative damage to your health, showering in chlorinated water is one of the most dangerous risks you take daily. Some believe that there could be short-term risks of irritation to our eyes, sinuses, throat, skin, and lungs. Long-term risks include free radical formation that ages you faster, higher vulnerability to genetic mutation and cancer development, and difficulty metabolizing cholesterol, which can harden arteries.

Your 24-Hour Turnaround

As you start Total Life Change 4, I want you to stop relying on your thirst mechanism—if you even have one! Many of us drink water only when we are thirsty, and this is especially true as we grow older. However, thirst is a poor indicator of when to drink water. If you depend on thirst alone as a stimulus for drinking, you will usually stop drinking liquids when you are still 1 to 2 percent dehydrated. Sadly, a dry mouth is the very last sign of dehydration.

HOW MUCH WATER?

We have all heard the old "8 glasses a day" standard from just about every expert. But consider this: Should a 110-pound female who doesn't exercise drink the same amount of water as a 190-pound man who exercises and drinks coffee and beer (all three of which dehydrate the body)? No. If you were to ask me to throw out a number that works for everyone, I would have to say 16 glasses of water a day! However,

I do have a formula that will come very close to your personal water needs, so get out your calculator.

Level 1. If you eat five servings of fruits and vegetables per day, then multiply your body weight by 0.55. This will equal the number of ounces of water you should drink each day. Divide this number by 8 (ounces in a cup) to get the total number of cups of water. Check to see how many ounces of water your water bottle and glasses hold since they all differ. Also note: If you don't consume at least five servings of fruits and veggies, you owe your body another 2 glasses of water.

Level 2. If your day includes 1 hour of the H.E.A.R.T. workout and five servings of fruits and vegetables, then multiply your body weight by 0.70 to find the number of ounces of water you should drink daily. Divide this number by 8 to get the number of cups of water.

Level 3. If your day (or the night before) included any of the following:
Air travel
Alcohol
Antihistamines
Caffeine
Extreme heat or cold
Many medications (stimulants in particular)
Nursing
Pregnancy
Sickness

add an additional .05 to the factor you multiply by for each condition that applies, to find your water needs for the day.

EXAMPLE

Following are Level 1, 2, and 3 calculations for a 135-pound woman. Level 3 calculations assume only one of the listed stressful conditions.

Level 1:

135 (body weight) × .55 = 74.25 ounces ÷ 8 = 9¼ cups minimum

Level 2:

135 × .70 = 94.50 ounces ÷ 8 = 11¾ cups minimum

Level 3:

135 × (.55 + .05) = 81 ounces ÷ 8 = 10¼ cups minimum

135 × (.70 + .05) = 101.25 ounces ÷ 8 = 12⅔ cups minimum

WATERLOGGED

"There's no way I can down ten glasses of water each day. I'd be hanging out in the bathroom instead of working and enjoying my life!" Suki, a health book editor from San Francisco, flatly refused to even try drinking enough water to keep her body energized and healthy—until she got a persistent bladder infection. Her doctor told her that drinking water, even 2 glasses an hour, at the first sign of pain might help to clear the urine and prevent the infection. While I'm not a medical doctor, I do know that Suki and many other clients have found that being "water-

---

IMMEDIATE BENEFITS OF DRINKING WATER

Reduced stress
Suppression of appetite
Reduced constipation
Increased energy
Better fat-burning
Hydration of brain and body cells
Hydration of skin
Greater muscle endurance

---

logged" keeps all the plumbing of the body functioning beautifully—without the need for antibiotics every time they feel a twinge or burning during urination.

Suki was convinced! Because this water cure helped her get well, she continued to drink water on the Turnaround schedule and found that she had increased energy and less stress, and even lost weight because she stopped snacking on junk food.

THE SPA HYDRATION SCHEDULE

I have many clients who are now convinced that water revitalizes aging bodies. When my clients come to Hawaii for a spa week, they are required to log everything that passes their lips, and the time of day as well. On a perfect day it would look something like this:

Rise-and-shine water. Consuming 16 to 24 ounces of tepid water (or herbal tea) with a fresh lemon twist first thing in the morning is one of the healthiest ways to cleanse your system and detoxify your cells. The fresh lemon aids in the cleansing and "detox" of the liver and colon while providing vital phytonutrients and beneficial natural enzymes. The juice of the lemon also contains potent antiviral and antibacterial agents that help fight off colds and other illnesses. Additionally, some studies have demonstrated that the scent of fresh lemon energizes you and lifts your mood *immediately*.

Water every hour on the hour. I recommend that my clients stay with an hourly (yes, on the hour!) hydration schedule. If you had tepid water at 7 A.M., then have your next 8 ounces at 8 A.M.

Water before, during, and after exercise. The requirement for water during exercise is 6 ounces for every 15 minutes of physical training. The water you drink during training replaces water lost through perspiration and does not count toward your hourly water. Stay on track. Your thirst factor is most likely to kick in after exercise, so take advantage of it and have extra!

FLUIDS AND MEALS

Water suppresses the appetite naturally, so adjust your hourly water to coincide with your meals and snacks. Always drink your water before eating for two reasons:

1. Drinking water before meals reduces food consumption and controls your appetite. The thirst signal, sent from the hypothalamus, is often confused with the hunger signal, making you eat when you're not really hungry or eat more than you should at meals.

2. Watery solutions help dissolve nutrients and carry them to all parts of your body. Through chemical reactions, your body can turn these nutrients into energy or into the materials it requires to regenerate and repair itself.

So by maintaining a well-hydrated body and drinking before your meals, you minimize this thirst/hunger confusion, help to dissolve and utilize nutrients, and save yourself from overindulging in the next 24 hours.

FOUR WINNING WATER TIPS TO KEEP YOU LEAN

1. *Drink before you eat.* Drink 1 or 2 glasses of water before each meal. Water can fill your stomach, calm the hunger pangs, and cause you to leave more on your plate.

2. *Freeze plastic bottles of water.* Leave a six-pack of plastic water bottles in your freezer. Take these instead of colas or snacks when you are driving on a trip or on the way to the grocery store. The cold water will quench your thirst without adding calories. This is also a great tip for exercise class.

3. *Order water when you eat out.* Get in the habit of just ordering water with lemon when you dine out. Alcohol, coffee, tea, and artificially sweetened sodas will only slow down your weight loss. Water is your weight-loss friend.

4. *Keep a glass of water on your desk while you work.* When you finish it, make a point of refilling it immediately. Aim for your individualized water prescription at the very least.

H_2O STATS

- About 75 percent of Americans are chronically dehydrated.

- In 37 percent of Americans, the thirst mechanism is so weak that it is often mistaken for hunger.

- Even *mild* dehydration will slow down one's metabolism as much as 3 percent.

- In a diet study at the University of Washington, researchers found that just 1 glass of water shut down midnight hunger pangs for almost 100 percent of the dieters.

- Lack of water is a key contributor to daytime fatigue.

- Preliminary research indicates that 8 to 10 glasses of water a day significantly eased back and joint pain in many sufferers.

- A mere 2 percent drop in body water can trigger fuzzy short-term memory, trouble with basic math, and difficulty focusing on the computer screen or on a printed page.

As you age, the body's ability to utilize the water you drink diminishes by as much as 50 percent. The solution? Drink twice as much! If you want to look and feel young, hydration is a crucial part of your antiaging program.

FOR YOUR KIDS

Make sure you share information in this chapter with your kids. While it's easy to give a toddler water, many older children and teenagers gravitate toward colas and sweet drinks.

Teach your kids how to use the formulas to figure out the minimum number of ounces they need, and then challenge them to drink at least that amount each day.

TRAVEL TIPS

1. *Consider your vacationing climate.* If you are from Boston and vacation in Tampa, Florida, you need to consider the warmer temperatures and adjust your water intake accordingly.

2. *Watch out for water when traveling abroad, as it may be contaminated with fecal organisms.* Buy bottled water to drink and to use for brushing your teeth. Do not use ice cubes made from the area's tap water. And avoid swimming in freshwater ponds, rivers, streams, or lakes to avoid infectious bacteria that may be in the water. Also avoid vegetables and fruits that cannot be peeled, as they may have been rinsed in the tap water.

We have contests in our house. (My kids especially love to do the urine test; I'm sure you'll get the report at your house too.) Make sure your children take water breaks every 20 minutes while engaging in a physical activity or playing in the hot sun. This is especially necessary in the summertime, when they can easily get dehydrated. Also make sure your children carry water in a plastic bottle when they play sports or have games. (Coaches aren't always hip to the hydration rules.) Save juice for a special occasion or a dinner out. Instead of carbonated drinks, serve refreshing and healthful water instead.

FOR YOUR HUSBAND

If your husband resists drinking 10 or more glasses of water daily, serve foods that are naturally rich in water. There are only three kinds on the planet: fruits, vegetables, and sprouts. Fruits are around 90 to 95 percent water and are the most perfect food for hydration. It takes the least amount of energy to digest fruits, and they give the body the most in return. The fluid contained in fruits seems to play a very important role in our hydration because it directly affects our digestion. As I've pointed out, it just so happens that the only food your brain can use is glucose. The

The older we get, the more the body's ability to conserve water is reduced. If you are over sixty-five, you may not know that you are thirsty. That's why a specific schedule of water consumption can help keep you well. Also, if you take diuretics (water pills), watch for signs of dehydration. When you are severely dehydrated, you will not feel thirsty at all. If you start to drink less water or if your diuretic dose is too high, you could become seriously ill, with a sudden drop in blood pressure and decreased oxygen supplied to the brain.

sugar in fruit is primarily fructose, which can be easily converted into glucose. That means that fruits are cleansing and energizing at the same time. Keep a large bowl of fruit on your kitchen table, and encourage your husband to pack several fruits in his lunch to ensure extra hydration when he's at work or traveling.

Young and Healthy Cells in Just 24 Hours

You cannot change your past hydration history. If you have avoided drinking ample water for fear of weight gain or being bloated, I hope this Total Life Change helped you see the facts—that water will help you to lose weight, feel more alert, resolve constipation, and stop bloating.

Start with the hydration Turnaround plan today and see an immediate result! Drink 10 or more glasses of water in the next 24 hours and every 24 hours after that. It will be easy to change your bad habits of just sipping water every now and then, especially when you experience the dramatic weight loss and antiaging benefits. Cheers!

Alcohol and
the Myth of Moderation

BUT MY DOCTOR said that moderate drinking—one or two glasses of wine each evening—will help me live longer and protect my heart." Claire, forty-three, loved her wine with dinner. It was difficult to convince her that this evening ritual was putting her at risk for serious illness and accelerating aging—not to mention that it was the probable reason for her 15-pound weight gain this year.

When you drink, even just one glass of wine, one bottle of beer, or 1 ounce of alcohol, your cells are depleted of much-needed water and key nutrients, and your mind, body, and mood will pay the steep price within 24 hours and for days and weeks to come. While you cannot always tell that your cells have been abused or even destroyed after an innocent cocktail or glass of wine with dinner, you will notice the effects in the way you sleep (fitfully) look (tired and older), or feel (fatigued or ill).

Some recent studies do suggest that having one or two drinks a day (a level of drinking referred to as *moderate*) is good for your health. Yet as I explained to Claire, if you want a good definition of the term *moderate* as it relates to alcohol, ask the National Institute on Alcohol Abuse and Alcoholism (NIAAA), the world's largest researcher on alcohol and the effects of its use. This watchdog agency defines *moderate* as one or two drinks per day, and it also reiterates that "moderate" amounts of alcohol are a contributing factor to a "moderate" incidence of cancer, "moderate" incidence of high blood pressure, and "moderate" amounts of liver damage. I don't know about you, but I'd rather *not* have any of those conditions, however "moderate."

What Your Doctor May Not Have Told You About Alcohol

The fact is, alcohol is *not* a moderate substance; it's a toxic drug and a deadly poison. No matter what you have read in slick magazine ads or what your doctor has shared—or *not* shared—about alcohol and your health, I'm going to be very straightforward with you: *alcohol is lethal.* Alcohol causes cancer. It also increases your blood pressure, causes fluctuations in your blood sugar levels, ages your skin, and contributes to weight gain and obesity. Alcohol metabolism is a total short-circuit to your body's normal mechanism for burning fat and building tissue, and just one drink will disrupt fat metabolism for two days.

1 drink = 2 days of backsliding on your Turnaround

I know you're probably skeptical of this dramatic stand against drinking, but read on, learn the facts, and make your own well-informed decision. Even with all the medical studies and media updates, confusion remains about what alcohol does to the body, how it affects our weight and health, and how it can negatively impact longevity. Before I go further, check out the following myths about alcohol and your health—along with some interesting scientific facts.

Myth. Wine is fat-free, and 4 ounces are only about 125 calories, certainly not enough to cause weight gain.

Fact. Alcohol causes weight gain by short-circuiting the metabolism of food. Let me explain. When you eat a serving of fish (about 125 calories and low in fat), it undergoes a long process of digestion before it can be used to build tissue or produce energy. It's mashed by your teeth, softened by saliva, attacked by stomach acids, and finally worked over by billions of bacteria in your intestines. Even after passing through the intestinal walls into your bloodstream, the digested food products (including fat) are subjected to a "first pass" through the liver. The liver scans for unwanted chemical signals (toxins, bacteria, and so on) and removes them from the stream of nutrients. You are what you eat—but only *after* it gets through your liver.

In sharp contrast to most foods, including the low-fat fish, alcohol requires *no* digestion. About 20 percent can pass right through the walls of an empty stomach directly into your bloodstream, and the rest is easily absorbed in the small intestine. From there it heads to the liver

(just like the fish). The liver's method of dealing with alcohol is to metabolize it for energy, creating glucose that's used to power your body. This becomes a top priority for the liver, which is smart enough to know that alcohol is a toxin. But smart as it is, the liver is fairly slow at turning the alcohol into energy. The alcohol that can't be used by the liver immediately enters the bloodstream, causing the blood alcohol level to increase within a minute after the first sip.

With this extra energy available from the alcohol—and this excess toxin to be removed—the liver becomes very preoccupied, leaving almost all other food that you consume to turn into fat. Shocking but true. These fats are then dumped into the bloodstream where they cause tissue damage, compromise immunity, and are stored in fat cells. The liver is still dealing with the alcohol even after your blood alcohol level is back to normal. It can take up to *48 hours* to return to the normal metabolism of dietary fat, during which time you will have reduced your chances of weight loss. In fact, you may be putting on a few extra pounds. Alcohol itself is rarely converted to fat. Usually it's the "sparing effect" described above that results in increased body fat.

I am simplifying the process a little, but you get the idea:

1 alcoholic drink → short-circuit in the metabolism of food → food is turned into fat → 2 days to recover = 0 weight loss

So before you have "just one" glass of wine with dinner, think of everything you eat in the next two days (including the big dinner that the wine accompanies) going straight into the fatty parts of your body, where you least want it to go. (Make sure you're following the Definition Diet to ensure *slow and steady* permanent weight loss.)

Myth. Having a few beers while playing volleyball on the beach is just part of the game.

Fact. Here are the real rules of the game, and they apply to *all sports:*

alcohol + sports = Turnaround loser

When you drink alcohol, it immediately affects the body's ability to turn food into energy. We need that energy (calories) available to burn when we exercise, especially if we want to lose weight. Alcohol also slows down our reaction times, increases loss of body heat, and reduces endurance. If you consume alcohol 24 hours before playing volleyball (or any kind of exercise), it dehydrates your body, and you are more likely to develop muscle cramps. After exercising, your body must be rehydrated, so those who insist on a few beers to cool down and celebrate are only adding fuel to the fire. And if you get hurt during exercise, drinking alcohol will slow down the healing process, leading to an increased recovery time from an injury.

Myth. To lose weight overnight, drink two beers, which act as a diuretic.

Fact. Sorry, but your overnight weight loss is just temporary. Drinking alcohol stimulates a system that causes the water to drain *out* of your cells, which is why women who drink usually have older-looking skin—as quickly as 24 hours later. Among the functions that alcohol suppresses is the release of antidiuretic hormone (ADH). This hormone causes the body to retain water by controlling urination. With ADH suppressed by alcohol, there is increased urination and dehydration. This explains why you may weigh less for a day or so after two beers or an all-out binge, but this is weight that is quickly regained once you hydrate your body. (To keep your body hydrated so fluid retention is not a concern, reread TLC 4.)

Myth. Having a drink before bedtime will help you fall asleep more easily and get deeper sleep.

```
┌─────────────────────────────────────────────────────────────────┐
│                        CALORIE COUNT                              │
│                                                                   │
│   ●  12-ounce light beer: 110 to 120 calories                     │
│   ●  12-ounce beer: 146 calories                                  │
│   ●  12-ounce piña colada: 592 calories                           │
│   ●  12-ounce frozen daiquiri: 633 calories                       │
│   ●  12-ounce wine cooler: 142 calories                           │
│                                                                   │
└─────────────────────────────────────────────────────────────────┘
```

Fact. While you may think an innocent cocktail will help you sleep, years of sleep research prove this is a myth too. A host of studies show that even one or two drinks in the evening or before bedtime can increase wakefulness during the second half of sleep. By the time this effect occurs, the dose of alcohol consumed earlier has already been metabolized by the body, suggesting a relatively long-lasting change in the body's mechanisms of sleep regulation. Even though that nightcap may have a lights-out effect, your chances for continued deep sleep are low to none. And as you will learn in TLC 6, deep sleep is the antiaging secret.

I realize that these facts may come as a surprise to those of you who really enjoy that glass of fine wine with dinner or popping open a cold one on a hot day. But eliminating alcohol is a Total Life Change you'll have to make to get the result you are looking for: a young, lean, and healthy body. If you have difficulty with this decision and continue drinking alcohol on a regular basis, I'll have to return to the advice in the introduction: close this book and put it back on the shelf. (But remember which shelf because sooner or later . . . you'll be back!)

Why Your Doctor May Not Have Told You About Alcohol

"Wait a minute! I trust my internist to give me the latest health advice. Why hasn't he given me all this information about the destructive side of alcohol?" Claire was caught off guard with these facts on the deleterious effects of alcohol on the body. It was difficult for her to realize that doctors are human too.

I explained to Claire that factors in the doctors' own lives seem to affect the kind of health advice they give their patients. I'll summarize the results of one

WANT GREAT SKIN? STOP DRINKING ALCOHOL!

Angelika Arseneau, a medical esthetician and leading expert on skin, said that she can tell if a client has been drinking alcohol from the blotchy or uneven skin tone. According to Angelika, "Alcohol expands your capillaries and creates a rosacea condition. It also promotes chronic acne with inflammation, redness, and pimples or papules. Alcohol dehydrates the skin's cells, and if the liver is subjected to continuous use of alcohol, it can no longer properly filter the toxins out of the blood. When the body is toxic, we immediately see the result in the skin."

When Angelika examines the skin of a drinker, she sees fine telangiectasis (dilation of a group of capillaries), which may occur in conjunction with persistent acne. Skin deterioration can be identified and corrected, but you must end even moderate alcohol consumption and use proper techniques to restore the health of the skin. Learn more in the chapter "Spa Secrets."

study, published in the December 17, 2000, issue of *Family Practice,* that involved about 500 Swiss physicians in general practice:

- Physicians who consumed three or more alcoholic drinks per day were 8.4 times as likely as those who drank less to "have a negative attitude" toward counseling against alcohol and smoking.

- Physicians who had a sedentary lifestyle were 3.4 times as likely as those who were active to resist recommending lifestyle interventions.

- Physicians who lacked national certification were 2.2 times as likely, and those who did not know their own blood pressure were 2.0 times as likely, to avoid the use of preventive health interventions.

In this study, researchers concluded that physicians' negative health behaviors could result in high-risk behaviors of patients and in the population as a whole. I believe this study means that we shouldn't count on all doctors for preventive health care involving lifestyle changes, especially if they engage in high-risk behavior (which you often have no way of knowing). It's your body, so take responsibility for your health. Seek information and answers that will keep it well—for the rest of your life.

More Serious Alcohol Concerns

ALCOHOL AND CANCER

The relationship between alcohol and cancer is just now becoming clear. Would it surprise you to know that in past studies researchers found higher rates of breast cancer among women who drank alcohol? For years cancer researchers have studied the effects of diet, exercise, family history, and alcohol on the body. Now, according to a comprehensive report on cancer and diet from the American Institute for Cancer Research, the findings suggest that the risk of breast cancer among women could increase 25 to 30 percent with only 1½ drinks a day. Women who have 6 drinks a day face *twice* the breast cancer risk of nondrinkers. Other studies reveal that 10 grams (⅓ ounce) of alcohol consumed daily increases the risk of breast cancer in women by 11 percent. (For a typical wine with 12 percent alcohol content, that's the amount of alcohol in only 3 ounces of wine.) Perhaps that glass of wine will taste different to you, knowing these facts.

For those women with a familial history of breast cancer, stopping alcohol is an excellent preventive measure. A 1998 study in the *Journal of the American Medical Association* revealed that when compared with nondrinkers, women who consumed 2 to 3 drinks per day and whose mothers had a history of breast cancer had a 50 percent higher risk of breast cancer mortality.

Increased risk in postmenopausal women. The studies on alcohol and breast cancer continue to disclose that this toxic drink changes the chemistry in the body. In a revealing study published in July 2001 in *Epidemiology,* scientists confirmed that postmenopausal women who drink more than ½ glass of alcohol per day and have low intakes of the B vitamin folic acid found in fresh fruits, vegetables, and lentils are at increased risk of breast cancer. In this study researchers found that these women were 60 percent more likely to develop breast cancer than those who did not drink alcohol and had the highest intake of folic acid. Because alcohol use has been linked to an increase in the risk for breast cancer, it is time to make

WHOLE FOODS HIGH IN FOLIC ACID

Lentils (cooked)
Chickpeas
Spinach (cooked)
Bananas
Black beans
Kidney beans
Oranges
Broccoli (raw)

the choice to eliminate it and protect yourself. Folic acid may play an important role in the body's capacity to repair the genetic damage that can lead to cancer. So stick with your Definition Diet, which contains many whole foods high in folic acid.

How alcohol leads to cancer. Get the facts now: alcohol is broken down in the body into a chemical called *acetaldehyde*, which has been shown to cause cancer and a host of other chronic and life-threatening ailments. While researchers contend that alcohol itself is not carcinogenic, we do know that it has tumor-promoting and carcinogenic properties. Scientists are unsure of the exact method by which alcohol leads to cancer. Some researchers believe that drinking alcohol reduces the intake and bioavailability of other dietary cancer-protective substances. In layman's terms, this means that when you drink, you often substitute alcohol for nutrient-dense foods high in antioxidants, phytochemicals, and flavonoids that protect against the toxins in alcohol. Or alcohol could in some way dilute the protective power of healthy foods. Other studies reveal an increased activation of "procarcinogens" (cancer-boosters), which are triggered by alcohol and a suppressed immune function. And some scientists hold fast to the theory that drinking alcohol causes direct local mucosal damage, which results in chronically increased cell division and thus an increased risk of cancer in the gastrointestinal system. Other theories include the following:

- Drinking alcohol decreases the level of folic acid in the body. Folic acid, among other B vitamins, protects against cancer.
- Alcohol leads to dehydration, which compromises the immune system.
- Drinking alcohol interferes with normal sleep and dream patterns, which also compromises immunity.

ALCOHOL AND BLOOD PRESSURE

Alcohol is a targeted culprit in boosting blood pressure, and if you've been diagnosed with hypertension (high blood pressure), stopping alcohol consumption is one proactive step that will save your heart. In women, hypertension increases the risk of heart attack and cardiovascular disease by 25 percent, and more than half of all women over age forty-five have it, including millions of women who have undiagnosed hypertension. Hypertension makes your heart work harder than normal, increasing the stress on your heart muscle and arteries, which leads to a thickening of the heart muscle, which in turn can cause irregular heartbeats (arrhythmias). High blood pressure can also lead to atherosclerosis (plaque buildup in the arteries), putting you at high risk for a heart attack or stroke.

In a study reported in *Hypertension*, researchers concluded that a reduction in alcohol intake among drinkers significantly reduced their blood pressure. They found that when alcohol consumption fell by 16 to 100 percent, there were significant drops in systolic blood pressure (the top number in a blood pressure reading). Diastolic blood pressure (the lower number) also dropped significantly in eight clinical trials. The greatest drop in blood pressure was seen among patients with the highest blood pressure before treatment and those who cut their alcohol consumption the most.

It makes you wonder why doctors recommend drinking alcohol to reduce the risk of heart attack, when it increases the risk of hypertension, a major factor in cardiovascular disease!

RED FLAG! HRT AND ALCOHOL DON'T MIX

If you are considering taking hormone replacement therapy (HRT) for menopausal symptoms, or if you are postmenopausal and already taking HRT, a study published in December 2000 in the *Journal of Family Practice* concluded that alcohol combined with estrogen replacement therapy synergistically enhances the risk of breast cancer. (Check out the natural alternatives to HRT in TLC 7.)

ALCOHOL AND INFERTILITY

If you're trying to get pregnant and still insist on a glass or two of wine each night to "relax," try replacing that alcohol with fresh water and you may be singing lullabies to baby soon. Alcohol is one proven risk factor for infertility that you can control. We know that for men, alcohol lowers sperm density, sperm motility, and the number of normal-appearing sperm. Low sperm count and poor motility are leading causes of male infertility. Some of these studies show that beer in particular may have a negative effect because the hops may alter hormones and lower the production of testosterone.

For women, alcohol is linked to irregular ovulation, increased chance of miscarriage, and a 50 percent reduction in fertility. Perhaps one of the most challenging study results came from the National University Hospital in Denmark, where researchers tested 430 couples ages twenty to thirty-five who were conceiving for the first time. They concluded that women who did not drink at all had the highest chance of conceiving in that menstrual cycle. (And, of course, once you get pregnant, continue to stay away from alcohol because it can increase your baby's chances of birth defects.)

You can wait for the warning labels to appear on alcoholic beverages, but don't hold your breath—remember how long the tobacco companies got away without labels? Or you can wait for even more studies to come out. My opinion? If you want to stay well and be lean, younger looking, and energetic, *do not drink alcohol.*

Physiology, Not Morality

Okay, before you decide that I'm a pious teetotaler, you need to know that I'm not coming from some moral high ground on the alcohol issue. I'm a fitness and health-care professional, and my advice is driven by physiology, not morality. I'm not a prude in a high-collared Victorian dress, and I will strongly recommend a pleasurable alternative to drinking alcohol: *have more sex.* Why not? Safe sex is almost always good for you, and I'm not being flippant. Orgasm increases your levels of growth hormone and other natural anabolic hormones that will keep you young and healthy. For men, increased sex helps to prevent prostate problems. And without alcohol in your system, there's a good chance you'll experience a noticeable increase in libido.

RED FLAG

Alcohol consumption can lower blood sugar levels to the point of hypoglycemia (low blood sugar), which causes symptoms like fatigue, disorientation, and dizziness (similar to being drunk). Alcohol can also cause blood glucose levels to rise, due to the carbohydrates in certain drinks, which can result in a deadly reaction.

THE FRENCH PARADOX

For those who hang on to the belief that wine has been proved to be beneficial for the heart and circulatory system, keep reading. The positive relationship between wine and cardiovascular health, often referred to as "the French paradox," *flies in the face of reason.* Let me explain. Researchers know how devastating alcohol is to human physiology, yet they find this curious positive relationship in certain populations, particularly French and other Mediterranean cultures. What's *really* happening in France, Italy, and other Mediterranean populations that associate daily wine-drinking with healthy hearts and longevity? Here's the skinny: it almost certainly has more to do with the abundance of antioxidants in fresh vegetables, the medicinal power of garlic, and the phytochemicals and phenols from the grape skins and grape oil.

You mean it's not the alcohol? Sorry! In fact, the healthy heart benefit in these countries could result from a cumulation of many factors:

- The grapes, which have a more powerful antioxidant than vitamins C, E, or beta-carotene
- The low-stress lifestyle

HORMONE HAVOC

Alcohol consumption by women (only two or more drinks a day) has been linked to an increased risk of menstrual problems and early menopause.

- Regular exercise, as villagers walk to market and jobs each day
- Strong social support—a compassionate network of family and friends close by

Each one of these factors has been scientifically substantiated to be good for your heart. While the French paradox is real, it is also misleading. There are a host of lifestyle habits that contribute to heart health, and to isolate wine-drinking as the reason for longevity is ludicrous.

Hello, are you there? It's the grapes. . . . Phenols in purple grape juice exert the same kind of protective effect as those in red wine. These compounds, found naturally in grape skins, have an anticoagulant effect. Like aspirin, warfarin (Coumadin), and other commonly prescribed anticoagulant drugs, they keep blood platelets from sticking together and forming the tiny clots that can be responsible for heart attacks and strokes. Some red wines contain salicylic acid, the active ingredient in aspirin.

Here's a 24-hour fact: the anticoagulant effect from grape phenols *lasts only 24 to 48 hours.* That's why the medical recommendation is for a "daily dose" of wine to get the promised result. But you don't need to drink toxic alcohol every day to get the good phenols. A glass of purple grape juice has the same benefit. In your Turnaround, I recommend eating fresh whole grapes, the way they were packaged by nature, with the skins still intact and all the phytochemicals unmolested by processing. If grapes aren't your thing, you can find similar phenols in fresh bilberries, blackberries, blueberries, garlic, and onions. (Does this suggest another reason for the French paradox?)

BONE ROBBER

Alcohol consumption is a risk factor for early fractures in women as well as men. Osteoporosis is found earlier in life in those who consume alcohol for a number of years; osteoporosis fractures can be found in people as young as thirty to forty.

ALCOHOL AND GERD

Regardless of the type and dose of beverage involved, according to a study published in December 2000 in the *American Journal of Gastroenterology,* alcohol facilitates the development of gastroesophageal reflux disease (GERD). Gastroesophageal reflux generally occurs at night when you are lying down. Normally a valve between the esophagus and the gastric system prevents stomach acids from backing up into the esophagus. In GERD, this valve does not work properly. The stomach acids reflux, or back up, into the esophagus, causing irritation and inflammation. Sometimes, if the acidic liquids are aspirated, the lungs can also become inflamed, and you can develop a certain type of pneumonia. Stopping alcohol consumption is one surefire remedy for ending GERD in some people.

Symptoms of GERD

Bad breath (halitosis) and a bitter taste in the mouth in the morning
Excessive, thick phlegm, particularly in the morning
Heartburn
Chronic throat clearing and tickle in the throat
Chronic irritating cough
Scratchy, sore throat, particularly in the morning
Chronic hoarseness
"A lump in the throat"
Excess mucus production
Prolonged vocal warm-up, with low or husky voice quality
Undependable voice—good one day and hoarse and tired the next
Vocal fatigue after short periods of singing or speaking
Trouble breathing or laryngospasm (closing off of the airway)
Regurgitation of food and liquids
Exacerbation of asthma, which is much more difficult to control when complicated
   by reflux

Mother Nature has provided us with a fruit that can keep us healthy—no toxins involved. Even in the popular diet books that praise the effects of red wine, you will always find a line, usually in fine print, that admits that the protective value of wine is merely speculative.

So why do the best-selling books say it's okay to drink alcohol if it's a proven body-buster? Probably because they want to be best-sellers. At this writing, when the evidence clearly states that alcohol is toxic, the question remains: Why is it still being recommended as a healthy alternative? In the United States, many guidelines and recommendations are influenced by what the authors think Americans are capable of doing and believing, and this includes government guidelines.

Using alcohol to cover up or resolve symptoms of diseases is like taking prescription drugs. There is always a consequence or side effect, and it usually involves adding another problem. Of course we need prescriptions when we are acutely or chronically ill with bacterial infections, degenerative diseases, or life-threatening ailments like cancer. But all these pharmaceuticals come with a written list of side effects. In other words, along with the healing effect, there will also be a negative effect. The good news is when you turn around your life and work to stay well and prevent illness, your new prescriptions of exercise, stress reduction, and the Definition Diet all have *no* negative side effects!

Grapes or Viagra? One of the more interesting phytochemicals in grape skin is resveratrol, which contributes to arterial health by scavenging free nitric oxide to prevent oxidative damage. Resveratrol relies on fermentation to move from the grape skins into the wine, so it is not present in most grape juices; you will need to eat grapes or take a resveratrol supplement. There is a company (Arkopharma of Wallingford, Connecticut) that sells a resveratrol supplement, called French Paradox, that is extracted from red wine.

Nitric oxide management is a key element of the physiological pathways that led to the invention of Viagra, first as a blood pressure drug and then as a sex aid. The link between dietary resveratrol and sexual performance has yet to be completely established (studies take years, even decades, to make conclusive statements). But what a shame that we mask this possible benefit of grape phytochemicals with the sexually debilitating effects of alcohol. I predict that someday when we know more about this benefit, your doctor's advice will be, "To increase sexual performance, try grapes for dessert."

EXPLODING THE FRENCH PARADOX

Alcohol is the basis of a huge global industry with a strong influence at all levels of the popular media, so the French paradox gets a lot of airplay. Perhaps the message you hear from the media—and your personal physician—should be more carefully worded and include all the facts. According to a study published in *The Lancet,* experts concede that much of the data upon which the French paradox is based should be studied further. For example, more investigation must be made into the control groups, who are nondrinkers. We need to know if these nondrinkers are really comparable in lifestyle to the drinkers in the study. Probably not, and here's why:

1. As we get older, there is a strong drift from heavy or moderate drinking toward nondrinking. Age is usually associated with declining health, so any research that does not allow for this will show a strong pro-alcohol bias.

2. Nondrinkers and heavy drinkers are often working-class men and women who are in relatively poor health compared with regular light drinkers. Regular light drinkers are usually from the healthiest and wealthiest demographic. Now here's the crux of the paradox: *regular light drinkers are part of the fittest group of people despite their alcohol consumption, not because of it.* This population has the best medical care, preventive medicine, and therapies, a more varied and nutritious diet, and fewer stressors than the nondrinkers or heavy drinkers. All of this must be studied carefully before we make the assumption that alcohol is the cure-all for what ails you.

Alcohol as a stress reducer? As you know, I am a big believer in stress reduction for an effective 24-Hour Turnaround. However, using alcohol as a stress reducer is a big mistake.

While drinking alcohol to relax is a common rationalization for addictive behavior, the result is temporary. On the one hand, alcohol may help someone reduce stress. But this generally results in a high-stress rebound when the numbing effect wears off. And as with most psychoactive substances, there can be a long-term adaptive response, requiring progressively higher doses to achieve the same result.

One glass may work the first week, but by week four, or with increased stress, you'll be downing two or three glasses of alcohol to gain the same benefit that you originally received with just one.

TURNAROUND FACT

For stress reduction, exercise and mind/body innercise (TLCs 2 and 8) work faster and longer than drinking alcohol.

FOR YOUR KIDS

Alcohol is gaining in popularity among young people in the United States. The PRIDE survey data, reported by teens in the United States, indicates a higher intoxication level than just a few years ago. Binge drinking is epidemic on college campuses, and parents may be shocked to learn that many teens as young as thirteen tell of drinking regularly.

If you have a daughter, read this: girls are less vulnerable and better able to make choices when they do not drink alcohol. In fact, alcohol is reportedly the most common drug in date-rape cases. Drinking can make a young woman less observant, less careful about how she gets home, and less able to defend herself in case of attack. Young women who drink are more likely to have early sexual experiences, to have sex with a greater number of partners, and to have unprotected sex—all deadly recreational practices.

Parents beware: alcohol abuse is at least or more prevalent in the athletic department as in other areas of student interest, if not more so. Hard to believe, but abusive use of alcohol by athletes often starts at the junior high level. The use of alcohol by athletes at the college level seems to be changing for the better; nonetheless, it is high enough for alcohol to have been named the most abused drug in collegiate sports by the NCAA and in professional and Olympic sports by the NFL and the NBA.

What do you tell your children? I believe we should let the facts speak for themselves. Give your child the facts about alcohol and its effects on health, weight gain, and performance. The effect of alcohol on sports performance is profound, and if our young athletes had counseling about the negative consequences, there might be a reversal in the numbers. Even with low to moderate use we see reduced grip strength, jump height, 200- and 400-meter run performance, and faster overall fatigue. Use of alcohol will result in decreased eye-hand coordination and a slower reaction time.

Realize that you are the best role model your kids have in life. Whether you consume just one glass or a bottle, it's all internalized by your child in the same way. I'll be frank in letting you know that our children have never seen my husband or me with a drink. Don't kid yourself. It does make a difference.

FOR YOUR HUSBAND

Many men, particularly those in the business world, find that eliminating the lunchtime cocktail and the "one to unwind" at night is a very effective way of losing weight. If your husband drinks—or if you drink—check out the following Tips for Drinkers to see how you can modify this destructive health habit.

Tips for Drinkers

I've already made it clear that if you're not willing to give up regular drinking, my office door will slam hard on your (paradoxically French) derriere on your way out. But here are some parting words of advice:

- Make sure you eat foods high in B vitamins like folic acid to give your body protection against the toxic chemical influence of alcohol.
- Favor younger wines—less than five years old. These may have some natural antioxidants still intact.
- Drink lots of water to help compensate for the dehydrating effects of alcohol and to speed up detoxification.

DEALING WITH DRINKING

Alcohol can easily become a serious problem, especially if you find yourself drinking more to get the same relaxed feeling you had previously. "It will never happen to me," "I don't have a problem," "I'll stop before it gets bad" are words spoken by people who are unable or unwilling to do anything about an alcohol problem that already exists. The self-deception commonly known as *denial* presents the major obstacle to recovery.

The truth is that anyone can get into trouble with alcohol. Some people are more at risk than others. For those who depend on alcohol to ease their inhibitions at a social engagement or to give them courage during tense moments or who find that they are drinking more frequently than ever before, the following quiz may help you recognize that there may be a problem and motivate you to seek solutions to stop drinking altogether.

ALCOHOL CONSUMPTION QUIZ

The following statements can help you to see if drinking is a problem in your life. Answer honestly, and then follow the Turnaround directive in the key. (On the quiz, a drink is 8 ounces of beer, 1 glass of wine, or 1 shot of whiskey or other liquor.)

Yes___ No___   1. I drink alcohol almost daily.

Yes___ No___   2. My drinking has increased in the past six months.

Yes___ No___   3. I sometimes need to drink in the morning, especially if I have a social engagement.

Yes___ No___   4. I frequently have more than six drinks on one occasion.

Yes___ No___   5. Sometimes I am unable to stop drinking until I black out (pass out).

Yes___ No___   6. I have sometimes forgotten to do what was expected of me because of my drinking.

Yes___ No___   7. The more I drink, the more I need to drink, and I feel it is out of my control.

Yes___ No___   8. Many times I cannot remember what I said after a binge-drinking episode.

Yes___ No___   9. My spouse or family members are concerned about my drinking.

Yes___ No___ 10. My need to drink alcohol stems from an intense craving, similar to craving a favorite food.

If you checked even one Yes on this quiz, you seriously need to consider seeking professional help. I'm not saying that you have a true drinking problem, but it is better to seek help before an alcohol problem progresses and robs you of quality of life. Talk to your personal physician, a licensed therapist, or call Alcoholics Anonymous (AA) for effective and inexpensive therapy. You can also check out websites on the Internet for the names and numbers of support groups in your area.

My Parting Shot (No Pun Intended)

Excess alcohol consumption kills more than 100,000 Americans each year. Let's review the facts. Alcohol:

- Decreases fat-burning for up to 48 hours
- Increases blood pressure and triglycerides
- Causes an imbalance in blood sugar levels, increasing the risk of diabetes
- Boosts the risk for osteoporosis, resulting in brittle bones and fractures
- Increases the risk of hemorrhagic stroke, pancreatitis, cirrhosis, and cancers of the liver, breast, mouth, esophagus, stomach, and possibly colon
- Adds calories with few nutrients
- Affects the absorption of many vitamins and minerals, notably folic acid and thiamine

When you consider all the health hazards associated with alcohol, and then realize that more than 16,000 people, including innocent children, are killed each year in alcohol-related accidents, it surely makes you rethink having that glass of wine with dinner, doesn't it?

"Is any consumption sufficiently moderate to protect us and others from the fruits of a dulled mind?"

—Gavin Harrison, my teacher and dear friend

TOTAL LIFE CHANGE 6

Sweet Dreams

I T ' S   C U R I O U S   H O W we never think about the importance of sleep—until we toss and turn all night long and awaken feeling exhausted the next morning. Laura was convinced that she needed little sleep. This thirty-seven-year-old artist always got a "second wind" late at night and bragged that she could get the most creative work done after midnight, when her family was asleep. The problem is that Laura also had to wake at 6 A.M. to get her kids up for school, and on most mornings she was irritable, exhausted, and felt as if she'd been "run over by a truck." As I explained to Laura, to ensure a good night's sleep, night owls should protect themselves by going to bed before that "second wind" comes blowing in.

One of the most common Turnaround stumbling blocks my clients have is getting proper sleep at night, especially in achieving deep level or stage 4 sleep. Not only does stage 4 sleep allow you to feel alert and energetic and be more productive, it is also vital for restoring your body—repairing tissues and skin, building bone and muscle, and strengthening immune function. I call it antiaging sleep.

What Gets the Blame?

While there are many reasons for poor sleep, here are some of the most common culprits.

THE LIGHT BULB

More than a century ago, Americans slept an average of 10 hours each night. But that was before Thomas Edison perfected his miracle: the incandescent light bulb. Since the invention of the light bulb in 1880, the number of hours Americans sleep has greatly declined. Today the average American sleeps 6½ hours. Not only can lack of sleep put undue stress on the body, releasing a torrent of stress hormones that interfere with the way blood sugar (glucose) is processed, but poor sleep affects our overall energy and makes us look older than we really are.

STRESS

Since the September 11 terrorist attacks, I've been inundated with calls from clients around the globe wanting help with sleep problems. One client, Sheila, a forty-two-year-old boutique owner in Paris, said she awoke every morning at 3 A.M. to check the world and national news and make sure another attack had not occurred. Not only was her anxiety level high for weeks, she was getting just a few hours of sleep each night and felt depressed and distracted. Another client, Judy, lives in Manhattan and continued to relive the terrorist attacks in her mind each night when she tried to sleep. This forty-nine-year-old real estate broker said the lack of sleep kept her from taking care of herself, and she gained 11 pounds over a three-week period from stress eating.

While 25 percent of Americans occasionally have insomnia, according to the National Library of Medicine, the September 11 terrorist attacks made this number skyrocket. In a recent survey from the National Sleep Foundation, a research institute in Washington, D.C., of the 993 American adults interviewed, 44 percent reported insomnia during the days immediately following the attacks. And women were more affected than men, no matter where they lived.

Whatever the crisis, chronic stress is guaranteed to ruin your sleep and make you look and feel old. Check out the list of side effects of poor sleep. If you experience more than one, take the steps recommended in this chapter to calm down, unwind, and prepare your body, mind, and spirit for healing sleep.

AGE

The older you are, the more problems you will have achieving restful and healing sleep if you don't take care of yourself. Declining sleep quality begins between the ages of twenty-five and forty-five, according to a study in the *Journal of the American Medical Association*. In this study, researchers at the University of Chicago evaluated sleep study data from 149 healthy men, ages sixteen to eighty-three, and found that sleep deteriorated at two points in their lives—between the ages of sixteen and twenty-five and again between the ages of thirty-five and fifty. Data from the University of Chicago study indicated that the time spent in deep sleep dropped from 20 percent in men under twenty-five to less than 5 percent in men over thirty-five. Researchers said that as deep sleep decreases, so does the secretion of human growth hormone (HGH), the antiaging hormone. By the time a person is thirty-five, HGH can decrease by as much as 75 percent. Quality sleep and exercise can decrease this number significantly! Studies have shown that HGH deficiency can lead to obesity, loss of muscle mass, and a reduced capacity to exercise. We want to do everything in our power to promote deep sleep and the production of HGH.

HORMONES

We are just beginning to collect data on deep sleep in women, who are trickier to study because of the effects of estrogen on their sleep patterns. For those women who find it difficult to sleep during the premenstrual period, you are not alone. Studies show that women have more awakenings, sleep disturbances, and vivid dreams during the premenstrual period than the rest of the month. Some women report feeling fatigued no matter how long they stay in bed. Menstrual symptoms such as bloating, headache, abdominal cramps, food cravings, irritability, and emotional changes all appear to contribute to the inability to get sound sleep. These problems generally disappear a few days after menstruation begins.

For women in perimenopause, or just prior to menopause, the declining levels of the hormone estradiol may increase your chance of poor sleep. In a study published in September 2001 in *Obstetrics and Gynecology,* researchers at the University of Pennsylvania Medical Center followed 436 women age thirty-five to forty-nine over a two-year period. About 17 percent of the women reported suffering from poor sleep throughout the entire study period. While researchers identified anxiety, depression, and caffeine consumption as factors that disturbed the women's sleep, they also considered low estradiol levels and hot flashes in older women aged forty-five to forty-nine as responsible for the sleepless nights, even though all women were experiencing regular menstrual cycles and had not yet entered menopause. The study concluded that the decline in estradiol that occurs with ovarian aging may, in fact, be associated with poor sleep in women. This sleep deprivation results in daytime fatigue and irritability and can even lead to feelings of depression. (It is hard to differentiate between poor sleep due to aging and poor sleep due to declining estradiol, as they happen at the same time. Or it could be the hot flashes themselves that trigger the loss of quality sleep.)

While many professionals recommend hormone replacement therapy to resolve sleep problems associated with the decline in hormones, I have found a safer way using a combination of exercise, diet, meditation, and alternative hormone care—all explained in TLC 7, on hormones. Whatever your female afflictions, the 24-Hour Turnaround will balance your hormones and provide you with the sleep your body needs.

SNOOZE YOU CAN USE

What happens if you try to relax and follow good bedtime hygiene yet still cannot achieve restful sleep? Talk with your doctor. If your doctor suspects that you may have a sleep disorder, you might be referred for a sleep study called a *polysomnography*. The sleep study will help determine if you have snoring, obstructive sleep apnea, restless legs syndrome, or some other problem. All these disorders require specific therapy that your doctor will prescribe.

YOUR MATTRESS, YOUR BED PARTNER, AND THE TICKING CLOCK

There are many reasons why we have disturbed sleep—from a mattress that is too hard or too soft, to the snoring of our bed partner, to the ticking of a bedroom clock or noises outside the bedroom window. No matter what awakens us and causes us to sleep fitfully, when the sleep cycle is disrupted, you won't wake up feeling well rested and energized.

In this chapter, we begin to understand why sleep is even more important as we age, to help balance hormones, keep our minds focused, fight disease, and prevent unnecessary aging. Some studies confirm that getting ample sleep at night may even help you lose weight!

Stages of Sleep

In adults, sleep is made up of distinct types or stages with specific characteristics defined by brain waves, eye movements, and muscle tension. The two broad categories of sleep include rapid eye movement (REM) sleep and non–rapid eye movement (NREM) sleep.

REM AND NREM SLEEP

During REM sleep you experience small, variable-speed brain waves, rapid eye movements like those of eyes-open wakefulness, and no muscle tension. We have almost all our dreams during REM sleep. REM sleep is associated with psycholog-

WHAT'S DISTURBING YOUR SLEEP?

Check the following problems that apply to you, and talk with your doctor if you feel that a serious sleep disorder might need further investigation.

___ Difficulty in getting to sleep

___ Many arousals during a night's sleep

___ Noise

___ Sleeping partner disturbs your sleep

___ Light in the room

___ Bruxism (grinding teeth)

___ Long awakenings (10 minutes or longer) during sleep

___ Restless legs or arms (jerks or movement) during sleep

___ Nightmares

___ Gasping, choking, or pauses in breathing during sleep

___ A feeling of creeping sensations in legs while lying down

___ Hot flashes

___ Difficulty in breathing

___ Tossing, turning, or an inability to relax

___ Awaken feeling exhausted and foggy

ical well-being and feeling refreshed upon awakening, and young adults spend about 25 percent of their sleep time in REM. By age sixty, REM sleep can be as low as 15 to 20 percent of sleep time. If you are deprived of REM sleep, you might complain of irritability and moodiness.

NREM sleep is composed of four different levels or stages—1, 2, 3, 4—and characterized by different combinations of brain waves, eye movements, and reduced but not absent muscle tension. Stages 3 and 4 are important as they are defined by relatively large, slow brain waves (called delta waves), absent eye movements, and reduced muscle tension. Stage 3 sleep is characterized by extremely slow (delta) brain waves interspersed with very quick brain waves; stage 4 sleep is made up entirely of delta brain waves. Recent studies have shown that delta sleep appears to be the most important for physical recovery.

DELTA SLEEP

Delta sleep, which occurs *mostly* in the first third of the night and makes up about 10 to 20 percent of total nighttime sleep in normal young adults, is affected by age, amount of prior sleep, various diseases, and physical or emotional trauma. Not surprisingly, young children have large amounts of delta sleep. During delta sleep, HGH is most abundant, so the rate of tissue repair and cellular growth is at its highest. If sleep disturbances occur during these stages, you will wake up feeling tired and may complain of muscular aches and pains.

SWEET DREAMS

Although it's possible to dream in any of the four NREM sleep stages, we dream mostly in REM sleep, which takes place mostly during the last third of your night's sleep and normally comprises 35 percent of the sleep period. During the dream sleep state, hormones from the brain stem effectively paralyze the entire

---

THE FIVE TYPES OF SLEEP

Stage 1—light sleep
Stage 2—moderate sleep
Stages 3 and 4—deep or delta sleep
REM (rapid eye movement) sleep or dream stage

---

skeletal muscle system, presumably to prevent us from hurting ourselves by acting out our dreams as we sleep. Eye muscles are the exceptions; the eyeballs move about just as if we were awake and active.

Theories vary about just what our brain is really doing during dreams. Because sleep deprivation impairs long-term memory, we tend to believe that the most likely role of dream sleep in adults is to reinforce the neural connections between brain cells that are necessary to make memories stick. Or, because we now know that new brain cells are always being made even in the adult brain, perhaps the brain growth function is really the same as in infants. Infants sleep 16 hours a day, 50 percent of them in REM. The stimulation during REM sleep is crucial to the growing and developing infant brain and to the development of new cells in the adult brain. All in favor of new brain cells should go to bed earlier.

Understanding Sleep

We spend almost one-third of our life in the restorative process of sleep. We know it can keep us well and let us live a long life. We also know that without ample sleep we are subject to fatigue, depression, forgetfulness, weight gain, illness, and probably a decrease in life span. But what is sleep, really?

While sleep is thought to be a period of rest and inactivity, it is hardly a "shutting down" of our bodies. Restful state? No way! When we sleep, many biological processes go into high gear, helping to revitalize the body, repair tissue and organs, and boost our memory storage. Even the nondreaming brain uses more sugar and oxygen during sleep than when we are awake. To see how alert the brain is during sleep, scientists have used a positron emission tomography (PET) scanner to scan the brains of people while they were sleeping. They found that the same areas that are involved in learning new tasks when we are awake are still rapidly processing information when we are asleep.

During sleep, your muscles relax, and sensual perceptions are disengaged from the brain (although hearing remains active above a certain threshold). Different hormones interact with the brain, placing a kind of screen between your brain and your consciousness.

SLEEP-WAKE CYCLE

Studies have demonstrated that we have a built-in cycle of sleep-wake times, which is actually 25 hours long. Since the cycle is longer than the 24-hour day, some factor must serve to synchronize the body's pacemaker with the external clock time. The most important and powerful cue is light.

Upon awakening at the dawn's early light, you continually feel more alert until about 1 or 2 P.M., when you begin to have a lull or sag in wakefulness. Although you may think this dip in alertness is due to that oversize bagel you ate for lunch, it's not so. The lull is a natural consequence of your circadian rhythm. Later in the afternoon your alertness improves again until late evening, when you start to experience a wave of sleepiness. With your Turnaround bedtime ritual, you will fall asleep until the next morning, when the cycle starts again.

ACTIVATING BRAIN HORMONES

For those who wonder why they are so exhausted the next day after missing just a few hours of sleep, a study published in the June 2001 issue of *Military Medicine* may give the answer, and it all points to melatonin. Melatonin, which is secreted by the pineal gland in the brain, is the hormone most closely linked to your circadian system.

Melatonin has been referred to as the hormone of darkness, as its secretion is activated almost immediately after exposure to darkness. Melatonin also accounts for almost half the body's temperature rhythm, signaling other glands that control the nighttime temperature drop required for sleep. In this study, researchers found that even one night of sleep deprivation causes an almost immediate rise in sleep-inducing hormones, which results in significant stress about 1:30 P.M. the next day, when you try to fight the forces of sleepiness. In the study, cortisol, the body's main stress hormone, rises as your body fights an overwhelming sense of fatigue. And just as with chronic stress, cortisol ages your body, inhibits the white blood cells (lymphocytes), and compromises your immune system. Other chemicals produced by the brain's autopilot—known as the autonomic nervous system—can similarly damage the cells that make up the immune system.

About forty years ago, pharmacological studies suggested that the hormone serotonin, a neurotransmitter in the brain associated with a calming, anxiety-reducing reaction, might have a role in sleep induction. Later on, experiments in animals showed that destruction of the parts of the brain that housed serotonin-containing nerve cells could produce total insomnia. Partial damage to these areas of the brain caused variable decreases in sleep. The percentage of destruction of these particular nerve cells correlated with the amount of slow-wave sleep.

It turns out that a nutrient, an amino acid called tryptophan, is a precursor in the synthesis of serotonin in the brain. Tryptophan is present in a variety of foods. Milk, a centuries-old remedy for curing insomnia, is one of them. When the body is deprived of REM sleep, the brain stem attempts to compensate with more serotonin. Serotonin depletion is thought to underlie the enormous increase in depression attributed to insufficient sleep.

PREVENTING JET LAG

On trips of only a few days, I have found that keeping my schedule as close as possible to Hawaii Time (my home time zone) keeps me on track. On longer trips I try to adapt to the new schedule the very first day. Travelers who get a lot of outdoor light adapt twice as fast as those who do not. If the new time zone requires earlier rising, exposure to bright light first thing in the morning will shift your internal clock to an earlier setting. Several studies have confirmed that melatonin helps with jet lag. Melatonin taken in late afternoon or early evening advances the circadian rhythm, convincing the body that night has fallen earlier.

SUPPLEMENTAL MELATONIN

Melatonin supplements are available over-the-counter in drug, grocery, and natural food stores and are used by many as sleep aids. Even though the supplement is not regulated by the FDA, it has been recommended by many researchers as a way to counter the effects of jet lag. In some research studies, scientists report that melatonin taken an hour before bedtime induces sleep more quickly and that sleep continues longer than with a placebo. Melatonin is said to be nontoxic, but use some caution when taking it. If you take it at the wrong time, such as during the day, it could make you sleepy when you need to be alert and awake.

Melatonin manufacturers recommend starting with a low dose (1 milligram) until you see how your body will react. Some people find that melatonin helps them get sounder sleep, while others report disturbed sleep, vivid nightmares, and an inability to think clearly the next day. Those side effects typically come when you take too high a dose.

The use of supplemental melatonin has been shown to raise brain serotonin levels. Melatonin is also responsible for helping us adapt to the day-and-night rhythms of our body, telling the body that night has arrived and the mental and physical restorative processes will begin.

NATURAL MELATONIN BOOSTERS

The production of melatonin increases with calorie reduction. Exercise also increases melatonin production, as long as you don't exercise late in the evening, which can boost alertness. More important, make sure the exercise is not intense. The more intense the exercise, the more you deplete your natural hormone production. Wearing your heart-rate monitor will keep you in your zone, protect your hormones, including melatonin, and encourage sleep.

Late to Bed and Early to Rise Makes You . . . Dysfunctional

"I sleep well on the weekends, averaging about eight hours each night. But on weeknights, forget it! I toss and turn while my mind is on red alert thinking of all the business decisions I must make. After a few hours of sleep, I awaken the next morning feeling achy, exhausted, and almost depressed, and then I have to get dressed, meet clients for breakfast, and be sharp. Not only am I sleep-deprived, but on the nights I can't sleep I crave junk food and I'm unable to deal effectively with stress."

Forty-six-year-old Liz, a CPA, poured her heart out about her problems in maintaining restful sleep. She said that during tax season, she gains about 15 pounds because of poor sleep and other bad habits—a more sedentary lifestyle and increased consumption of high-fat foods. As we talked about why Liz was having sleep difficulties, she mentioned that worries about her business kept her from relaxing, and even the slightest noise or smallest flicker of light at night disturbed her sleep quality.

Liz is not alone. Many of us claim to have poor sleep, especially when life's stressors interrupt our daily routine. But disturbed and poor-quality sleep can have very serious health implications, especially as we age, because sleep predicts our susceptibility to disease and correlates with life expectancy.

FIVE SERIOUS SLEEP ALERTS

As you read this chapter, keep in mind that adequate sleep is *not* negotiable in the 24-Hour Turnaround. Getting at least 8 hours of sleep each night is as important to your program as your H.E.A.R.T. workout, the Definition Diet, the 2-minute meditation, and drinking 10 or more glasses of water each day. If you have to wake up using an alarm clock each day, then you should take to heart all the latest studies that I will share, along with sleep strategies to help you relax and easily drift off into a deep sleep. But before I get into what you can do to guarantee sweet dreams, let's look at some serious problems associated with sleep deprivation.

1. Lack of sleep increases the chance of accidents. More than just making you tired and crabby, sleep deprivation has some dangerous physiological consequences (high blood pressure or heart complications) and psychological consequences that can result in serious—even deadly—accidents. For instance, both the Chernobyl and Three Mile Island nuclear disasters occurred in the early morning hours, when the body wants and needs sleep. And while most people think that a captain's drunkenness caused the *Exxon Valdez* oil spill, the National Commission on Sleep Disorders says otherwise. The real problem was the severe fatigue of the ship's third mate, who was in charge at the time of the accident.

Activities that involve total concentration, such as driving a car, are much riskier because of the tendency for a sleep-deprived person's attention to wander without diversion or constant stimulation. It's interesting that the National Commission on Sleep Disorders concluded that drunk driving causes fewer fatalities than sleepiness! In fact, the foundation estimates that 100,000 traffic accidents and 1,500 fatalities occur each year due to driver fatigue. Studies reveal that the day following the switch to daylight savings time, when an hour of sleep is lost, traffic accidents increase by 7 percent. When we later gain the hour back going off day-light savings, we see the opposite—a 7 percent decrease.

2. Lack of sleep affects your mood and motivation. I'm sure you've felt the irritability that goes hand in hand with lack of sleep. I have a family member who can go from Jekyll to Hyde after missing only a few hours of sleep. Some research reveals that sleep deprivation degrades your mood even more than it reduces your ability to function, meaning that you may get through the day, but you won't have many friends. This impact on mood is not limited to chronic or long-term lack of sleep. Missing an adequate amount of sleep tonight can make you more sensitive to criticism, more volatile, and even more depressed-feeling tomorrow.

3. Lack of sleep results in decreased immune function. Sleep plays a big role in regulating your immune system, and a weakened immune system leaves you vulnerable to illness. You've probably caught a cold or gastrointestinal virus the day after a late night out. That's because your immune system was in a weakened state from missing quality sleep, making your body easy prey for a virus.

From a host of scientific studies, we know that exposure to viruses and bacteria does not result in health problems if your immune system is strong. Yet when faced with sleep deprivation, the immune system cannot work at full capacity. When your immune system malfunctions, it yields to autoimmune diseases such as some types of arthritis, allergy, or asthma. If your immune system is depleted, your body can be overwhelmed by bacteria, viruses, or toxicity, which can result in cancer or other life-threatening diseases.

4. Lack of sleep makes you old before your time. Even more compelling data come from research involving sleep, disease, and longevity. In one study, rats died of massive bacterial infections after being deprived of sleep for sixteen days. Bacteria appeared in the lymph nodes of the rats as early as four or five days.

In another study, the rats were allowed to sleep but not allowed "dream sleep," or the REM sleep usually associated with dreaming. These dream-deprived rats died of bacterial infection after forty days. What's interesting here is that they did not become dysfunctional due to sleep-deprived rat psychosis, but they died of infections.

Enough about rats, let's talk about the humans! Scientists know that sleep is possibly one of the most important predictors of longevity. Some researchers even suggest that it is more important in predicting how long you live than well-known risk factors like smoking, high blood pressure, and high cholesterol levels. After conducting a major six-year study that involved more than a million people, researchers at the American Cancer Society concluded that sleep time had the greatest correlation with longevity. The data are quite revealing:

- People who slept the *fewest hours* had the *greatest risk* of dying prematurely.
- People who averaged *4 hours* of sleep or less had the *highest death rate.*
- Those who averaged *8 hours* had the *greatest longevity.*

The short sleepers in this study were reported to have the highest rates not only of cancer but also of fatal coronary heart disease and stroke. A good reason to move the TV out of the bedroom!

5. Lack of sleep can affect production of human growth hormone. Human growth hormone (HGH), secreted by the pituitary gland of the brain, is one of several endocrine hormones, like estrogen, progesterone, testosterone, and DHEA, that decline in production as we age. Located at the base of the brain, the pituitary is the master gland that regulates the entire hormonal system. A microscopic protein substance, HGH is secreted in short pulses during deep sleep and after exercise. The decline of HGH with age is directly associated with cardiovascular disease, increased body fat, osteoporosis, gray hair, wrinkles, decreased energy, reduced sexual function, and other symptoms. Many of these symptoms have been found in younger adults who have HGH deficiencies. Increasing deep sleep to promote an increase in HGH can prevent or even reverse many of these conditions.

SIGNS OF SLEEP DEPRIVATION

Many of my clients have more on their plates than even a superhuman could handle. They have taken on new responsibilities and commitments in their complex lives and actually deducted time from their amount of sleep to get it all done. But most of my clients have no idea how tired they really are until they take a vacation at the spa and begin to experience true feelings of rest and relaxation.

I explain to them that long-term sleep deficit compromises their immune systems, makes them accident prone, and quickly accelerates aging. Fatigue is actually an extreme symptom. That's why it's important to recognize the more subtle signals that you need more and better sleep before you feel all-out exhaustion. Read the following list and check the ones that apply to you.

___ The children are twice as annoying after 3 P.M.

___ You cannot function without your morning coffee, followed by another cup after 10 A.M. to make it to lunchtime.

___ You fall asleep at meetings, in movie theaters, or while enjoying a symphony orchestra.

___ You fall asleep when you are a passenger in the car.

___ You sometimes become overwhelmed with drowsiness when you are driving.

___ You cannot wake up without an alarm clock.

___ When the alarm goes off, you stop it and drift back to sleep.

___ When you sit down to watch television with the family after dinner, you fall asleep on the couch.

___ You have trouble concentrating.

___ You always seem to have a cold, sore throat, or some type of virus.

___ Your skin looks sallow and pasty.

___ Your eyes are dull and listless.

___ You look older than your age.

___ You're putting on weight despite a proper diet and quality exercise.

If you checked three or more of these signs, it's time to take a very serious look at your sleep schedule.

The 24-Hour Turnaround

As I explain to all my female clients over forty: it's not enough just to get sleep. You have to get enough of the *right kind* of sleep. That means *deep sleep,* which supports HGH release as well as the repair and regeneration of body tissue and immune cells. So let's look at some ways to enhance deep sleep and also boost HGH starting tonight.

EXERCISE

Exercise is one of the best antidotes for fatigue and has been proved to be the fastest way to improve sleep. At the spa, we see that clients who exercise regularly rarely have difficulty getting to or maintaining deep sleep, and they're also more energetic during the daytime hours.

The type of exercise you do can boost your energy and help you sleep better or take away all your energy and disrupt your sleep patterns. Exercising in Zone One of your H.E.A.R.T. workout increases your total hours and quality of sleep. The simultaneous performance of specific-intensity aerobic exercise and resistance training sends a strong signal to the body's tissues to be metabolically active and stimulate the production of HGH.

Try to avoid exercising within 2 hours of bedtime; some people find it difficult to unwind after exercise. Also watch out for signs of "overtraining," which can affect both your body and your mind. With overtraining, you will feel tired all the time yet have difficulty getting to sleep or maintaining deep sleep.

EAT RIGHT

It sounds simple enough, doesn't it? But eating to improve sleep isn't easy, especially for those who work late and eat heavy meals after 7 P.M. Heavy, fat-laden dinners make you drowsy, but they won't help you sleep through the night. Heavy and/or spicy meals stimulate prolonged digestive action, which can keep you awake. Eating gas-forming foods or eating too fast can also interfere with sound sleep.

- *Follow the Definition Diet.* The Definition Diet, outlined in TLC 3, combines the right balance of carbs, protein, and good fats to give your body a hormone-friendly environment. When your hormones are balanced, you will experience fewer symptoms (including sleeplessness) from premenstrual syndrome, perimenopause, and even menopause.

- *Do a meal Turnaround.* Stay with the 3/500 Rule you learned about in TLC 3. Focus on keeping your evening meal the same size as your breakfast and lunch rather than having a large, 1,000-calorie dinner. Your pituitary gland secretes less HGH if you eat a large meal right before bedtime or if you have a processed carbohydrate snack, such as cookies or cake, or drink alcohol, late at night.

- *Change bad dietary habits.* Several dietary habits—including consumption of coffee, a heavy and/or spicy evening meal, and even quick-weight-loss dieting—could keep you tossing and turning. Try reducing the caffeine in your diet if you suffer from insomnia. My clients have had immediate results by cutting back to no more than 2 cups a day and using 1 P.M. as their coffee "last call."

- *Avoid additives.* Foods seasoned with monosodium glutamate (MSG), a taste enhancer often added to Chinese food, are notorious for causing sleep disturbances. Other food additives, such as aspartame, can have similar effects, causing vivid dreams and restless sleep. In fact, the higher the amount of additive, the greater the likelihood of a sleep reaction, especially in allergic or sensitive people.

- *Watch your snacks.* Eat less sugar, which can cause sudden rises in blood sugar. This may then cause you to wake up in the middle of the night when your blood sugar drops below normal. Also, avoid salty foods. Following a reduced-sodium diet helps some insomniacs sleep more soundly.

- *Add supplemental vitamins.* Elevated requirements for several of the B vitamins have been linked directly to sleepless nights. Your Definition Diet supplies adequate amounts of Bs in the whole grains that you eat. Other nutrients are indirectly linked to sleep-and-wake patterns. For example,

HIDDEN ADDITIVES CAN DISTURB SLEEP

Many processed foods contain monosodium glutamate (MSG) and aspartame—both additives that are associated with interrupted sleep. While eliminating these additives is difficult, you should be aware of processed foods that contain them, even though they may be listed under other names:

- Autolyzed yeast
- Calcium caseinate
- Gelatin
- Glutamate
- Glutamic acid
- Hydrolyzed protein
- Monopotassium glutamate
- Monosodium glutamate
- Sodium caseinate
- Textured protein
- Yeast extract
- Yeast food
- Yeast nutrient

calcium and magnesium work as a team to relax and contract muscles and to stimulate and subdue the nerves. Deficiencies of either mineral can cause muscle cramping and abnormal nerve function that theoretically might affect sleep. You will find these minerals in a good multiple vitamin. Check my website.

- *Eat foods to raise levels of tryptophan.* You can self-regulate your natural tryptophan level by eating a small whole-carbohydrate, low-protein snack 1 or 2 hours before bedtime. (Please, nothing sweet!) A carbohydrate snack such as a sprouted-wheat bagel raises brain levels of tryptophan, which in turn increases brain levels of serotonin. Consequently, pain tolerance

EAT TO SLEEP

1. Avoid beverages, foods, and medications that contain caffeine.
2. Split your calories evenly between breakfast, lunch, and dinner to avoid overeating at dinnertime. Be sure to keep protein servings small at the evening meal.
3. Avoid spicy foods at dinner if they affect your sleep.
4. Check all labels for MSG-containing foods and avoid them. At Chinese restaurants, ask your server for "no MSG, please."
5. Eat slowly and chew your food thoroughly.
6. Follow the Definition Diet. Overeating protein puts a huge added demand on your body that interferes with sleep.
7. Consume a small complex-carbohydrate-rich, low-protein snack 1 or 2 hours before bedtime.
8. Try a cup of warm milk at bedtime.
9. Skip the alcohol and other stimulants.

improves, insomnia is reduced, and mild depression is often alleviated. Keep the snack small, since large meals or volumes of liquid just before bed can disturb sleep.

SKIP ALCOHOL

We have already agreed to skip the alcohol today to be better fat-burners; now we will be better sleepers as well. A nightcap may make you sleepy at first, but you'll sleep less soundly and wake up more tired as a result. Alcohol and other depressants suppress REM sleep, the time when most dreaming occurs. Less REM sleep is associated with more night awakenings and a more restless sleep.

DESTRESS

By controlling the source of your stress, you can improve or completely eliminate your sleep problems. Ironically, sleep deprivation increases stress and also interferes with your ability to solve problems, thus speeding a downward spiral unless you can intercede to stop the process. Read TLC 8 for easy ways to identify life's stressors and mind-body exercises that work in easing their impact on your life—and sleep.

If you wake up and can't get back to sleep, don't lie in bed tossing and turning. It will only frustrate you and make it even more difficult to get to sleep. Get out of bed and go into another room. Do something monotonous, such as reading a boring book, knitting, folding clothes, or listening to soft music. Avoid watching television because it may increase alertness if the program is stimulating. Stay up until you are sleepy again, and then go back to bed.

A major difference between good sleepers and poor sleepers is not what they do at bedtime, but *what they do all day.* Good sleepers are more likely to be physically active. The physical activity helps them cope with daily stress and tires the body so it is ready to sleep at night.

SIX SIMPLE STRATEGIES TO CHANGE SLEEP HABITS

I'll have to admit that my clients who live in New York seem to have the hardest time getting enough sleep. Not only do they work long hours in the corporate world, but evening activities keep them up well after 10 P.M., which is the bedtime I recommend.

But no matter where you live or what your career, it's important to start somewhere to adjust your habits to increase healthy and healing sleep. Eliminate a late night dinner (and the calories) twice a week. Get together with those clients or friends for lunch or at the club or gym on the weekend. In a perfect world, your sleep routine would include the following:

1. Perform a relaxing ritual or routine before you get into bed. Leave your worries and the stress of the day through a breathing, prayer, or meditation practice. Some of my clients find that yoga before bedtime is very helpful in preparing their bodies and minds for sleep.

2. Avoid using the bedroom for anything but sleep and sex. Keep the TV in another room since it stimulates the brain and arouses the nervous system. Make family decisions and argue, if necessary, in a common family area, and avoid any major decision before bedtime.

3. Try to be in bed and on the way to sleep by 10 P.M. as many nights as possible. Start tonight.

4. Keep the bedroom temperature around 67°F (19°C) to naturally lower your body temperature and slow your metabolism, both necessary to achieve a dormant physical state.

5. Make sure your bedroom is protected against sound. Wear earplugs, if you are bothered by noises while sleeping. Some people find that it helps to hear white noise from a machine that produces a humming sound or by turning the radio to a station that has gone off the air.

6. Keep a regular waking time—even on weekends—helping to strengthen circadian cycling. Make sure you get some early morning light when you first awaken to help set your body clock and keep the melatonin production normal.

KEEP A SLEEP JOURNAL

If your journal does not have a section to record sleep patterns, you can copy the one on page 19. I want you to record the number of hours you sleep each night, as well as how well you slept. Did you toss and turn? Were you in a light sleep, or did you sleep soundly? Keeping a journal will enable you to see patterns that can correlate your sleep with your activity level, eating habits, amount of daily stress, and other pertinent factors.

While many of us might have objections to the structure and organization required to keep a daily journal, including logging every hour of sleep, keep in mind that the real purpose of it is to make it easy for us to recognize our individual differences. The journal is not a conforming influence, it's a tool to discover your individuality and to help you figure out how to fine-tune the tools you have available to make them work more effectively for you. A detailed journal will help you discover and correct the real factors that might be contributing to your poor sleeping habits.

A WARM BATH WILL INCREASE DROWSINESS

A warm bath or soak in a hot tub or Jacuzzi will make you drowsy by drawing blood away from the brain and toward the skin's surfaces. The warm soak also relaxes tense muscles, reduces pain, and allows for easier movement when you exercise the next day. After a leisurely warm bath at night, sleep can easily follow the cooling phase of your body's temperature cycle. Be sure to keep the temperature in your bedroom cool to see if you can influence this phase. Some studies show that warm, moist heat may raise levels of endorphins and decrease levels of stress hormones. I can personally confirm this, because my husband has problems sleeping, especially after working on a big project. A hot bath with ten drops of lavender essential oil puts him out for the night.

According to research published in the *Journal of Geriatric Psychiatry and Neurology,* a warm bath (about 100°F or 38°C) can induce drowsiness even in people suffering from insomnia. Filter your tub water so you are not breathing or soaking in chlorine (see TLC 4).

WHAT ABOUT DARK UNDER-EYE CIRCLES?

There are many triggers of dark under-eye circles, from alcohol consumption to smoking. If you have allergies, chances are that you live with permanent under-eye circles called *allergic shiners.* With an improvement in allergies, the under-eye circles disappear. And sometimes no matter how long you sleep, your genes are to blame for the tendency to have dark circles. (Just look around your family dining room table to see the strong family resemblance.)

If you have under-eye circles, make a point to get at least 8 hours of sleep each night to see if this condition might improve. Also watch what you eat, sticking to the Definition Diet and drinking at least 10 glasses of water each day. According to Asian facial diagnosis, dark circles under the eyes may be related to a weakness in the kidneys. Because many of the herbs prescribed for the kidneys can have a

YOGA OCEAN BREATH

The yoga ocean breath practice can help relax your body and mind and prepare you for a peaceful night's sleep. Follow these easy steps:

1. Sit in a chair or on the floor with your spine straight. Lift your right palm in front of your mouth and imagine that it's a mirror. Inhale through your nose, and then exhale through your mouth, making a *haaa* sound to fog the imaginary mirror. Next, inhale through your nose and, closing your mouth as you exhale, imagine that you are fogging a mirror in the back of your throat with the same *haaa* sound.

2. Place your hand in your lap or at your side, and repeat the inhalation and the *haaa* exhalation with your mouth closed. Notice the slight constriction in the back of your throat. Allow yourself to become absorbed in the sound you're making.

3. Keeping your mouth closed, lengthen your exhalation. Inhale for 4 counts; exhale for 5 to 8 counts.

4. Imagine the ebb and flow of ocean waves washing away your tension. Practice with your eyes closed for 20 slow breaths. Be patient; this technique takes practice. Soon it will feel natural and you can increase your practice time.

diuretic effect, you should see an herbalist for the proper dosage. Talk to your doctor if you have a family history of allergies or are concerned that the circles may stem from a health problem.

MORE SERIOUS SLEEP PROBLEMS WITH AGING

Snoring is one common sleep disturbance that affects more than forty million people. While more than 60 percent of all men age thirty-five to sixty-five snore, women are not immune from this nocturnal singing. In fact, more than 40 percent of all women age thirty-five to sixty-five snore. This is a number that soars dramatically at menopause as levels of estrogen decline.

This low-frequency noise occurs as a result of airflow limitation and the associated vibration of the soft tissues in the back of the throat. While snoring is annoying and causes poor sleep, it can also be a symptom of a very serious medical condition and sleep interrupter called obstructive sleep apnea (OSA).

OSA involves severe narrowing or occlusion of the airway with cessation of airflow. With OSA, your lungs do not get enough fresh air, so the brain wakes you up just enough to catch your breath and unlock the air passage. OSA can lead to severe cardiac and pulmonary problems, even death.

While OSA needs professional attention, both snoring and OSA can usually be resolved with weight loss. Talk to your doctor about your condition and see if the Definition Diet, H.E.A.R.T. workout, and other Total Life Changes may help to resolve these conditions.

FOR THE KIDS

How would you rate your family's sleep score? Are the kids falling asleep in the classroom and searching for chocolate or colas at three or four in the afternoon? Have their grades dropped for no apparent reason, while the television and computer are both on until midnight? Are your kids catching colds more often than usual, feeling irritable, having difficulty making friends?

I think this chapter should be mandatory reading for anyone over the age of twelve. Hopefully, you can still influence the younger children's bedtime. But as a mother of three, I know that by the age of twelve, homework gets more time-consuming and after-school activities take up a bigger chunk of the day, moving the bedtime later and creating chaos in the most stable families.

Ten years ago, when my boys were in their teens, much of the most important sleep research was new, and I'll confess that I did not place as much emphasis on sleep as I do now. On a typical evening, my boys would have a large dinner, talk on the phone, hang out, and do anything but homework. From nine to ten each evening, they looked as if they could pass out from exhaustion, but at ten they got a sudden burst of energy that allowed them to do another hour or two of homework, and sometimes hit the fridge just one last time.

The problem with getting into this new cycle of energy is that it almost becomes addicting, and it becomes virtually impossible for teens to switch back into a normal bedtime pattern. Teens need proper sleep to secrete the HGH desperately needed for their growing bodies, and moms and dads must take charge at home.

Encourage your children and teens to complete most of their homework before dinner or immediately after you eat. Set a time for them to be in their rooms preparing for bed, and work toward meeting this goal. Then, as a family, set a time for "lights out," so everyone gets in bed (training the body to prepare for sleep) and awakens fresh and in a great mood the next day. I recommend that preschoolers be tucked in by 7 P.M., elementary age children by 8 P.M., and teenagers no later than 10 P.M. Of course, your children may need an earlier bedtime, depending on their personal sleep requirements. These bedtimes sound early, don't they? We have become a society of night owls. At the same time we are a society with high rates of disease, depression, obesity, and premature aging.

FOR YOUR HUSBAND

Some sleep experts contend that sleep deprivation may affect men's hormones, possibly causing a deficiency in HGH. This loss of HGH, called *somatopause,* may need treatment, but the studies so far are few and inconclusive. I believe we should take active steps before we start losing HGH, and one step is to get more sleep. This goes for women, men, and kids. Ask yourself the following questions, and then find workable solutions to help your husband feel great.

- *Is he falling asleep during meetings and reviving himself with coffee, caffeinated colas, or candy bars from the vending machine?* Give him some power-packed options that will keep his eyes open and his mind alert. Pack his briefcase with Zip-Lock Snacks (see the recipe chapter), which include foods such as dried fruits, nuts, and whole-wheat pretzels, that help increase alertness but don't cause great increases or drops in blood sugar levels. Also, encourage him to forgo the coffee and drink bottled water.

- *Does he have trouble sleeping at night?* Explain to him the benefits of having a larger lunch and a lighter dinner, and do a menu turnaround. The lighter dinner meal will be easier to digest and help him feel drowsy and sleep soundly. Be sure he has a light snack high in carbohydrates before bedtime to help boost serotonin levels, and ask him to make the "no alcohol" commitment with you.

- *Is he unable to get out of the office for lunch?* Pack him several minimeals to keep at his office. (Pack your minimeals at the same time!) He can eat these on days when meetings last longer than expected and he cannot leave for a nutritious meal. (Check out our "wraps" in the recipe chapter.)

- *Does he have trouble falling asleep after a stressful day?* Teach him how to do the 2-minute meditation on page 35 or the heart-rate biofeedback in TLC 8. Encourage him to use this technique both midafternoon, after a stressful meeting, and again before bedtime. Also make sure he knows the stress-reducing benefits of the H.E.A.R.T. workout, which is guaranteed to help him sleep like a baby!

Lights Out!

Now you are beginning to understand the real meaning of the 24-Hour Turn-around and how it works to benefit your mind, body, and spirit, transforming who you are right now into the new you. Your own Turnaround can begin tonight with this Total Life Change. You will feel the difference by this time tomorrow—and as you can now realize, all 24 hours of every day are important, even those during sleep.

By the way, if you are reading this book in bed, please turn the lights off right now and *get some sleep*!

Balancing Hormones

WHEN I STARTED to have hot flashes, unpredictable mood swings, and other symptoms of menopause at age forty-eight, I was devastated. Yes, I had pored over all the research. Yes, I had counseled thousands of women on lifestyle changes to enhance their health and emotional well-being through the years. Yes, I saw incredible results in my clients. No, I was not ready to do it myself. My daughter, Riley, was six; my sons, Dustin and R.J., were in high school and college; and my husband was convinced that we should have another baby.

What did I do? I immediately started eating two servings of soy a day. I used a natural progesterone cream twice daily. I called my Transcendental Meditation teacher from college (I had forgotten my mantra!) and resumed my meditation practice. And I went to bed half an hour earlier than usual. Within one cycle, all my symptoms were gone. I continued to menstruate for another year, and then one month, without notice, I stopped. No hormone replacement therapy, thank you, only safe and natural Turnaround strategies.

I am here to tell you, years later, that I have *not* fallen apart. (No, I did not have another baby!) My bone density is that of a twenty-five-year-old woman, and my heart health is excellent because I do H.E.A.R.T. workouts daily. My skin looks healthy and young because I eat nutritious, whole, living food. I have not gained weight, because my hormones are in balance, and I get the sleep required to stimulate human growth hormone (HGH). You can do the same, no matter what stage of your life cycle you are in. The younger/sooner you start, the better the result. Start right now, and 24 hours from now you will feel younger than you've felt in years.

I am not an expert on hormones, but I will share what I have learned from studies and the experts on natural care. I will also let you know what I have learned from my personal experience using natural hormone alternatives as well as reading stacks of scientific research and working with tens of thousands of women over the past twenty-six years.

Hormones 101
(The Short Course—Mandatory Reading!)

Before I explain some natural therapies for "harmonious" hormones, I need for you to understand exactly what hormones are, what they do, and how they can make you feel incredibly energetic, sexy, and alert—or lethargic, moody, and irritable. Hormones are minute chemical messengers that are carried by the bloodstream to relay information from one part of your body to another. At the cellular level, hormones are used for communication between body tissues, including the brain, organs, glands, and muscles. Our growth, mood, digestion, respiration, sense of thirst and hunger, sexual functions, fat metabolism, and most other bodily functions are all triggered by hormones. In most situations, hormones are not physically directed toward any specific site or organ but travel in the bloodstream throughout the entire body searching for a home. The hormones eventually end up in the organs and cells that have special receptors "tuned" to respond only to that particular hormone. Much as you tune a radio to pick out only one station from a large number of signals, the receptors for a hormone ignore everything except that hormone.

It may seem inefficient to send all the hormones everywhere, but consider how low the concentrations can be: one part hormone to *five trillion* parts of blood, in some cases. That's like a single salt crystal dissolved in a large swimming pool. Nature had this balance figured out until recently when man (clever creature that he is) invented synthetic hormones. Because of the extremely low concentrations of our own hormones in our blood, there is a danger of overexposure to the hormones found in food or in the environment. Imagine the mayhem in your body if you suddenly found yourself with the hormonal profile of a cow or a sheep, not to mention the effects of artificial hormones widely used in commercial meat, dairy, and chicken production. Add to that the daily exposure to hormonelike substances in chemicals and plastics, and suddenly it becomes clear why our own hormones are often confused.

Fortunately, our digestive system has a built-in safeguard called *first-pass removal*, a firewall between the hormones in our food and the hormones in our blood. First-pass removal means that everything we swallow is broken down and absorbed through the small intestine into the bloodstream, but this blood doesn't go anywhere until it makes a pass through the liver. There, *most* foreign hormones and chemical signal molecules that survived cooking and stomach acids are removed or deactivated. *Most* is the operative word here, because some of the foreign material sneaks through the firewall. The pharmaceutical companies had to figure out how to get past it to deliver synthetic hormones to the bloodstream. It was overcoming this obstacle—creating an oral formulation of hormones that could survive both gastric digestion and first-pass liver removal—that made birth control pills a reality in the mid-twentieth century.

First-pass removal is the reason for the increased popularity of transdermal (through the skin) and sublingual (under the tongue) delivery systems for drugs, vitamins, and food supplements. Surprisingly large hormone molecules can pass directly through the skin into the blood, bypassing the liver entirely. In the Turnaround strategies, I'll tell you about natural hormones that can be put into a cream, rubbed on your body, and effectively delivered to the proper cell receptors. No worries about trying to trick the first-pass removal system with these effective hormone stabilizers.

Understanding the Sex Hormones
(Important Information About Your Body)

Ask people about hormones, specifically the sex hormones, and they will probably say that testosterone is the male sex hormone and estrogen is its female counterpart. They will understand that testosterone is produced in the testes, while estrogen is made in the ovaries. They also might know that women lose their ability to produce very much estrogen at about age fifty, and that doctors often prescribe supplemental estrogen in the form of hormone replacement therapy (HRT).

When we fill in the details, however, we begin to realize that this simplistic view can easily lead down the wrong path. To begin with, estrogen and testosterone are not really opposites. Estrogen, which can be produced in the body's peripheral tissues, such as the liver, fat, and muscle, usually refers to an entire class of related hormones, including estradiol, estrone, and estriol. Estriol is made from the placenta and is important only during pregnancy. Estradiol is the primary estrogen of childbearing women and is formed from the developing ovarian follicles. While weaker than estradiol, estrone is widespread throughout the body and is the most abundant estrogen after menopause. Estrone is usually produced in fat cells. Estrone acts as an antiestrogen, stopping the full action of estradiol. Testosterone, on the other hand, is one of a class of male hormones called *androgens*. It is far more correct to say that androgens and estrogens are opposites.

WOMEN PRODUCE ANDROGENS AND ESTROGENS

In women, androgens are produced by the ovary and the adrenal glands. The adrenal glands also produce hormones such as estrogen, progesterone, steroids, cortisol, and cortisone, as well as chemicals such as adrenaline. These gland's help regulate chemical balance by supplementing estrogen as other sources start to diminish. The adrenal glands help regulate metabolism as well.

Stress plays an important role in the severity of short-term estrogen loss. This is because the adrenal glands can make up for some of the lost estrogen, but if you are stressed, your adrenal glands make hormones to react to the stress, and the production of estrogen is stunted.

While all women produce androgens, elevations in androgens can interfere with normal egg development and release, causing menstrual irregularities and infertility. In severe cases, excessive androgen production can cause unwanted facial or body hair (hirsutism).

We also produce *dehydroepiandrosterone* (DHEA), a weak androgen, in our adrenal glands. DHEA aids in the production of sex hormones, particularly testosterone and estrogen. While it's plentiful during youth, DHEA subsides as we age. In cases of androgen excess, you may have excess DHEA coming from the adrenal glands.

Pregnenolone, a sex hormone precursor to DHEA, is often called the ultimate steroid hormone because all steroid hormones in the body (including cortisone, testosterone, estrogen, progesterone, DHEA, and others) are produced from pregnenolone, which in turn is synthesized from cholesterol.

While *testosterone* is usually associated with men, in women this hormone is released into the bloodstream by the ovaries in relatively small quantities. Most testosterone binds to sex hormone binding globulin and remains inactive. High levels of testosterone are common with polycystic ovarian syndrome (PCOS), a common but treatable hormonal problem among women of reproductive age that results in obesity, excessive hair growth or thinning, problem skin, and menstrual irregularity.

It is estradiol, the principal estrogen during reproductive years, that separates men from women. You can thank estradiol for your female characteristics, but it's also the source of most gynecologic problems such as endometriosis, fibroids, and even cancer. All estradiol is produced from testosterone, the principal male hormone, and if there's a block in the conversion of testosterone to estradiol, you will have reproductive or gynecologic problems.

PROGESTERONE PLAYS A KEY ROLE

To complicate the situation further, there are really *three* major categories of sex hormones, not two. Progesterone is the third, and it plays an important role in both female and male physiology. This naturally occurring hormone reaches high levels after ovulation in a normal menstrual cycle. Synthetic near copies (pill forms) of progesterone include progestins and progestogens, often loosely referred to as progesterone. There is a great deal of confusion about the correct use of some of these terms. In this book, I'll use *progesterone* to refer to natural human progesterone, or the exact substance found in many plants. *Progestins* will refer to the class of synthetic hormones that are almost, but not quite, the same as natural progesterone. The difference is vitally important, as we will discover.

Environmental Estrogens or Xenoestrogens

We live in a world of petrochemicals and come in contact with hundreds if not thousands of these products in our everyday lives. Our homes are heated with petroleum oil, and our cars run on petroleum fuel. Plastics, medicines, and food containers all contain petroleum by-products. The problem is that some of these petrochemicals, called *xenobiotics,* can act similar to and thereby interfere with our own female hormones, altering the way we grow and reproduce.

The majority of xenobiotics mimic the action of estrogen and are called *xeno-estrogens.* We touch them, wear them, eat them, sleep in them, and breathe them daily; now we are seeing the unfortunate results: an epidemic of reproductive abnormalities, including increasing numbers of cancers of the reproductive organs, infertility, and low sperm counts. There is also speculation by some researchers that xenoestrogens might have a role in the feminization of males.

There are about 100,000 registered chemicals in the world that have hormonal effects in the body, as well as carcinogenic and toxic effects. In theory, first-pass liver removal should take care of any stray hormones we eat. But first-pass removal is not totally effective, and with hormones, a very little bit can go a very long and negative way. The bad news? Many of the harmful hormonelike substances that we absorb from the environment are hard to avoid.

Why do some petrochemicals behave like potent estrogens? Something in their molecular structure contains the basic "key" that fits in the hormone receptor of the cell, switching on hormonal action. In a May 1993 article in *The Lancet,* researchers in Scotland and Denmark hypothesized that xenobiotics are responsible for the steadily declining sperm count in men. One Dartmouth University study showed that plastic wrap (a petrochemical product containing xenoestrogens) heated in a microwave oven with vegetable oil had 500,000 times the minimum amount of xenoestrogens needed to stimulate breast cancer cells to grow in a test tube.

Xenoestrogens, in addition to being highly estrogenic, are fat-soluble and non-biodegradable. That means they are here to stay; you can't get them out of your

LIMIT YOUR FAMILY'S EXPOSURE TO XENOESTROGENS

t's important to reduce your family's exposure to xenoestrogens. Here are some practical measures you can take:

- Avoid using pesticides.

- Minimize your use of plastics.

- If you must eat meat, stop your consumption of commercial meat and purchase hormone-free meat.

- Eat organic produce. The most expensive food you can buy is far cheaper than any illness you can imagine. *Do not attempt to economize on the quality of your food.*

- Use "green" products for detergents and household cleaners, and when possible, use natural rather than petrochemical products. Earth-friendly products are sometimes more expensive, but in the long run you will save on pain, misery, medical bills, and the horror of seeing your child face a debilitating disease.

body (or off planet Earth). Fact is, the major sources of xenoestrogens are red meat and dairy products.

Xenoestrogens accumulate in our fatty tissues (breast, brain, and liver) and cause "estrogen dominance," with all its symptoms and diseases. And billions of pounds of these substances are applied to our fruits and vegetables every year in the form of chemical fertilizers and sprays. Because xenoestrogens do not go away, when you eat the fruit or vegetable you generally get a small amount of these substances. This is why I suggest that everyone eat organic fruits and vegetables as much as possible.

Dr. John Lee, known for his landmark clinical research on reversing osteoporosis with natural progesterone, reports that daughters of mothers who had been given diethylstilbestrol (DES), a synthetic hormone, during pregnancy are more likely to develop vaginal and cervical cancer. Due to the bombardment of xenoestrogens, we are seeing earlier menstruation in our daughters. As you know, the long-term consequences of early menstruation are a lengthy lifetime exposure to estrogen, with an increased risk of hormone-driven cancers such as breast and uterine cancer.

Seeking "Harmonious Hormones"

Popular recognition of the important influence of hormones on our daily quality of life has been slow in coming. Medical recognition has perhaps been even slower. Interestingly, in 1931 the first scientific description of premenstrual syndrome (PMS) came on the scene. What did they call it before 1931? Nothing. Our naturally nourished female ancestors, for the most part, did not have this bevy of symptoms (and neither should a modern woman who practices a healthful lifestyle). When the symptoms did occasionally appear in women of previous generations, they were written off by physicians as just another manifestation of feminine frailty rather than recognized as a very real and correctable medical condition.

I've consulted with hundreds of women who've complained of dramatic changes in hormones that caused uncomfortable symptoms such as water retention, bloating, cramping, violent mood swings, headache, and sadness. In fact, it is estimated that 80 percent of women in their childbearing years suffer from PMS, recognized as an emotional and physical disorder that affects a woman's ability to function. While researchers don't know why the intense mood and physical symptoms occur right before a period, they do know that normal cyclical changes in a woman's hormones may interact with neurotransmitters, including serotonin, which is associated with a calming, anxiety-reducing reaction. This may result in the emotional and physical symptoms of PMS. No matter what causes your hormonal imbalances, the holistic strategies in this Total Life Change will help get them on track again.

MENOPAUSE

I can't remember my mother or her friends ever discussing menopause. Now this ongoing natural process of physical change is a household word. The nightly media give health tips to millions on innovative ways to control night sweats, hot flashes, mood swings, and loss of libido, while Internet health sites describe the latest scientific breakthroughs in understanding this phase of life. Slick magazine advertisements tout the latest hormone replacement therapies (HRT) and even offer coupons to use with any new prescription.

After menopause, total androgen levels may drop, while ovarian testosterone may slightly increase because of the elevated gonadotropins. But it's during the four to five years before menopause, a period called perimenopause, when estrogen levels are declining and menopausal symptoms send women to their doctors, begging for answers. At that time, some doctors recommend HRT to alleviate menopausal symptoms and to prevent bone loss after menopause.

Please listen carefully! While estrogen used to be the most common prescription doctors wrote for women ages forty-five to fifty-five, we now know that taking estrogen after menopause may do far more harm than good. The problem with using a synthetic near copy of a hormone to treat menopausal symptoms is that we are looking at tiny pieces of a much larger picture—and covering up symptoms instead of correcting the hormone loss or imbalance. This is dangerous and irresponsible, in my opinion. While HRT may control hot flashes or vaginal dryness, it's important to consider the more serious and even life-threatening effects of synthetic hormones:

- *Breast*—The risk of breast cancer is increased with supplemental estrogen or HRT: estrogen is believed to increase the amount of dense tissue in the breast, making it difficult to correctly identify abnormalities on mammograms.

- *Uterus*—HRT increases the risk of uterine cancer.

- *Heart*—The American Heart Association advises that HRT should not be initiated solely for its potential protective effects against cardiovascular disease. The new position, reported in July 2001 in *Circulation,* is based upon recent scientific studies with conflicting results about the role of HRT in reducing the risk of coronary heart disease in postmenopausal women.

  Another new study, published in February 2001 in *Arteriosclerosis, Thrombosis, and Vascular Biology,* suggests that HRT does *not* slow the progression of atherosclerosis—a buildup of fatty plaque in the arteries—particularly in postmenopausal women at increased risk. Researchers involved in this study found that heart disease in women appeared to worsen when they were given HRT shortly after a heart attack. Other studies of healthy women, such as those participating in the long-term Nurses' Health Study, concluded that women who had taken long-term HRT were relatively protected against heart disease. But wait! There was a big problem in this study in that the women who participated were health-care professionals who were thought to have healthy lifestyles.

- *Hypertension*—HRT may increase blood pressure as a result of fluid retention.

- *Gallbladder disease*—This condition is worsened by supplemental estrogen or HRT.

- *Migraines*—HRT may either improve or worsen migraines.

- *Liver function*—HRT worsens liver function in those who have impaired liver function.

- *Hypertriglyceridemia*—Triglyceride levels above 300 may worsen with supplemental estrogen or HRT.

- *Asthma*—HRT may worsen.

- *Thromboembolism*—HRT increases the risk of blood clots in women at risk.

- *Weight*—The effects on weight of taking synthetic estrogen and progestins are far greater than most people ever realized, and that includes our medical community. Has anyone ever told you that taking estrogen will probably cause you to gain weight? Many of my clients found that out the hard way.

Osteoporosis

Sarah, a sixty-two-year-old client from the Midwest, had taken early retirement from her government position and was looking forward to traveling around the world with her husband on his business trips—until she broke her hip while walking down a flight of stairs. She underwent surgery followed by a long and painful rehabilitation that extended for more than a year. She is now doing her Turnaround to keep fit and, more importantly, to halt osteoporosis and keep her bones strong. She vows never to suffer another fracture.

WHAT'S IN A WORD?

Perimenopause (climacteric): the four to five years before menopause during which time there is a natural decline in ovarian estrogen production.

Menopause: a natural process that occurs when the estrogen production of the ovary is insufficient to stimulate the development of the uterine lining and bleeding stops.

Estrogen replacement therapy (ERT): the use of supplemental synthetic estrogen to replace what is lost by the body.

Hormone replacement therapy (HRT): the use of supplemental synthetic medications—usually estrogen, progestins, and androgens (again, man-made pharmaceuticals)—to compensate for what is lost by the body either naturally at menopause or surgically through hysterectomy.

Estrogen dominance: a condition in which a woman's progesterone levels are too low in relation to her estrogen levels. It does not mean, however, that she has too much estrogen. A transdermal progesterone cream can be used to bring the hormones back into balance. Symptoms that can be caused or made worse by estrogen dominance include accelerated aging, fat gain, osteoporosis, PMS, uterine and breast fibroids, water retention, and memory loss.

Why talk about a bone disease in a chapter on hormones? Because osteoporosis, a debilitating bone loss disease that afflicts the majority of postmenopausal women in North America, is one of the major (but questionable) justifications for HRT.

Osteoporosis is a quiet and accomplished thief—there are no visible signs until fractures occur. Your body can harbor it quietly for years. Then suddenly, normal stress on bones from sitting, standing, coughing, or hugging a loved one can cause fractures that lead to chronic pain and immobility. With repeated fractures, this condition gradually leads to more pain, disfigurement, and immobility.

PREMARIN STANDS FOR *PREGNANT MARES'* UR*INE*

Premarin is a drug made up of estrogens obtained from the urine of pregnant mares. It's used to reduce menopausal symptoms and lower the risk of osteoporosis, and it's given to women who have had a hysterectomy. It's the bestselling drug in the country—the one that doctors often automatically prescribe. It is not identical to the estrogens your body makes and therefore may cause changes in your liver or cause cancer.

To make Premarin, pregnant mares are kept tied up indoors for at least six months out of the year. These mares are impregnated, fitted with urine collection devices, and normally kept throughout their pregnancy of eleven months in stalls just 8 feet long, 3½ feet wide, and 5 feet high! In most cases they are impregnated within two weeks of foaling and returned to the production line again. (Mares that do not become pregnant within a very short time are often sent to the slaughterhouse.) Foals are taken from the mares, fattened, and sold for slaughter. A colt foal has less than a one-in-fifty chance of living. Please check out www.premarin.org before taking Premarin.

THE LIFE CYCLE OF BONE

Bone is complex living tissue. Our bodies constantly break down old bone and rebuild new bone (a process called *remodeling*). In children, more bone is built than is removed, so bones become larger and stronger. The skeleton contains about 95 percent of its peak amount of bone by age twenty. Our bones then maintain their strength until we're age thirty or thirty-five. Then the amount of bone our bodies break down begins to catch up with the amount they are building. Sometime during this period the bone removed *equals* the bone built. Usually after age forty the mass of bone removed *surpasses* the amount of bone built. It is then that osteoporosis can disrupt the natural bone-building cycle, resulting in a decrease in the amount of bone in our bodies. There are many factors that can cause early bone loss, including strict dieting, lack of menstrual periods because of strenuous exercise, lack of calcium in the diet or poor calcium absorption, early surgical

VEG OUT FOR WRINKLE PROTECTION

Want to stave off wrinkles associated with aging and the reduction of female hormones? Then you may want to watch what you eat. A study published in April 2001 in the *Journal of the American College of Nutrition* revealed that what you eat could show up on your face—either in wrinkles or in smooth skin. In the study, Dr. Mark L. Wahlqvist of Monash University in Melbourne, Australia, found that people who ate plenty of wholesome foods but avoided butter, red meat, and sugary foods were less prone to wrinkling. Because the skin is a major target of oxidative stress, the authors speculate that some foods protect the skin because of high levels of antioxidants such as vitamins A, C, and E. Some of the skin-boosting foods included green leafy vegetables, beans, nuts, and multigrain breads.

menopause (hysterectomy) without estrogen supplementation, illness, and medications such as corticosteroids, to name a few. Then comes menopause. At this normal life stage, hormonal changes disrupt the bone-building cycle again. Specifically, the natural decline in estrogen at menopause speeds up the breakdown of bone. In the five to ten years after menopause, there is a greatly accelerated loss of bone mass in women. Many women lose a startling 25 percent of their bone density within five years after menopause.

I know that if you are active, it's hard to imagine that your body is undergoing any negative changes. Fewer than 10 percent of those who have osteoporosis actually know they have it and are treated. If the decline in bone density continues over a period of ten to twenty years, your bones become thinner and easier to break or fracture. When bones are fractured, though painful, they will eventually heal, if you are lucky. For the not so fortunate, the result is immobility or even death.

GET OFF THE DIETING MERRY-GO-ROUND

If you have a history of yo-yo dieting, it's time to get on the Definition Diet—once and for all—if you want your bones to stay strong. In a study published in 2001 in the *American Journal of Clinical Nutrition,* researchers sought to find out if post-menopausal women lost bone during periods of calorie restriction (dieting). They concluded that even moderate energy restriction (dieting) is accompanied by a noticeable increase in markers of bone metabolism (breakdown of bone) in postmenopausal women. This important study has vast public health implications concerning weight loss and risk of osteo-porosis due to the incessant dieting of many women. The moral of the story is to achieve your ideal body weight, using the Definition Diet and the other TLCs, and *stay there.* The more times you gain and lose—and lose and gain—the more at risk you are for bone loss, as well as other degenerative diseases.

We know that more than thirty-eight million women are over fifty right now, making this the largest group in history to hit menopause. We know that many of these women will live at least one-third of their lives after menopause. Soon one person out of six will be over age sixty-five. The number of hip and other fractures will only skyrocket unless we all take personal responsibility and action to stay strong and healthy. You can take steps at any age to prevent bone loss, and the younger you start, the better for your bones. In fact, it's best to build strong bones during childhood and early adulthood, while bone density is naturally increasing, and then continue to strengthen your bones throughout your lifetime. Share this information with your daughters and sons—osteoporosis affects men as well.

Bone-Boosters

Synthetic hormone replacement is *believed* to halt and even reverse bone loss and reduce the incidence of fractures. I say *believed* because the data are somewhat inconsistent, depending on what you read and whom you ask. Some studies report only a slight bone-strengthening effect; others show a 50 percent reduc-

EIGHT WAYS TO STOP PMS

PMS symptoms may include mild breast tenderness, fluid retention, anxiety, dietary cravings, irritability, and an inability to concentrate.

1. **Avoid alcohol.** Alcohol is a mood-altering drug and can compound feelings of depression and hopelessness. Furthermore, many women have a decreased tolerance for alcohol prior to their period and may become intoxicated quickly.

2. **Follow the H.E.A.R.T. workout.** Exercise reduces stress and keeps your body fit. A daily H.E.A.R.T. workout regimen can decrease PMS symptoms by increasing endorphins in the body. H.E.A.R.T. exercise also increases your sense of well-being and decreases fluid retention.

3. **Reduce or eliminate caffeine consumption.** Studies show that the symptoms of PMS increase with the consumption of caffeine-containing beverages. In one study, women who totally abstained from caffeine during the PMS period had a complete resolution of symptoms.

4. **Avoid foods high in sodium.** Sodium retention can contribute to PMS headaches, bloating, edema, and fluid weight gain during the premenstrual phase of your cycle. The best approach is to eat foods naturally low in sodium, including fresh fruits and vegetables, legumes, and whole grains. Also avoid using table salt.

5. **Take a high-quality acidophilus supplement.** These "friendly bacteria" help to suppress yeast infections, which contribute to bloating.

6. **Avoid diuretics, as they contribute to PMS headaches.** Use herbal diuretic teas instead. Your local health-food store will carry a variety to choose from.

7. **Take B vitamin supplements (especially B6).** Or be sure to eat lots of uncooked whole foods that are high in B vitamins, such as grains, cereals, and sprouted grain bread.

8. **Eat high-carb meals.** In a study done at the University of Tennessee Health Sciences Center, researchers reported that women with PMS who had a meal high in carbohydrates were happier and more relaxed within an hour. In contrast, women who ate a high-protein meal felt angry, sad, and more tense. Within 3 hours the carb group was back to baseline and needed to eat. Conclusion: PMS sufferers should eat smaller and more frequent meals that include carbs. Also, avoid sugar and white flour. Hint: include a couple of Zip-Lock Snacks (see recipe chapter) when you are away from home.

tion in hip fractures. At the 2001 Annual Meeting of the American Society for Bone and Mineral Research, researchers concluded that osteoporosis therapy using pharmaceuticals is limited in that increases in bone mineral density are responsible for only about 20 percent of the fracture risk reduction seen with current therapies. In a study published in the August 15, 2001, *Journal of the American Medical Association,* researchers found that HRT has significant bone-strengthening effects in very old, physically frail women. However, it was noted that the fracture risk in very old women is due to multiple factors in addition to low bone density, including sensory and neuromuscular impairments, medications, and environmental hazards. The study concluded that further research is necessary to clarify the effectiveness of HRT in reducing fracture rates and postponing disability. In my opinion, HRT is not only unreliable but a tremendous health risk.

Even if the effectiveness has the potential of being 50 percent, what about all those hip fractures that have not been prevented? In another recent study published in 2001 in the journal *Maturitas,* it was shown that participation in training programs (such as the H.E.A.R.T. workout) undertaken regularly by older women was associated with better postural stability. In the study, women who participated in an exercise program were compared with women who took HRT and did not exercise. As one would expect, postural stability in HRT users did not improve. The women who exercised were stronger, more coordinated, and had better stability—all factors that prevent fractures. Researchers found that poor postural stability, reduced lower limb strength, and decreased reaction time were important risk factors for falls and hence for fractures. In my opinion, the biggest plus for exercise as opposed to HRT is the absence of dangerous side effects. After starting exercise to prevent fractures, your second line of defense should be eating soy products. High consumption of soy products is associated with increased bone mass and is a natural method for preventing the effects of low estrogen.

PMS HEADACHE RELIEF

When migraine headaches occur with regularity in women only at premenstrual times, they are most likely due to estrogen dominance. Estrogen causes dilation of blood vessels and water retention, which contribute to migraines. One of the many positive effects of natural progesterone is that it helps restore normal vascular tone, counteracting the blood vessel dilation that causes the headache. Again, hormone balance is the key.

SIX NATURAL BONE-BOOSTERS

1. Use a natural progesterone cream. I find it curious that we are told that HRT (or estrogen replacement) prevents osteoporosis when this bone-robbing disease begins in the mid-thirties, before we experience any major decrease in estrogen levels. Many doctors still believe that prevention of osteoporosis "requires" pharmaceutical estrogen, sometimes augmented by a synthetic progestin. But are we replacing the right hormones? There is a more effective and safer way to prevent bone loss, and that is using a natural progesterone cream, steering well clear of the popular estrogen and estrogen-progestin regimens.

You can stimulate your own hormones to start working for you again and bring them into balance without taking dangerous supplemental estrogen that has possibly deadly side effects such as breast cancer. In fact, hormones from the natural progesterone cream can show up in the saliva just *hours* after putting it on your body, so you know it's working for you almost immediately.

HERBAL RESCUE FOR PMS

I n a study published in July 2000 in the British *Journal of Obstetrics and Gynaecology,* researchers found that Saint-John's-wort, an herbal remedy used to ease feelings of sadness or depression, may help women with PMS by easing nervous tension, anxiety, and insomnia. Saint-John's-wort is taken daily by more than twenty million Germans and has become quite popular in the United States, where it is available without a prescription.

In the four-month study at the University of Exeter, women with PMS kept track of their daily symptoms and took psychological tests to assess their emotions and physical state. During months three and four, women were given 300 milligrams of hypericin, the active ingredient in Saint-John's-wort, and continued to chart their symptoms. Treatment with Saint-John's-wort for two menstrual cycles resulted in significant improvements in PMS symptoms, greatly reducing symptoms such as nervous tension, insomnia, crying, and depression.

2. Eat foods high in phytoestrogens. Again, go soy—but this time to keep bones strong. Reduced sex hormones may be a contributing factor to osteoporosis, but it is only one of many factors. And it's a deficiency that is much better addressed by natural phytoestrogens, the estrogen-like substances found in plants. Unlike the xenoestrogens that are part of the witches' brew of the petrochemical industry, phytoestrogens have been part of the human food environment for millions of years. Our bodies know how to use them to our advantage.

Phytoestrogens are adaptogenic. That is, they tend to suppress estrogen function when it is too high and supplement estrogen when it is too low. Soy products are a great source of beneficial phytoestrogens. As I said earlier, eating two servings of soy daily helped to eliminate my menopausal symptoms and has kept my bones strong. In a study on postmenopausal women who weren't taking HRT, the group that received the most isoflavones (from soy) increased their bone density by 3 percent. In another study published in the December 8, 2001, *American Journal of Clinical Nutrition,* researchers had perimenopausal women supplement their diets with soy. These researchers suggested that isoflavones decreased bone loss from the spine in perimenopausal women who were estrogen-deficient. Premenopausal women may be expected to lose bone at an annual rate of 2 percent per year if they do not take precautions with bone-boosting foods and exercise.

3. Eat plenty of green, leafy vegetables and other food sources of calcium. No, you do not get much calcium from milk. Milk has a lot of calcium in it, but for an adult human, this calcium is almost entirely unabsorbable. I explain this fully in TLC 3; you may want to reread it to see why dairy is one of the biggest hormone offenders.

The cow pumping out all that calcium is not drinking milk or taking calcium pills. The cow is eating grass. We can do

BONE MINERAL DENSITY TESTS

Bone mineral density tests are painless, noninvasive tests (similar to an X ray) that accurately evaluate bone density, a measure of your bone strength. With the information obtained from this test, your doctor can predict the likelihood of future fractures. Whatever the results of this test, the Bone-Boosters in this chapter can help you turn around bone loss and increase strength and density. Check with the National Osteoporosis Foundation (202-223-2226) for information on testing.

the same. Leafy green vegetables are the most absorbable form of calcium for both cows and humans. Just as important is that the leafy green plants permit the uptake of calcium from the digestive tract and its placement into the bone structure. (It doesn't do any good eating calcium if you can't use it.)

Not only is calcium necessary for strong bones as we age, but this mineral may also help keep blood pressure low and play a role in preventing colon cancer. You can easily boost bone strength the natural way by eating calcium-enriched foods and calcium-containing vegetables such as artichokes, broccoli, brussels sprouts, cabbage, carrots, snap beans, spinach, and Swiss chard.

Aging plays an important role in the efficiency of calcium absorption. The older we get, the less able our bodies are to absorb nutrients. This is why for every 24 hours that pass it becomes even more important to eat a varied diet of calcium-rich foods to ensure proper absorption and utilization of this bone-boosting mineral. Eat as many veggies as you can raw. The live enzymes in raw veggies provide you with a 24-hour Turnaround in nutrient absorption.

4. Follow the H.E.A.R.T. workout plan. To keep placing calcium into the bone structure, you need to exercise. Read that sentence again. Doesn't that appear to be the answer to your bone loss situation rather than dangerous drugs? Mild to moderate exercise stress (muscles pulling on bones) activates the mechanism that builds bones. Some revealing studies have shown that a marked decrease in physical activity, such as being confined to bed rest, results in a profound decline in bone mass. A prime example is seen in the bone disorders of astronauts. Tests on those who experience weightlessness show the necessity of physical activity in keeping bones strong.

After age forty, many women become less active. Planning time to do your H.E.A.R.T. workout is crucial to maintaining bone strength.

5. Watch out for bone robbers. While eating calcium-rich foods can build bone, other foods can decrease bone, robbing you of strength. Red meat and carbonated sodas are both bone robbers and should be eliminated from your daily diet. Stomach acids are necessary to move dietary calcium into the blood, and both of these foods interfere with this mechanism. Alcohol is another major bone robber. In fact, the reduction of bone mass with age is related to the amount of alcohol you drink.

6. Be sure you have an adequate supply of vitamin D and phosphorus in your diet. You can get these nutrients from supplements or preferably from the fresh foods in the Definition Diet. They are both a necessary part of the process of placing calcium back into bone.

FACTORS THAT AFFECT CALCIUM ABSORPTION

INCREASE ABSORPTION	DECREASE ABSORPTION
Vitamins A, C, D	Aging, menopause
Adequate protein intake	Too much protein—especially animal protein
Low-fat diet	High-fat diet
Lactose	Fast-moving intestinal tract
Gastric hydrochloric acid	Low stomach acid
Amino acids (lysine and glycine)	Stress
Exercise	Lack of exercise

Breast Cancer

Contrary to popular belief, new reports show that women with a family history of breast cancer are not likely to develop breast cancer at a young age. Most women with affected relatives who get breast cancer themselves develop the disease after the age of fifty. But listen to this and believe it: in a study published in October 2001 in the British medical journal *The Lancet,* researchers found that eight of nine women who are diagnosed with breast cancer—regardless of age—do *not* have an affected mother, sister, or daughter. So, what then? If it's not genetic, it's lifestyle and environment—two risk factors for serious diseases that you can control—today—by starting your 24-Hour Turnaround.

One of the biggest choices you can make to protect yourself from breast cancer is to eliminate alcohol from your life—totally. Carefully read TLC 5 before having your next glass of wine.

Keep in mind that the choice to use HRT is just that—a choice. A revealing study about this concern was published on June 9, 1999, in the *Journal of the American Medical Association.* In this publication, researchers involved with the Iowa Women's Health study, an ongoing study of 41,837 postmenopausal women who have been followed since 1985, concluded that long-term, postmenopausal use of HRT appears to increase breast cancer risk. More studies are beginning to surface indicating the same. And to complicate the link between HRT and breast cancer, concern is now coming from the most conservative medical community about HRT and its effect on breast screening. The *British Medical Journal* reported that in many women, HRT increases breast density, which reduces the sensitivity and specificity of breast screening. (The effectiveness of breast screening depends on the *decreasing* breast density normally seen with age.)

Progesterone and Transdermal Creams: The Natural Way

When you read or hear the term *progesterone treatment,* beware because it often refers to synthetic progestin rather than natural progesterone. *Natural progesterone* is derived from wild yam or soybeans and is formulated from the plant

- A woman *had* one chance in twenty of getting breast cancer in 1950.
- A woman *has* one chance in eight of getting breast cancer today.
- Breast cancer is the most common type of female cancer.
- Each year 182,000 American women are diagnosed with breast cancer.
- Each year 46,000 women die of breast cancer.

source (diosgenin) in a laboratory. This always made me suspicious until I learned that diosgenin is identical to the molecule found in the human body. *Synthetic progestin* resembles our progesterone and is also produced in a lab, but trust me, your body will be able to tell the difference between the synthetic and the real thing. Progesterone is the primary building block for all the other steroid hormones, including estrogen, which distinguishes natural progesterone from synthetic progestin. The synthetic cannot do this job.

One similarity between synthetic and natural forms of this hormone is that they both trigger uterine bleeding similar to menstrual flow. When this occurs with the use of natural progesterone, however, it is usually a needed "cleaning out" process and rarely continues beyond a single cycle.

Natural progesterone is usually supplied in the form of a transdermal cream that is applied to the skin on a schedule synchronized with the menstrual cycle. Some of the products provide a significant dose of natural progesterone itself (usually derived from soy or Mexican yam), while other products only carry the precursors. The precursors-only variety encourages your body to figure out what to use and what to ignore; the body will make its own progesterone in the right proportions if it has the materials to work with. The stronger formulas, creams that contain natural progesterone, can be tried if your symptoms persist. Check my website for a list of companies that make a natural product.

Natural hormones are not the same as pharmaceutical hormones. Your body has the wisdom to take substances from nature, use them for energy, maintenance of health, and repair of tissues, and then eliminate them. But the opposite happens when synthetic, chemically altered hormones are sent to your cell receptors. The message they carry may be different, even contrary to that of the hormone they are meant to simulate. The results? A host of negative side effects such as weight gain, bloating, tumor growth, high blood pressure, unwanted hair growth, and cancer.

A synthetic drug is made in a laboratory and usually not found in nature. In the late 1800s, laws were passed in the United States that allowed medicines to be patented only if they were substances not found in nature. So if a drug manufacturer discovered a natural substance from leaves, herbs, plants, animals, or natural medicine, there was a strong incentive to isolate the "active ingredient" (a clever name created by the drug

industry) and modify it into an unnatural form in order to obtain a patent. Without the patent, another company could sell that same substance. I think it's safe to say that drug companies have zero interest in naturally occurring medicines.

Nature has great wisdom that humans, to date, have not been able to duplicate with synthetic drugs. The history of creating synthetic drugs repeatedly reveals that separating the active ingredient from the rest of the plant to create a new miracle drug almost always creates harmful side effects. It is becoming more and more apparent that HRT is not what it purports to be.

Which is best: cream or pill? After looking at all the available information on natural progesterone pills vs. natural progesterone cream, I will have to go with Mother Nature's opinion. That is, the ovaries never put their hormones into the stomach! You have to take 100 to 200 milligrams by mouth to get the required 20 milligrams you get by using a cream. Why? The liver does its job and removes "foreign" material on the first pass. When you use a natural progesterone cream, your body will use what it needs to replace progesterone and to make the other needed hormones. The creams contain the same safe amount that your own body is supposed to make every day. The good news about natural progesterone cream is that there are *no* known side effects.

You can find natural progesterone creams at any health-food store. They are usually sold in a tube instead of a jar, reducing their exposure to oxygen and ensuring that they retain potency over time. Keep in mind that not all labels claiming "wild yam extract" actually contain any progesterone. Be sure the cream you buy has at least 400 milligrams of progesterone per ounce.

A word of caution: even when a cream contains progesterone, it will not be effective if it isn't suspended in the proper medium. Products containing mineral oil will prevent the progesterone from being absorbed into the skin.

Testing your hormone levels. The most common way to test hormone levels has been with a blood test. This is typically the method that doctors use to determine if HRT is for you. But these tests can be unreliable because they do not give your "biologically active" hormone levels.

Hormones made in ovaries, testes, or adrenals are wrapped in protein envelopes so they can be carried in the blood. These protein-bound hormones are not fully biologically active. The more important and relevant hormone levels are the 1 to 10 percent that are unbound and biologically active. (Saliva contains only the unbound, biologically active hormone molecules.) When progesterone is absorbed through the skin, it is not coated with protein and is carried in the blood's fatty components. Even though progesterone from the skin creams is slow to appear in blood serum, it is found to be present within hours in saliva, indicating that it is well absorbed and available to cells in biologically active form.

Saliva testing is quicker, less expensive, less invasive, and less painful than blood tests and is a reliable way for you (or your doctor) to measure your hormone levels and test for hormone deficiencies. Home tests can be ordered through your health-food store or on the Internet. The test will indicate whether the hormones you are taking are being absorbed and utilized. It doesn't involve a trip to a lab or drawing blood, and it's inexpensive enough that you can do a number of tests, over several days or a month.

We know that hormones change from second to second as they are altered by food, stress, exercise, the environment, medication, the plastic and petrochemical products around you, and many other things. The test you take today can have completely different results from the test you take tomorrow. That's why it makes sense to do several saliva tests if you're looking for accurate feedback.

TURNAROUND STRATEGIES FOR A
HORMONE MAKEOVER

I've given you plenty of reasons to start today to balance your hormones, from avoiding life-threatening diseases such as breast cancer and osteoporosis to keeping irritating menopausal symptoms at bay. As you incorporate these Turnaround strategies in your daily routine, keep in mind that I'm a fierce proponent of using natural therapies as opposed to the latest pharmaceuticals, which come with a bevy of side effects and contraindications. I believe life should be lived to its fullest—naturally—with the optimal nutrition, exercise, and health strategies presented in *The 24-Hour Turnaround.*

To keep your hormones working for you—not against you—begin today with the following Turnaround tips to help you stay youthful, lean, and active—whether you are twenty-two or seventy-two.

Tip 1: Try a natural progesterone supplement. Make sure you have a good supply of all the necessary progesterone precursors, including a nutritious whole food diet, plenty of sleep and exercise, and living in a clean environment. If lifestyle changes don't seem to make a noticeable difference in the way you look and feel, then a natural progesterone supplement can often work wonders. (I know because it helps me and many other women feel great!)

Tip 2: Keep your digestion working well by eating plenty of fiber. If you minimize the work your digestive system has to do, then you maximize the efficiency of all other systems, including hormone production and regulation.

Tip 3: Take a balanced supplement that includes calcium and digestive enzymes. Enzymes help extract the maximum number of nutrients (from your food and supplements) for hormonal health.

Tip 4: Minimize external sources of estrogen-like artificial substances found in commercial meats, plastics, and other foods.

Tip 5: Destress using mind-body innercise (TLC 8). Stress activates your adrenal glands, which emit chemicals like cortisol that can give you the "altered state" feeling when you have your period or in a menopause moment. If you keep your adrenal glands healthy, they will help make extra estrogen as yours starts to diminish.

Tip 6: If you smoke cigarettes, stop *today*. Your day may be somewhat uncomfortable, but your hormones will be calmer with each passing hour. If you have an addiction that is difficult to break, seek help now through the American Lung Association, a community organization, or your physician.

Tip 7: Get at least 8 hours of sleep each night. Women who secrete the highest amount of stress hormones have the hardest time sleeping, which is likely to lead to depression and even osteoporosis. There is also a risk of high blood pressure associated with fragmented sleep.

Tip 8: Have more sex. Hormones associated with female orgasm are likely to contribute to vascular health, among other beneficial effects.

Tip 9: Eat hormone-friendly foods like soy, yams, almonds, and sunflower and pumpkin seeds.

Tip 10: Get control of your blood sugar. High and low levels of glucose can make hot flashes worse and cause mood swings. Eliminate refined sugar and white flour, and consume plenty of whole grains, legumes, fish, fruits, and vegetables. In other words, follow the Definition Diet.

Tip 11: Schedule a spa getaway in Hawaii ASAP! I'm right here waiting to help you with a hormone "makeover."

SOY PROPAGANDA?

It's hard to argue with hundreds of years of incredible good health in Asian countries where the people eat a soy-based diet. But there are some researchers who have hired high-powered public relations firms to try to discredit soy. You may ask why. What did that little old soybean do to upset someone? The reason is simple—and disturbing. There are several billion-dollar industries out there that stand to lose when more people switch from HRT and beef-eating to a soy-based diet. If you take a closer look at some of these so-called studies, perhaps you too can detect some manipulation of facts.

In one study, "The Modest Hormonal Effects of Soy Isoflavones in Postmenopausal Women," *Journal of Clinical Endocrinology and Metabolism,* October 1999, the data suggest that effects of isoflavones on plasma hormones per se are not significant mechanisms by which soy consumption can exert estrogen-like effects in postmenopausal women.

Fact 1: In the study, volunteers were given soy powder, not tofu, soybeans, or other pure soy products. One might ask: What additives were in the soy powder? Who was the manufacturer? How many isoflavones were in each serving? Ironically—or sadly—none of these facts were reported. Remember, it's the isoflavones in the soy that have the estrogenic effect on the body.

Fact 2: Eighteen women participated in the study. Any scientist knows that a scientific study needs thousands of subjects to have any validity at all. The Nurses' Health Study had more than 122,000 respondents. Now that is a credible study.

Fact 3: The length of the study was ninety days. A credible study goes on for years or even decades. The Nurses' Health Study was started in 1976 with funding from the National Institutes of Health and is still going.

Get SOY Strong

If you want to stay strong and young after menopause, head to your local supermarket or health-food store and stock up on soy products. Soybeans are a rich source of isoflavones, a class of phytoestrogens (plant estrogens) that mimic the female hormone estrogen. Isoflavones, found predominantly in legumes and beans, reduce and often erase menopausal symptoms. High consumption of soy products will help you increase your bone mass and reduce the effects of low estrogen. Plant estrogens have been shown to completely stop or at the very least minimize menopausal symptoms by making up for the body's diminishing supply.

There's no word for *hot flash* in Japanese. PMS? Not a problem. With a diet high in soy, Japanese women have blood levels of phytoestrogens that are ten to forty times higher than those of their Western peers. In fact, breast cancer rates for the Japanese are four times lower than those in the United States. Research findings published in January 2001 in *Obstetrics and Gynecology* suggest that a diet rich in soy may help women retain strong bones and reduce the risk of painful and debilitating fractures. In a study in Japan led by Dr. Yoshiaki Somekawa, researchers found that women in both the early and late postmenopausal periods who consumed the highest level of isoflavones in foods such as tofu, boiled soybeans, and soy milk had significantly thicker bones than women who consumed the lowest level of isoflavones. Women in the early postmenopausal period also had significantly fewer backaches and aching joints. Soy is perhaps a far safer "treatment" for osteoporosis than HRT, with no risk of breast or uterine cancer. I believe that the natural use of phytoestrogens should be the preferred treatment for all women.

FOR YOUR HUSBAND

A study reported in the *Journal of the American Medical Association* concluded that a lack of deep sleep actually increases fat in men aged thirty-five to fifty. They may experience an increase in weight gain, loss of muscle mass, and reduction in exercise capacity because of decreased levels of human growth hormone. How can they remedy this? Start the H.E.A.R.T. workout and heart-rate biofeedback, and set the clock for an earlier bedtime. Make sure your husband is not at risk.

FOR YOUR KIDS

Protect your children's hormones by feeding them organic, hormone-free foods. The soy and plant phytonutrients are just as important for them as they are for you, maybe even more so because building strong bones is especially important during childhood and adolescence. Be sure to feed your kids vegetables that are loaded with calcium, to ensure bone strength now and in later life.

TEN VEGETABLES LOADED WITH CALCIUM

1. Artichokes	6. Celery
2. Broccoli	7. Lima beans
3. Brussels sprouts	8. Snap beans
4. Cabbage	9. Spinach
5. Carrots	10. Swiss chard

Be Your Own Bodyguard

I believe that in most cases, natural relief for unbalanced hormones is best. In many cases, natural progesterone replacement in a cream formulation has been shown to be more effective than estrogen replacement, without the negative side effects. If you choose to let a physician manage your hormones, seek a doctor who has a strong background in nutrition and who is willing to help you the natural way. Your doctor should also be your guide to decisions regarding diagnostic testing for prevention purposes. If your health plan doesn't allow a wide enough range of choices, be prepared to spend some money for a qualified practitioner. Keep in mind that even the most enlightened physician can only aim you in the right direction. Once you understand what you have to do, the physician's role becomes less important and those out-of-pocket consultations will become much less frequent.

I urge you to become your own bodyguard as you seek the latest health information, particularly the new studies on hormone replacement and menopause, and then learn to follow the natural path when at all possible. In short, we all have to be our own doctors at some point in life in order to prevent diseases, seek treatment when necessary, and experience optimal health.

Destress with Mind-Body Innercise

MY OFFICE PHONE rang off the hook after the September 11, 2001, terrorist attacks. Clients on the East Coast told of having overwhelming feelings of anxiety, nervousness, and fear—and rightly so. Not only did the horrific attacks cause loss and distress, but going to bed each night with the unknown, thinking of what might happen, greatly accelerated these emotions. Many of my clients admitted to stress eating, especially high-calorie foods loaded with fat and sugar, along with decreased exercise and less restful sleep.

"Life is so out of control and unpredictable that my heart races all the time." While Kate, fifty-three, said that this described her life after a turbulent divorce and cross-country move, I've heard similar words from other very successful clients, including those who are happily married. We all find life to be overwhelming at times.

Doesn't it seem as if things that used to last a lifetime now change overnight— careers change, you move to a new home or another state, kids grow up too fast, adult children move out and then move back home again? In the midst of all these changes, we hurry to keep up, thinking that if we're running hard and doing all the right things, we can stay in control of our lives. *Wrong!* Control is about staying focused on the major goals and letting go of things outside your control, realizing that you cannot alter many of life's challenges. Whether from an illness in the family, relationship troubles, a job crisis, or even more monthly expenses than money to cover them, life will throw unexpected stumbling blocks our way. I'm not by any means a proponent of taking a backseat approach to life. I think we all have to operate at 200 percent of our ability and do the best we can. But that's where it must end. If you are stressed about a situation, ask yourself if there is *anything* you can do to alter the circumstances. If the answer is yes, then take those proactive steps. If the answer is no, openly acknowledge that you cannot influence the situation, and then use one of the Turnaround techniques in this chapter to resolve your tension and unhealthy anxiety. Staying centered even when the world around you is falling apart will help you stay healthy and avoid the negative impact of stress on your mind, body, and spirit.

Stress and Your Health

The truth is that when outside demands exceed your ability to cope, it creates stress. Many of my high-profile clients live in a world of continuous stress. I have seen it weaken their immune systems, with consequences such as hypertension, irritable bowel syndrome, constant infections, skin problems, and many types of cancer. Stress can create symptoms, such as the racing heart that Kate felt, or it can exacerbate existing medical conditions such as diabetes, hypertension, or asthma. Intense and/or ongoing stress wreaks havoc on your body and is a key trigger in many diseases—not to mention that stress *makes you look and feel old.*

CHRONIC STRESS LEADS TO ILLNESS

In the 1930s the Austrian physiologist Hans Selye first introduced the general adaptation syndrome (see page 298). Selye theorized that when we encounter a stressor, specific physical changes take place in the body. These changes allow us to react quickly and to gather all the body's resources to cope with that stressor. This adaptation involves drawing on resources within the body to provide the energy and oxygen your body needs to either "fight or flee." The changes that occur in the body can be helpful or harmful depending on your particular response, how long the changes last, and the coping strategies you use to combat stress.

When you find yourself in a stressful situation, one of the first things that happens is activation of a pair of tiny glands in the body called the *adrenals*. The adrenal glands are controlled by brain cells, and their primary mission in life is to produce a chemical, or hormone, called cortisol, which converts stored energy into usable energy. Without this chemical, which signals the fight or flight response, you could not possibly survive an emergency. Today our stressors come in the form of perpetual voice mail, E-mail, and junk mail, telephones, cell phones, pagers, and faxes 24-7—all while we're juggling marriage, kids, and other commitments.

If you have an acute, stressful emergency that lasts for only a short time, no permanent physical damage is usually done. (In biological terms, a short time would be a few hours, perhaps even a couple of days.) Yet if the stress becomes chronic and lingers for weeks or months, then problems arise and processes that are essential to your health become impaired. (For some of us, even daily short-term events are too much!) This is because the same chemicals, including cortisol, that help mobilize resources within the body during the emergency are also capable of damaging certain systems. For example, elevated levels of cortisol for extended periods of time will inhibit the ability of white cells to combat viruses or bacterial infections. When memory centers within the brain become bathed in high levels of cortisol, it's more difficult to encode information into memory, and you become forgetful. If the autonomic nervous system, which controls various functions such as heart rate, blood pressure, and intestinal movement, gets out of balance, problems within the cardiovascular and gastrointestinal systems may very well occur and you may experience heart palpitations or diarrhea. How can stress influence the likelihood of becoming ill? If stress weakens your immune system, you will be more likely to develop an illness. If you look back over a period of sev-

SELYE'S GENERAL ADAPTATION SYNDROME

The general adaptation syndrome is the predictable sequence of reactions (stages) that we show in response to stressors.

Stage 1: Alarm. You sense danger, and adrenaline begins to flood the bloodstream. This causes your heart rate to quicken and your blood pressure to rise, increasing blood flow to the muscles so you can "fight or flee." A lump develops in your throat, which helps to contract throat muscles and open airways to the lungs.

Stage 2: Resistance. The body tries to recover from the alarm of the first stage. The heart rate and breathing slow down; muscles relax. This normal body state is called homeostasis (balanced). If you have good coping skills, you will bounce back and stay stress-free. If your coping skills are not developed, you may have further distress. I'll show you how to develop those skills later in this chapter.

Stage 3: Exhaustion. If stress is chronic (long-term), your body will pay the price with overtiredness. You may require more sleep yet feel fatigued and have no energy for things you enjoy. Or you may get sick easily. If your coping strategies are not strong, in extreme cases this stage can cause serious illness and even death.

eral years, you may find that the times you developed a cold or flu were right after a stressful event in your life.

Given the evidence that stress contributes to illness, it seems logical to presume that decreasing stress can modulate illness. The most convincing evidence appears in two small but well-done studies by researchers at the UCLA School of Medicine published in *Archives of General Psychiatry*. One six-month study found that patients with malignant melanoma who were trained in relaxation techniques, such as the ones I explain in this chapter, showed significant increases in the number and activity of cancer-slaying natural killer cells. The recently published six-year follow-up found higher mortality (death) among the untrained group.

This is where mind-body "innercise" can help. Most relaxation therapies are based on the premise that the mind and body are interconnected to an extent far surpassing previous assumptions, and physical health and emotional well-being are closely linked. Not only can relaxation therapies increase endorphins so that you experience a positive feeling about the moment, but there are fascinating reports that these therapies can enhance feelings of calmness and that the benefits of these techniques extend throughout the entire day.

In harmony with that belief, we all know that when we have peaceful thoughts, we tend to have comparable emotional and physiological reactions as well—we feel in control of our life and our health. When we have angry or anxious thoughts, we tend to be emotionally aroused, and consequently our physiological reactions are more dramatic and we are prone to making bad health choices. An increasing number of physicians, psychiatrists, and psychologists acknowledge that the way we think, feel, act, and react can be a powerful determinant of physical and mental health.

STRESS ACCELERATES AGING

Over time, stressful or anxious moments accumulate, creating a long-term negative impact on our health, increasing our susceptibility to obesity and a host of lifestyle diseases, such as diabetes and hypertension. According to researchers at Wake Forest University School of Medicine, when we fail to practice a form of stress reduction, the ongoing, sometimes unavoidable small stresses of everyday life accelerate aging.

STRESS TRIGGERS WEIGHT GAIN

Does stress interfere with our ability to make good food choices, or does it actually change our physiology and increase our appetite? From my professional and personal experience, I would respond: both! Let me explain. When our adrenal glands release cortisol during stress, this hormone has a direct impact on the body's blood sugar levels, then triggers the flow of insulin, itself a potent appetite stimulant and fat storage hormone. We know that high levels of cortisol result in increased appetite and fat deposits, typically in the cervical area, trunk, and abdomen, producing the "spare tire" phenomenon.

Stressed spelled backward is desserts. The brain has two energy sources: carbs and water. When stressed, the body becomes dehydrated. Like a hungry newborn, the brain screams to be fed. Most people make the wrong choice and go for food. However, when the food is eaten, only about 20 percent of the energy (calories from the food) reaches the brain. The rest of the calories end up on your hips. This is an important reason to exercise—not eat—when you're stressed. Now if you choose water instead as a source of energy for the brain, this fat storage won't happen because water is calorie-free.

So there you are in a stressful situation, with your appetite increased, and what sounds good? As you may have experienced, it is *not* a salad of fresh field greens but rather the doughnuts in the coffee break room or the double-fudge icing-filled cookies that you bought for your son's lunch. Some stress eaters can't stop until they find foods containing sugar, especially chocolate. Others prefer salty or high-fat foods, such as pizza and cheeseburgers with fries. Then there are the stress eaters who enjoy crunchy foods like chips and granola (that would be me!). In other words, most of us are not immune from choosing the wrong foods or too much food when stressed.

Nancy, an E-mail client, sends me her weekly log every Saturday. One time, she wrote that she'd had "a very stressful eating day." Does this stress-eating pattern look familiar?

Breakfast: ½ grapefruit, 1 slice whole-wheat toast, 5 egg whites, 1 cup soy milk
Lunch: small portion lean steamed fish, cup of spinach, herbal tea, 1 Hershey's chocolate Kiss
Afternoon snack: the rest of the Kisses in the bag
Dinner: bottle of wine (½ each of red and white), garlic bread, pizza
Dessert: ½ pint of Häagen-Dazs Chocolate Brownie with Fudge ice cream (eaten directly from the container)

The obvious answer to stuffing your face when you're stressed is to comfort yourself with an alternate source of relief. For me, exercise helps put my worries in perspective, especially when I exercise outside, where the light gives my mood a boost as well.

Stress-busters. Make a list of favorite workouts and other activities (stress-busters) in your Turnaround Journal. You might include walking your dog, playing outside with your children, gardening or yard work, taking a nature hike, or biking. Some women like to clean their houses when they are super-stressed. If you get aerobic—bend, push,

> ## STRESS RX: SEEK SUPPORT
>
> Overwhelmed? Call a friend. Everyone needs someone to talk to—someone who will listen to your problems, joys, and concerns. Professional therapists can offer support, as well as your peers who are undergoing similar stresses. Often, close friends or family members can assist you in stressful times, but only if they will listen without giving unsolicited advice.

pull, reach—you'll not only have a clean house, but you'll feel less anxiety and be able to face life more positively. I personally believe that an active stress-buster works better than an inactive stress-buster; having a cup of tea to calm down allows your mind to wander back to the Kisses calling your name from the half-empty bag.

I find that it's better to make this list when you're *not* stressed, so you can unemotionally think of healthy choices. Then promise yourself that you will choose exercises from this list the next time stress begins to intrude into your somewhat controlled, hopefully peaceful life.

The Facts on Coping

Whether stress will affect your memory or make you ill depends in large part on the amount of different hormones produced by the body, which influence the immune system. You can counteract the production of these hormones by developing better coping skills. While you cannot change the stressor, you *can* change how you respond to it, as I explain with the following Turnaround strategies.

PERCEPTION

Turnaround Fact 1: We all perceive stress differently.
Turnaround Strategy 1: Change your perception to be positive and resilient.

Stress can be as simple as the way we perceive life. Dr. Dean Ornish tells the story of the father and son who come to the railroad track crossing and are forced to stop because there is a train coming. The father says, "Oh damn, I'm already late, and now I have to wait for this train." The young son responds, "Oh, Dad! We get to watch a train go by!"

Nowadays, it's hard to know exactly what constitutes stress. I mean, what may be painfully stressful for you may not seem like stress for someone else. For instance, fifty-one-year-old Bette from Switzerland loves challenges and has been skiing since childhood at the resorts of the Jungfrau region. But Bette cannot swim and is deathly afraid of the water. When she came to the spa, she said her fear of water created tremendous stress for her because she had to fly over the ocean to get here. On the other hand, I have clients from sunny California who virtually live in the water. Yet if they were to join Bette on the slopes, they would be a disaster waiting to happen. While a Pollyanna attitude may not seem realistic, it may help you move beyond negativity and fear. When fears and doubts creep into your mind, replace these negative thoughts with positive words such as *I can, I will, I am.*

- *Visualize a happy and successful person in your mind.* Know that you are that person.

- *Think you are great; be great.*

- *Take baby steps.* If your perception of a task causes nervousness and trepidation, tackle it one step at a time. For instance, at the spa, we encouraged Bette to start by sticking her feet in the pool while sitting on the side. Then she splashed water all over her body and enjoyed the cooling sensation. Finally, she was able to stand in the shallow end of the pool at about 3 feet deep without trembling. At the end of her spa trip to Hawaii, Bette was in the ocean (with a cute beach attendant), learning to tread water. While this may be easy for you, for Bette it was a major accomplishment. Who knows? Next year she may be snorkeling with the turtles or scuba diving with the tropical fish!

CONTROL

Turnaround Fact 2: Having a sense of control helps buffer stress.

Turnaround Strategy 2: Set a few goals, stay the course, and focus on your Turnaround to feel in control.

When you sense that you have no control in life, emotional excitement (positive feeling) becomes anxiety (negative). For instance, imagine that your life dream was

HOT FLASH!

Morphinelike endorphins are released during exercise that make today's mountains look like molehills. The good news is these mood-elevating nerve chemicals are also linked to appetite control. They may be responsible for a feeling of euphoria and satisfaction; they can also boost tolerance to pain and stress. Your H.E.A.R.T. workout in Zone One will accomplish stress reduction on demand. See TLC 2.

to fly your own plane. Your friend gives you flying lessons for your fortieth birthday, and without hesitation you begin the training classes. Yet on the day of your first solo flight, all the feelings of anticipation and exhilaration have turned to panic and apprehension. Why? You feel insecure and helpless about flying a plane alone.

Feeling a sense of control in life is vital for optimal health, and staying focused on personal and career goals is how you maintain a sense of control—even when everything else looks bleak. It's also important to know your stress point—the load in life that you can handle—and eliminate any obligations or pressures that take you over this mark.

- *To find* your *stress point, make a list of stresses in your life, including obligations and commitments.* Some of these responsibilities you must live with, such as being part of a family, going to work, and paying bills. But there are some obligations you can eliminate if they are overloading your system.

- *Eliminate any controllable situation in your life that causes you stress.* For instance, avoid stressful situations such as heavy traffic, loud noises, large crowds, long lines at the grocery store, or making hasty decisions when you feel uptight.

- *Accept those pressures that you cannot escape—such as illness in the family, a limited budget, or problems with a coworker—and learn to live with them.* Acceptance will enable you to deal with the moment and unleash pent-up emotion in a positive manner.

- *Focus on the tangible things in life that you do have complete control over—*things like choosing healthy foods, exercising in the morning, drinking water all day, and eliminating alcohol. Taking control of your health translates to feeling in control of your life.

COPING STYLES

Turnaround Fact 3: Personal coping styles determine how stress will affect us.
Turnaround Strategy 3: Learn new coping styles so that stress does not overwhelm you.

How we cope with stress is an important factor in how it will affect our health. We all have different coping mechanisms for dealing with stress—some better than others. Naturally, the better you are at coping, the less likely chronic stress will affect your body in a negative way. For instance, my husband, Michael, waits until the very last minute to finish a project. He thrives under pressure and does a superb job, and it causes no undue stress on his body. In contrast, I must plan my projects carefully and allow time for completion—ahead of the deadline. I know that for me the stress from waiting until the last minute would result in some negative effects. To learn new coping styles, try the following:

- *Avoid negative thinking.* Instead of thinking, "Why should I start exercising again? I'll just stop after a while and gain back the weight as always," analyze and counter the negative thought. You can change this thought to: "My Turnaround seems easy to implement, and wearing my heart-rate monitor will keep me at a pace that feels good to me. If it feels good, I'll stay with the plan."

● *Consider: "What's the worst that can happen?"* So many women—mostly perfectionists—anguish over all that can go wrong when they apply for a new job, change their hairstyles, or start a new eating plan. When you feel stress beginning to build, I want you to write down the worst that can happen. Chances are that *none* of these outcomes will occur at all, but you'll know that you've considered the worst—and tackle the project with a positive outlook. I always say to my kids, "A few mistakes are worth making on the road to a new and better existence."

PERSONALITY

Turnaround Fact 4: Personality type has a profound impact on our susceptibility to illness.

Turnaround Strategy 4: Identify your personality type, and work on negative attributes that could make you sick.

If you are a perfectionist, high achiever, and march to the beat of a fast drummer, chances are that you have a Type A personality. Type A is usually a slave to the clock and rarely stops to "smell the roses," or enjoy life. Mindfulness has little meaning for Type A people—they are forward-thinking, futuristic, and running fast to get there before anyone else.

Type B? You are simply the opposite of Type A. You are just as bright and successful, but you know when to turn off the lights and get in bed, and chances are that you've also finished that novel you were reading and had quality time with your family today.

There are other personality characteristics that can become barriers to your ability to deal effectively with stress, setting you up for all sorts of physical and emotional problems. Someone with a Type C personality is extremely passive, seeking to please everyone. Studies show that Type C personalities are more vulnerable to infections and illness because they allow their actions to be dictated by others and feel little control over their own destiny. In fact, the Type C personality has been correlated with some types of cancer.

Type T—thrill-seeking—is still another personality type. The biggest reason that Type T people have a decreased life span is not because they are passive or have little control; it's because they are daring and take risks, either with drugs or alcohol or with physical actions.

No matter what type of personality you have—and you may be a composite of all four types—understanding why you make the choices you do is important. Check out some ways to modify these personality traits:

- Type A's can recognize the warning signs of too much pressure and intentionally slow down using the Total Life Change suggestions (the relaxation response, deep breathing, meditation, yoga, or heart-rate biofeedback). Make time daily—or several times a day—to quiet your inner storm.

- Type C's can identify their likes and dislikes and become more assertive in sharing these with others, particularly when placed in a situation where they need to give their honest opinion.

- Type T's must evaluate lifestyle habits that put them at high risk for illness or that may harm them, such as elicit drug use or risky sexual behavior. It's hard to deal with life's stressors if you are not balanced 99 percent of the time.

Whatever your stress response, you can learn to manage daily stress just as you do other areas of your life. The key to reducing stress lies in recognizing its visible and invisible signs and taking active steps to reduce the stress before it further injures your health, self-esteem, and relationships.

_____

Mind-Body Medicine

Many people think that psychology (the mind) and physiology (the body) are separate, but research now shows a biomolecular basis for our emotions and provides the scientific explanation for the mind-body connection. Years of study in the relatively new field of psychoneuroimmunology (PNI) continue to document the two-way communication. Interest in the mind's role in the cause and course of cancer has been greatly stimulated by the discovery of the complex interactions between the mind and the neurological and immune systems. Many areas of both medical and psychological research are participating in the exciting field of PNI.

STRESS RX: LEARN TO SAY NO

Saying no, when appropriate, can bring your stress to a manageable level and give you some control over your life. Write down several polite ways you could say no to a friend. For example, you might say:

"No, I'm in over my head at work already."

"No, I don't feel comfortable doing that."

"Yes, I do want to help at school, but I've planned to take some necessary time out for me this weekend."

When you are able to follow through with your commitments, you can live your life without undue pressure and stress. In other words, sometimes saying no is the best weapon against feeling overwhelmed.

The clinical name for this new research is mind-body medicine. Most traditional Eastern medical systems make use of the connection between mind and body and the power of each to affect the other. Science now realizes that therapies, interventions, and lifestyle changes do not have impact on just the mind or just the body—mind, body, and spirit are one entity.

Although there is some belief among the most conservative Western health-care professionals that alternative therapies should be separate from mainstream medicine, there are many renowned medical schools that now teach varied types of alternative therapies. I know that 75 of the 125 medical schools in the United States—60 percent—now offer courses in alternative medicine. Duke University's Department of Psychiatry currently has a $4.3 million grant to study the herb Saint-John's-wort. The Center for Aging at Duke receives significant funding to study the effects of spirituality and religion on health. In related clinical research, the Durham Veterans Administration Medical Center is sponsoring the MANTRA project, in which patients undergoing cardiac catheterization are randomized to a control group or one of four complementary therapies, including meditation, imagery, healing touch, or remote prayer by several off-site prayer groups from around the world. Other well-known medical schools, such as Harvard and Stanford, are also integrating alternative therapies into their conventional medical curriculum.

Scientific evidence has established that many diseases result from repeated exposure to stress and that between 60 and 90 percent of visits to physicians are prompted by stress-related conditions. With all these statistics available, I have great hope that doctors and insurance companies will continue to support more alternative therapies for us in the future.

The Placebo Response

Even though scientists don't agree about the validity of the placebo response, it continues to play an interesting role in research into mind-body interplay. Placebos are usually viewed as fake treatments (like sugar pills) that doctors use to calm anxious patients or indulge insatiable ones. In controlled studies, scientists and researchers give placebo pills or interventions to one group of subjects, leading them to believe that they are getting the cure. The other group gets the real thing. In a "double-blind" study, the doctor is not aware which subjects get the placebo. It has been found that a placebo produces a beneficial effect on most common ailments, including asthma, headache, gastrointestinal problems, angina pectoris, herpes simplex, and duodenal ulcer. Three elements are involved in this effect:

1. Positive belief and expectations by the patient
2. Positive belief and expectations by the physician and/or health-care provider
3. A good relationship between physician and patient

It has been found that 30 to 40 percent of those treated respond to a placebo, and 55 percent respond to a placebo that's given for pain relief. How can anyone discount a mind-body connection with such a high success rate? Use this connection for wellness and stress reduction whenever you can.

The placebo effect relies heavily on your belief system as well as on an intimate relationship between doctor and patient. It also reflects the ultimate confidence we place in a physician's advice. Perhaps it should be mandatory that the medical community give further training to doctors on understanding the placebo effect and how to use it to keep us well.

> ## STRESS RX: YOUR H.E.A.R.T. WORKOUT (TLC 2)
>
> Continue to do your H.E.A.R.T. workout in Zone One during times of chronic stress. Exercise improves your mood, lowers your heart rate, and helps reduce stress hormones like cortisol, which damage your body and age you on a minute-to-minute basis. Aerobic activity can reduce anxiety, tension, and stress while it promotes clear thinking.

Not only has the placebo effect been ignored by conventional medicine, the therapeutic effect of a regular spiritual practice has been neglected in the teaching and practice of modern medicine. Although this area is just now being investigated by scientists and doctors such as Larry Dossey, Andrew Weil, and Herbert Benson, until there is conclusive evidence that can be seen under a microscope, we may not be hearing much about it on CNN. Of course, the link between spiritual health and physical health is spelled out loud and clear in religious texts that have been around for thousands of years.

Mind-Heart Energy

Molecular biologists, neurocardiologists, and biophysicists have discovered the power of the heart as a viable force on our mind, body, and spirit. Combined research in these fields is pointing to the heart as a major center of intelligence in human beings.

Molecular biologists have discovered that the heart is the body's most important endocrine gland. In response to world experiences, the heart produces and releases a major hormone, atriol neuriatic factor, which profoundly affects every

> "Great men are they who see that spiritual is stronger than any material force, that thoughts rule the world."
> —Ralph Waldo Emerson

operation in the limbic structure, or what is referred to as the *emotional brain*. The limbic structure is located just below the cortex of the brain.

Neurocardiologists have found that from 60 to 65 percent of the heart cells are actually neural cells, not muscle cells, as was once believed. These neural cells are identical to the cells in the brain. Quite literally, there is a "brain" in the heart that is linked to every major organ in the body and to the systems that enable humans to express their emotions. The emotional brain evaluates our experiences and instantly sends its opinion to the heart. In return, the heart advises the brain as to the appropriate response. In other words, our heart seems to be contributing to the decisions we make.

Biophysicists have discovered that the heart generates the strongest electromagnetic field produced by the body—forty to sixty times greater than that produced by the brain. When you are in a loving or caring state this field becomes stronger and can extend out 8 to 10 feet, positively affecting those around you. Try it right now. Put your arms around a loved one, and send a loving thought from your heart.

Make an effort to use mind-heart energy when you have conversations with family members, good friends, or even strangers. As you speak, shift the source of energy for your words from your brain to your heart. Give the conversation your undivided loving and caring attention, and you will both benefit greatly. Practice spending the majority of your day listening to the information your heart is sending to your brain. It is within our power to create a joint venture between head intelligence and heart wisdom and live a more balanced, healthy, and effective life.

Studies of practitioners who use therapeutic touch and other forms of energy-based healing, such as Reiki, have demonstrated increased rates of wound healing, hemoglobin levels, pain control, and reduced mental (and heart) stress. By practicing regular meditative activity, cultivating meaningful social support, adopting a positive attitude, and exercising mindfully, we can begin to make a greater connection.

In Hawaii it is customary to hug, hold, and kiss everyone when you greet them and say good-bye. You can fully experience mind-heart energy right now by touching and being touched. Have (or give) a massage, hold your children, and hug everyone.

The 24-Hour Turnaround

While stress does give us an adrenaline boost to perform at our best, most of us become so used to living with high levels of adrenaline that feeling frazzled *feels very normal*. Although stress begins in the mind, it winds up in the body, causing all sorts of detrimental physical symptoms and ultimately leading to burnout and serious illness. When this harried pace continues unchecked day after day, your nerves become hypersensitive, making you irritable and reactive to any additional stress that perhaps you hadn't planned on. You may become plagued by poor concentration, forgetfulness, insomnia, and chronic anxiety.

USE AN INDIVIDUALIZED APPROACH TO HALT STRESS

Trust me, there is a better way. Life is too short and precious to be lived this way, especially with all the new research on stress and related symptoms. But destressing must be individualized. Starting today, you can do something positive to counteract your body's reaction to stress *before* your nervous system goes into high gear.

All the mind-body innercise techniques in this chapter focus on the breath to relax your mind. Some techniques, such as meditation, are more spiritual than others and require a greater amount of time to learn and practice. Other innercise techniques, like deep breathing, can be learned quickly and used anytime, even in a stressful client meeting or when you're stuck in traffic during rush hour, as you quietly change the way you breathe to calm the body and mind.

Choosing the mind-body technique

STRESS RX: TAKE A TIME-OUT

Before you reach your breaking point from life's unending stressors, take a time-out for solitude. Being alone does not mean feeling lonely, for we can feel lonely in the midst of a crowd or even sitting with our family and friends. Being alone can help you find meaning in your life. Take time to nurture yourself away from the cares and responsibilities of the world. Find time to create inner strength and mind, body, and spiritual healing.

that works best for you is basically trial and error—trying the different exercises and finding the one that fits best with your philosophy of life and daily schedule, and that provides the greatest stress reduction or healing benefit. Props are not a necessity for deep breathing, meditation, yoga, or other stress-reduction techniques, although some people may choose to include incense, candles, music, or religious symbols to help put them in a meditative mind-set.

At the spa we offer many wonderful techniques for stress reduction and anti-aging. If you want to learn to meditate or practice qi gong, we have private and group sessions. If you are a golfer, the "Inner Game of Golf" will teach you mental focusing techniques to use on and off the course. The oceanside yoga class has changed the path of many, and the heart-rate biofeedback technique is a lifesaver for both acute and chronic long-term stress relief. I assure you, the magical tropical setting and the ions from the crystal blue water are enough to help you forget the stress you left behind.

Until you come to Hawaii and check into the spa, I can only counsel you on how very important this Total Life Change will be to your 24-Hour Turnaround. Until then, consider the following destressing tips from the spa's experts. Explore the options that appeal to you, and take advantage of the potential to enhance your health and happiness.

THE RELAXATION RESPONSE

The relaxation response is the opposite of the fight-or-flight response. The relaxation response is essentially a decrease in sympathetic arousal that can be elicited by many different interventions, such as meditation, breathing exercises, prayer, and other techniques that are easy to learn.

In 1974 the Harvard cardiologist Herbert Benson, M.D., author of *The Relaxation Response* and founder of the Mind-Body Medical Institute, showed that experienced meditators could produce dramatic changes in their physiology while meditating. Specifically, they were able to decrease their pulse and respiratory rates, decrease oxygen consumption, and change EEG patterns. Benson termed the combination of these physiological changes with a decrease in anxiety and hostility *the relaxation response.*

There are two steps necessary to elicit the relaxation response:

1. The repetition of a word, sound, or prayer
2. A passive return to the repetition when everyday thoughts or worries interfere with the practice

Here's how you can produce the relaxation response:

1. Set aside a period of about 20 minutes that you can devote to relaxation practice. Remove outside distractions that can disrupt your concentration: turn off the radio, the television, even the ringer on the telephone.

2. Lie flat on a bed or the floor, or sit comfortably so that your whole body is relaxed, relieving as much tension or tightness in your muscles as you can. You can use a pillow or cushion under your head if this helps.

3. During the 20-minute period, remain as still as possible. Focus on a word, sound, or line in a prayer, and ignore any outside thoughts that may compete for your attention.

4. Concentrate on breathing evenly. As you exhale, picture your muscles becoming even more relaxed, as if you were somehow breathing the tension away.

5. After 20 minutes, take a few moments to study and focus on the feelings and sensations you have been able to achieve. Notice whether areas that felt tight and tense at first now feel more loose and relaxed, and whether any areas of tension or tightness remain.

DEEP BREATHING

OXYGEN DELIVERY AND THE H.E.A.R.T. WORKOUT

The circulatory system is made stronger and more efficient by the H.E.A.R.T. workout. Use your heart-rate monitor and your Zone One prescription, and eliminate high-intensity exercise, which promotes oxygen deficit (lack of oxygen).

Breathing is the way you oxygenate your body and stimulate the electrical processes of your cells. The bloodstream is the circulation system that transports oxygen to all the cells of your body. Blood is pumped from your heart through your arteries, carrying oxygen and nutrients to the capillaries, which deliver both to the cells. The cells take what oxygen and nutrients they need and then excrete toxins, some of which go back into the capillaries. The rest of the toxic material must be removed by the lymph system. Deep breathing activates the lymph system. The body's cells depend on the lymph system as the only way to drain off the large toxic molecules and excess fluid, which restrict the amount of available oxygen. Deep breathing and exercise can accelerate this entire process by as much as fifteen times.

Dr. Otto Warburg, Nobel Prize winner and director of the Max Planck Institute for Cell Physiology, studied the effect of oxygen on cells. He was able to turn normal, healthy cells into malignant or cancerous cells simply by lowering the amount of oxygen they received. (Decreased oxygen to the cells can also result from high-intensity exercise.) Remember that the quality of your health is only as good as the quality of your cells. Fully oxygenating your system should be a number-one priority, and breathing effectively is certainly the place to start.

● *Turnaround Fact: Breathing helps to control your appetite.* I'm sorry I can't patent that concept and sell it! Researchers theorize that when the cells' craving for the most important nutrient (oxygen) is satisfied, the appetite is diminished. There is also a psychological link between deep breathing and the desire for food. For instance, when people get stressed or worried, many tend to reach for food as a comfort. By using deep breathing to reduce your stress level, you more effectively disengage the emotional link between food and appetite. The H.E.A.R.T. method is an "oxygenated" workout, which is one of the main reasons it is guaranteed to decrease your appetite and trigger weight loss. So—go for the oxygen and zero calories!

- *Turnaround Fact: Breathing affects your health.* We know that illness can be directly related to shallow, inadequate breathing patterns. Getting oxygen to the cells by deep breathing is the simplest, most fundamental method of giving those cells what they need. When used in combination with diet and exercise, deep breathing can have a very positive effect on your heart and your general health.

- *Turnaround Fact: Breathing influences your emotions.* Your brain and respiration are linked neurologically. Emotions, memory, and even motivation are affected by the limbic center of the brain. This part of the brain is connected to the lungs and diaphragm through the vagus nerve. In fact, this is the mechanism that accounts for yoga's profound effect. Yoga uses deliberate breathing patterns to influence the mind-body connection and heighten emotional well-being. Deep breathing (like that practiced in yoga) quiets your mind and brings about calmness. Calmness also increases mental and visual acuity and improves memory.

- *Turnaround Fact: Deep breathing improves your sleep.* It does this by slowing many of the body's metabolic processes, such as blood pressure, pulse rate, and brain wave activity. To fall asleep faster, focus on your breath and breath deeply. (This is a great time to read your CVEA script— TLC 1—for a 24-hour motivation boost.)

Learn TLC breathing. There is an old proverb that states, "Life is in the breath. He who half breathes, half lives." Breathing can alter your psychological state, making a stressful moment accelerate or diminish in intensity. Think about how your respiration quickens when you are fearful or in great pain and how taking a deep, slow breath can be calming and reduce stress.

Use TLC breathing anytime you feel tense, anxious, or need to boost your inner confidence, such as before you give a speech, during an important meeting, or when you're waiting in a long line of people (or cars). As you learn to do the TLC breathing, you will gain control over basic physiological functions, helping to decrease the release of stress hormones and slow down your heart rate during anxious moments. Also, by adding oxygen to the blood, you cause the body to release endorphins—the hormones that give you a greater sense of well-being and contentment.

1. Sit upright in a comfortable chair with your feet on the floor. Or sit on the floor with your legs crisscrossed and your feet as close to your groin as possible. Rest your hands on your knees with the palms facing upward. (If you're at the office, rest your forearms on your desk.)

2. With your eyes closed, inhale slowly through your nose by using your diaphragm. Let the air expand your belly, and keep your chest quiet. (You can place one hand on your chest and the other on your abdomen to make sure the abdomen is rising but not the chest. The chest should remain still to do this correctly.)

3. Once your lungs are full, hold your breath (comfortably) to fully oxygenate the blood.

4. Exhale for twice as long as your inhalation count. The exhalation phase is the most beneficial to the mind and body because this is when the endorphins (the "feel good" hormones) are released. The exhalation provides the most relaxation. Exhaling for twice as long also eliminates toxins by way of your lymphatic system. (Try using this breathing cycle with your heart-rate monitor—biofeedback—and kill the proverbial two birds.)

Ch'i **breathing.** *Ch'i* breathing is more spiritual than TLC breathing and can be used to strengthen the powerful connection between your mind, heart, and the universe. Because *ch'i* is the power of all life that is within you, use *ch'i* breathing to take time out for personal healing, reflection, and meditation. *Ch'i* breathing will help you find comfort and reassurance as you get in touch with your inner spirit.

1. Stand up tall. Think of your heart/chest as being lifted. Keep your lips touching, and breath only through your nose. Place your left hand below your navel with your thumb in your navel. Place the other hand on your heart.

2. Inhale through your nose, breathing in *ch'i* from the universe, and expand the diaphragm and lower abdomen while pushing on your hand. Your chest and shoulders should not move.

3. Exhale through your nose. Imagine the *ch'i* power and light within you traveling from your abdomen up your spine, past your heart, over the top of your head, and out through your nose.

4. Continue the practice until you feel the *ch'i* power within you. You will be calm and confident and feel a sense of warmth. Your health and well-being increase with each *ch'i* breath.

MEDITATION

Part of the New Age culture in the past decade has been a proliferation of meditation practices introduced in the West. Meditation, a way of relaxing the body and quieting the mind, came from Eastern spiritual traditions. However, meditation, prayer, and reflection are the foundations of all the great spiritual traditions. For instance, Christianity, Judaism, Buddhism, and Islam all use repetitive prayers, chants, or movements as part of their worship rituals. The Catholic practice of using rosary beads while saying the "Hail Mary" is a familiar example.

Health benefits. Meditation is easy to learn and can be practiced individually or in groups. It requires no change in your belief system and does not conflict with any religious practice. During the past fifteen years, it has been explored as a way of reducing stress on both mind and body. A landmark study of patients with heart disease, conducted by Dr. Dean Ornish, was one of the first to document significant health improvements when meditation was combined with diet and exercise. A comprehensive study reported in the American Heart Association's journal *Stroke* concluded that meditation by itself reduced the incidence of arteriosclerosis even when subjects made no changes to their diet and fitness routine.

Research has shown that meditation can save millions of dollars in health-care costs annually. A six-year study of Canadian citizens in Quebec who were enrolled in the government health insurance program showed that those practicing Transcendental Meditation for just 20 minutes daily required less care by their physicians than the control group. This translated into savings of more than $300 million over the course of six years for the province's health insurance company.

Effects on aging. While modern science tells us that the aging process is not reversible, at least three scientists have demonstrated that, contrary to conventional wisdom, physical aging can be slowed down and even reversed. In 1978 R. Keith Wallace, a UCLA physiologist, demonstrated the direct effects of meditation on aging. He measured three biological markers: blood pressure, vision, and hearing. Those who had practiced meditation for less than five years had an average biological age (according to physiological tests) that was functionally five years lower than their chronological age would indicate. But those who had practiced meditation for more than five years tested up to twelve years younger in functional biological age. In other words, regular meditation lowers your functional age, making you in effect younger.

Deepak Chopra, M.D., and his colleague Jay Glaser, M.C., also demonstrated that meditation reverses biological aging. As described in Chopra's book *Ageless Body, Timeless Mind,* in 1988 he and Glaser conducted a research project to study the effects on aging of the hormone DHEA, a hormone that reaches its highest levels in our bodies when we're twenty-five. Whenever you have a stress reaction, a portion of your DHEA supply is used up to make various stress-related hormones, such as adrenaline and cortisol. Thus DHEA levels are reliable markers for the body's exposure to stress over time. In the study, Glaser examined the DHEA levels of 328 meditators and 1,462 nonmeditators. In all the women's groups, DHEA levels were higher among meditators; the same was true in eight out of eleven of the men's groups. Glaser and Chopra concluded that meditation reduces biological aging as measured by DHEA levels. The most pronounced differences showed up in the older subjects. Meditating men over age forty-five had 47 percent more DHEA than men and women five to ten years younger. These levels were independent of diet, exercise, weight, and alcohol consumption. Yes, you can stop the clock and halt or even reverse the signs of aging!

Mindfulness. So many people these days feel blown around like a leaf in the wind by their thoughts, emotions, and difficult circumstances that arise in everyday life. Mindfulness meditation practice is concerned with developing the capacity and strength of mind to be more present with what arises moment to moment in the living of life and less reactive to whatever life brings us. It is a simple yet effective stress-reduction technique that teaches people to acknowledge fears and worries, yet keep them in balance with more positive feelings.

Mindfulness may be considered a philosophy as well as a meditation practice, its principle: being in the moment. I often find myself trying to get two things done at once. Talking on the phone while doing dishes is normal for me. And here's a confession: eating and writing this book is another. (*Jay, practice what you preach!*) Mindfulness is the antithesis of living on "automatic pilot." Strength and maturity of mind are called mindfulness. The ultimate goal of mindfulness meditation is to be more aware of whatever is happening with your body, mind, and spirit at this moment in time and to accept it.

> ## HEALTH BENEFITS OF MEDITATION
>
> Increased longevity and quality of life
> Reduced appetite
> Increased sexual function
> Reduced chronic pain
> Reduced anxiety
> Reduced serum cholesterol level
> Reduced substance abuse
> Increased intelligence
> Reduced post-traumatic stress disorder
> Lower blood pressure and blood cortisol levels
> Reduced aging hormones

With mindfulness, your goal is to develop a mind that is present, spacious, loving, and accepting of what is. In his book *In the Lap of the Buddha,* Gavin Harrison says, "In meditation we cultivate a new relationship with what is happening in our lives. Meditation does not take away or add anything to our experience. Rather it offers the possibility of finding balance and equanimity in all the changes."

"Thought is the seed of action."

—Ralph Waldo Emerson

How to meditate. My favorite place to meditate is outdoors in a very quiet place. There's something about being in nature that helps me connect to the bigger picture instead of merely focusing on my personal existence. It also seems to validate that I *am* a part of the big picture.

As you practice mindfulness meditation, choose a place that is comfortable and quiet. Try sitting on the floor Indian-style, upright with your back straight (a pillow

ONE IN SPIRIT

Realizing that we are more than a physical body enhances our Turnaround. How many times are we so inundated with life's stressors that we forget about the important aspect of human development called spirituality? By spirituality I mean the inner search for a sense of connection and meaning in life, a sense of optimism and hope that can carry us through difficult times. Spirituality gives you a sense of consciousness, insight, and perception, not only into your own feelings and personal beliefs but into the lives and needs of others—family members, friends and enemies, colleagues and coworkers, even strangers on the street. Spirituality also helps shape your approach to all aspects of life, including your personal and career goals and daily choices. And spiritual maturity brings with it important core values—self-respect, tolerance, responsibility, integrity, morality, honesty, and benevolence. It is a key factor in how you cope with the trials and tribulations of life. In my experience and observations, I know that spiritual poverty can leave a grave emptiness and loneliness, especially during rough or frightening times. No matter what you are faced with, an inner spiritual strength will sustain you.

is optional). Or sit on a chair with your feet flat on the ground and your hands relaxed on your knees or lap.

Begin your meditation with your eyes closed, focusing on your breath and the sensations of air passing in and out of the nostrils—the movement of the breath. You may passively observe flows of thought that occur during the meditation. It is entirely natural to have a stream of thoughts as you sit quietly. Watch each one nonjudgmentally as it comes and goes, like a movie, bringing your attention back to breathing. Don't ignore them, but rather treat them like background noise. Make a mental note (I'm "thinking"), as though the thoughts were something you might want to come back to later. Then return to your breath. A key to mindfulness meditation is the ability to accept rather than judge the wandering thoughts; that is, to let go of anxiety about meditating "correctly." The willingness to go back to the breath again and again is vital. The meditation can end in a certain time frame or when you feel ready to return to activity. Remember that consistency is more important than duration with mindfulness meditation or any relaxation technique.

In one study, people who underwent mindfulness meditation training experienced a 38 percent decrease in their psychological distress levels as well as a 34 percent decrease in depression and a 44 percent reduction in anxiety levels. In another study, medical symptoms were reduced by 46 percent (with no side effects).

HEART-RATE BIOFEEDBACK: THE "QUICK FIX" FOR STRESS RELIEF

I love my yoga practice, yet I rarely have the time to do a full session. So I integrate yoga into the cooldown and stretch after my H.E.A.R.T. workout. I make time to meditate or pray *almost* every morning, whether I'm doing a seminar in Europe or visiting clients in Manhattan. I encourage you to learn one of the relaxation or meditation practices in this chapter. However, one of the principal dilemmas some of my clients have with using their relaxation or meditation training for immediate stress relief is lack of time and lack of transference. That is, techniques that may work well when you're alone for 20 minutes at home are difficult to apply to situations in your busy schedule. It seems all but impossible to calm down when you're hit with problem after problem all day.

Neuroscientists agree that the most effective way to counteract stressful situations is to learn how to respond immediately—stop stress in its tracks! It's much more difficult and time-consuming to reverse tension than to deal with it and put it to rest. This is exactly the reason why I recommend heart-rate biofeedback: it works spontaneously and produces a 24-hour result.

Heart-rate biofeedback is a therapeutic practice that uses your heart-rate monitor to give you instant feedback during your stress-reduction training. Heart-rate biofeedback teaches you how to "relax on demand." If the thought of figuring out how to reduce stress tends to stress you out because it sounds time-consuming to learn to meditate or practice yoga, get out your heart-rate monitor, and I'll teach you a proven technique in 5 minutes.

If you haven't got a heart-rate monitor for your H.E.A.R.T. workouts, you now have two good reasons to get one today. Check my website for the latest monitor recommendations.

Learning heart-rate biofeedback. Learning heart-rate biofeedback takes seven days, but the first session can produce a 24-hour result. The first day takes 5 minutes; the last day takes only 1 minute. The learning curve is zero, the cost is nothing, and everyone in your household or office will benefit.

DAYS 1, 2, AND 3—AT HOME

1. Choose a time when you know you will not be interrupted, and turn off the phone. Put on your monitor and observe your heart rate. Lie down on the floor with something under your neck (a pillow or towel) to relax the neck area and put your spine in a neutral position. You might want a pillow under your knees as well, especially if you have back problems.

2. Rest the watch of your monitor where you can look at it occasionally. I like to rest my hands on my chest with the watch in one hand.

3. Continue by relaxing all the muscles in your face—around your eyes, your jaw, and your forehead. Make sure your teeth are not touching. Take the deepest breath you have ever taken and exhale. On that exhale relax every muscle in your body. Feel your heart rate slowing.

4. Continue to breathe deeply and slowly. Check to see if you can feel your shoulders, back, hips, and legs on the floor. They should feel heavy.

5. Observe your heart rate. As you begin to relax, your heart rate will go down. Repeat steps 3 and 4. Every time you look at your heart rate, it should be lower. If you get anxious or the number goes up, start over. End the session after 5 minutes regardless of the outcome.

DAYS 4 AND 5—AT HOME

1. Choose a time when you know you will not be interrupted, and turn off the phone. Put on your monitor, and observe your heart rate. Sit in a chair with your feet flat on the floor.

2. Rest your hands on your lap with your shoulders relaxed. Hold your monitor watch in your hand where you can see it.

3. Start by relaxing all the muscles in your face—around your eyes, your jaw, and your forehead. Make sure your teeth are not touching. Take the deepest breath you have ever taken and exhale. On that exhale relax every muscle in your body.

4. Continue to breathe deeply and slowly; scan your body and relax all your muscles.

5. Observe your heart rate. Repeat steps 3 and 4. Every time you look at your heart rate, it should be lower. If you get anxious or the number goes up, start over. End the session after 3 minutes.

BIOFEEDBACK SUCCESS STORY

I have a client who runs a huge corporation in New York. He has mastered the biofeedback technique to the point where he can lower his blood pressure and heart rate in the middle of a board meeting by just pausing between comments and taking a long, slow breath. His cardiologist is extremely impressed because it has been only one year since his last heart attack. By the way, he has been off his blood pressure medication for six months.

DAYS 6 AND 7—AT WORK OR DURING A STRESSFUL TIME OF DAY

1. Choose a time when you know you will not be interrupted, and turn off the phone. If you're not in an office or at home, go to a quiet place or your car. Put on your monitor and observe your heart rate. Rest your arms on your desk or your lap with your monitor watch in front of you. Your arms need to feel heavy in order to relax your neck.

2. You should now be able to do your relaxation exercise in 1 minute with your heart rate dropping after the first few exhales.

3. Practice your biofeedback at any time of the day that you feel stress coming on. Eventually you will get so good at "relaxing on demand" that you won't need to put your monitor on.

YOGA

I have a good friend and client who was very inflexible (in more ways than short muscles). I suggested that he try yoga, and I found a highly recommended teacher who could go to his home. Upon her arrival, he said, "You know, I'm only doing this so I can be more flexible for tennis. I don't care about the rest of the stuff." To that she replied, "Well, that is a *very* good place to start."

This ancient Indian practice allows you to experience your body (life force) from the inside out. The Western traditions typically look at the body from the outside in, taking it one layer at a time, believing only what can be seen, measured, and proved in randomized, double-blind tests. The East treats the person; the West treats the disease. Yoga is holistic, integrating the body, breath, and mind. Some people use it for stretching purposes only, while others prefer the more aerobic yoga positions to get a good cardiovascular and stretching workout. Many use yoga for stress reduction.

It has been eighty years since health professionals in both India and the West started investigating the therapeutic life change potential of yoga. Thousands of research studies have shown that with the practice of yoga you can learn to control your heart rate, brain wave patterns, blood pressure, respiratory function, metabolic rate, skin resistance, body temperature, and many other bodily functions.

Regular yoga practice has also been shown to reduce cholesterol levels (when combined with a low-fat diet and exercise) and increase cardiovascular circulation. Exercise in general activates the flow of lymph through the body, speeding up the filtering process, but yoga in particular promotes the draining of the lymph. Yoga has helped people stop smoking and has been successful in preventing and treating arthritis, among other ailments.

Dr. Dean Ornish is convinced that adherence to a yoga and meditation program is strongly correlated with changes in the amount of artery blockage, as is adherence to a very-low-fat diet. In 1998 Ornish published a study in the *American Journal of Cardiology* stating that 80 percent of the 194 patients in an experimental group were able to avoid bypass surgery or angioplasty by adhering to lifestyle changes, including yoga.

Yoga or Prozac? The pharmaceutical industry is making billions by promoting the concept that our "problem" is altered brain chemistry, and if we take a pill, we'll be okay. Consider that $44 billion is spent annually on Prozac and other antidepressants. Researchers tell us that Prozac or one of the other selective serotonin reuptake inhibitors can increase the amount of serotonin in our brains, and we may feel better.

But what affects the balance of serotonin in the brain? You guessed it: stress. It's obvious to me that the stress that comes along with our modern culture is the reason we have a "national serotonin deficiency," causing depression or at the very least bad moods in epidemic proportions.

Inverted postures in yoga have been used for thousands of years to alter mood. I have prescribed yoga to hundreds of my clients who are on Prozac for the following reason: the inverted positions alter the blood flow. With increased blood flow to the brain comes the availability of glucose (carbs). In the upside-down positions we produce our very own neurotransmitters, which by the way have no side effects. Both yoga and meditation can be practiced to increase your own production of serotonin. Forward-bending poses also massage the organs in the neuroendocrine axis, alleviating mood swings and insomnia associated with menopause and PMS.

How to start a yoga practice. There are many styles and methods of yoga to choose from. If you have never done yoga, you are considered to be a beginner (Level 1). I learned this the hard way! Years ago, prior to starting my yoga practice, I visited a popular yoga studio in California and chose a Level 3 class, thinking, "No problem, I'm very fit. Of course I can easily do this." Out of fifty people, I was the *only* student who could not hold the poses. The message? Start at the beginning. Learn how to do each pose correctly. Take several classes from different teachers and find a style that you like. Some are geared toward strength and stamina; others toward relaxation. I do not recommend learning yoga from a book, although there are some good books for people who already have yoga experience. There are also many good tapes and CDs available, which I list on my website.

I realize that there are only so many hours in the day, and yoga can be time-consuming to learn and practice. If you are short on time, start with a 10-minute routine in the morning or evening hours. (Be sure to watch for our *Yoga Stretches for the Office* offered on my website.)

Integrate yoga and H.E.A.R.T. exercise. After you finish your H.E.A.R.T. workout, replace your stretching with the sun salutation, a series of yoga postures linked together as one fluid movement (see pages 116 to 118). The sun salutation includes a standing stretch for your legs and upper body. End with a 5-minute meditation, and your inner and outer workout will be complete. Find a trained yoga instructor to show you the sun salutation postures to make sure you do them correctly. Most yoga studios have instructors who can teach this ancient discipline.

FOR YOUR HUSBAND

Given all the cold hard facts about stress, it would seem that it's important to learn to relax on demand—even if it means actively ignoring the source of your stress. I know it's hard to convince a man to do this; I'm married to a man who cannot relate to this concept. So . . . the next best thing is to tell your husband that he can learn a quick and easy technique to reduce or reverse stress and give him your heart-rate monitor to use. (C'mon, we all know that men love toys.) Tell him that heart-rate biofeedback takes just 5 minutes to learn. He can skip the commercials during the football game, or you can offer to trade off and do the dishes tonight. Heart-rate biofeedback is an incredible destressing technique your husband can use at work in between meetings or phone calls. It could save his life.

FOR YOUR KIDS

Studies have found that music therapy is effective as a relaxant and anxiety reducer for infants and children and that certain music increases the ability to focus and learn. There are several companies that make CDs that can help you improve your ability to focus, learn, and reduce stress. Check my website.

If your children seem interested in learning how to meditate or initiate social change and are looking for other young children with the same interests, there are some unique camps that you can contact:

- Insight Meditation Society—www.dharma.org
- Yes! Action Camps—www.yesworld.org
- E.A.R.T.H. summer camp—www.camppage.com/silverwater

Focus on Your Inner Spirit

Studies show that when you create a strong mental image using mind-body interplay, you can move beyond destructive habits and become centered in a world of health and healing. As you begin to incorporate stress-reduction techniques into your daily regimen, I urge you to include your spiritual side. This force can stem from a belief in God or another external guiding force, or perhaps from resources deep within.

Whether your spiritual belief is based upon the Bible, the Torah, the Koran, the Four Noble Truths of Buddhism, other learned social-cultural codes of behavior, or Nature and Goodness, including this powerful force as you focus on innercise techniques will help you cope with life's adversities while achieving health and happiness.

Namaste—the divine in me bows to the divine in you.

You *Can* Turn Back the Clock: Rewriting the Rules on Aging

ANTIAGING IS A COMMON term today, especially with the millions of baby boomers hitting fifty. But antiaging is *not* just a matter of simply living longer. Antiaging means intentionally *living better*—looking lean, defined, and young, enjoying optimal health and youthfulness no matter what your chronological age; feeling sexy, alert, and energetic; being active, involved, and able to do the things you enjoy. At the top of the list—antiaging is disease prevention. Now that you've made a commitment to the eight TLCs, I want to give you some more information on how they all work together to accomplish your Turnaround antiaging program.

When Rebecca walked into my office last summer, I could hardly believe she had just celebrated her thirtieth birthday. This young mother of twins could easily have passed for forty or even older. Rebecca said that she wanted to lose weight and get back in shape. Having gained more than 60 pounds with her recent pregnancy, she admitted to feasting on powdered sugar doughnuts and corn chips, her "comfort foods," after the doctor ordered her to bed at six months because of complications.

But it wasn't just the weight gain that added years to Rebecca's chronological age; she looked and felt old too. She complained of feeling tired all the time, and her body lacked youthful tone, muscle, and definition. Her eyes were dull and sunken from lack of sleep, her skin tone was red and uneven, and her hair thin and dry. I knew Rebecca had a big challenge ahead to recapture her youthful good looks, but she was committed. She said that she'd felt like this long enough and was ready to make a change. I gave her all the information she needed to start turning her weight and biological age around that very day. The last time I saw Rebecca, she had dropped her weight and looked like the young mom she was so happy to be.

I consult with hundreds of men and women each year, and I'll admit that these days chronological age is sometimes hard to guess. I am always surprised when a client like Rebecca is much younger than her appearance, but I'm never shocked when a client's actual age is years older than she looks. Instead I'm thrilled.

Take Jill, for example. I'm pretty intuitive, and when I first met Jill, I pegged her at around forty. With fierce blue eyes but a calm demeanor, Jill looked extremely healthy, and her skin was taut, without wrinkles or blemishes. When Jill first walked into my office, she dropped her keys and immediately bent over to retrieve them. She was agile, flexible, and had perfect posture when she stood up again.

When I reviewed Jill's records during the consultation and saw that she was fifty-eight years old—almost twenty years older than I had guessed—I was pleasantly surprised. This mother of three and grandmother of eight was actively living *all* her life—looking strong, lean, and healthy. By taking care of herself, Jill was already enjoying both the great looks and the health benefits associated with anti-aging. By adding the 24-Hour Turnaround, she was able to increase her lean muscle mass and strength and ensure herself the protection from several diminishing hormones.

Live Longer, Live Better

Aging, as you may think of it in terms of youthfulness, has *nothing* to do with chronological age or the passing of time. And I will go to my grave maintaining this! While aging is a natural process that happens to everyone, it can be greatly accelerated when we're hit with life's interruptions, including job and marital stress, financial worries, health problems, even raising kids or caring for aging parents. During these periods of chronic stress, most of us tend to sleep less, eat more, and exercise little or not at all. Negative habits like cigarette smoking, snacking on sugary or high-fat foods, or a sedentary lifestyle are also common as we seek comfort and consolation for our woes, *but the clock is ticking, and time is not on our side.* While you may rely on your genes and get to thirty-five or even forty without many visible signs of aging, for most of us genetics subside around midlife and our negative lifestyle habits take over, wreaking havoc on our mental and physical health and our outward appearance. Is it any wonder that:

- Eight million women in the United States have heart disease, and more than 500,000 women die of heart disease each year.
- More than half of all women over forty-five in the United States have hypertension.
- An estimated 8.2 percent of all women in the United States have diabetes, which is associated with obesity.
- A woman's chance of getting breast cancer is one in eight; a woman's chance of dying from breast cancer is one in twenty-eight.
- Thirty million Americans have osteoporosis, a debilitating weakening of the bones that leads to fractures and disfigurement, and 80 percent are women.
- More and more women are experiencing unnecessary skin wrinkling and sagging accompanied by adult acne or rosacea.
- Many women now have prematurely graying and thinning hair associated with poor health.

The statistics are startling. We now know that many chronic diseases and superficial signs of aging once thought to be consequences of growing older are *not* normal progressions and can be prevented with simple changes in lifestyle habits, including diet and exercise. Only 30 percent of the characteristics of aging are genetically based—the remaining 70 percent are not. That means that even if your parents had a chronic illness, you are not destined to *if* you take care of yourself. You will fail from the get-go if you're carrying around the belief that you will get cancer because your father had it or hypertension because your mother was diagnosed with it. If your mother had wrinkles at fifty, it does not have to happen to you. If your older sister has cellulite on her thighs, yours do not have to follow the same course.

Studies on twins make it possible to estimate how much inherited genes contribute to the development of malignant diseases. A Swedish study of 44,788 pairs of twins published in the *New England Journal of Medicine* in 2000 was one of the most elaborate ever performed on the contribution of environment and heredity to the most common forms of cancer. This study demonstrated that inherited genetic factors contribute only slightly to *susceptibility* to most cancers (the findings indicate that the environment is the principal cause of most common forms). However, the researchers also found that a few cancers did have a principal heredity factor, particularly prostate and colorectal. These might be explained by the "hereditary" nature of diet, as families pass dietary, culinary, and a host of other lifestyle habits from one generation to the next, and there is no shortage of carcinogenic habits passed along with them. Obesity and unnecessary aging get passed along with the negative lifestyle habits. In human studies it becomes impossible to separate "nurture" (our food environment) from "nature" (our inherited genetics).

Another superb study published in *Ethnicity and Disease* in 2000 showed that shared environmental factors are important in explaining familial similarities, particularly when coronary heart disease runs along family lines. The genes in our cells determine the hereditary aspects of life, including *susceptibility* to disease. Environmental factors, such as diet and lifestyle and even belief, modify these genetic patterns. The specific actions outlined in the Total Life Changes will help you change destructive lifestyle habits and reduce biological aging along with your risk of disease.

Since we may be spending more time in the "gray zone" than any former generation, staying healthy is more important now than ever before. I know I don't want to live my senior years unable to be active, or dependent on medications to function. That's why it's important to understand up front that *antiaging and disease prevention are one and the same.*

Let's Rewrite the Rules on Aging

Did you know that there are people who live to be ninety or even a hundred without great decline in physical or mental capabilities? On the Japanese island of Okinawa, the residents have the highest proportion of centenarians in the world—33.6 per 100,000 people. A 1999 study reported in the *Johns Hopkins Medical Letter* revealed that Okinawans have 80 percent fewer heart attacks and 75 percent fewer cancers of the breast, ovaries, and prostate than North Americans. Not only are they healthy, they are active, lean, and young-looking people. We know that Okinawans eat twice as much fish as other Japanese citizens, which gives them a hefty dose of heart-healthy long-chain omega-3 fatty acids. The Okinawans also eat two or three times more vegetables than the mainland Japanese. And although the

Okinawans consume fewer calories, they have the highest consumption of soy protein of any population in the world.

"Sure, I'd like to live to be one hundred," Teresa said honestly, "but only if science could promise me good health." Teresa's mother, aunt, and grandmother all developed breast cancer in their forties, and she was desperate for ways to stay well and decrease her risk of this deadly disease. For years most of us have been like Teresa, trusting science, the latest medical data, and cutting-edge research on anti-aging products to determine our longevity and youthful appearance.

I believe it's time to rewrite the rules on aging. While we can learn a great deal from science, it's also important to take personal responsibility for yourself—particularly when it comes to the physical and mental well-being associated with aging. The Okinawans don't rely on science and medication, and if you take care of yourself, you won't have to either.

Defining Aging and Disease

Disease, defined as "lack of health," results when any system, organ, or group of cells is not functioning well due to trauma, toxicity, or stress (physical, emotional, or spiritual). As I tell my clients, we don't "catch" a disease or illness, *we earn it*—and knowing what we do about lifestyle and heart disease, you could say it is a "disease of choice." Even a contagious disease can usually be avoided *if* we take care of our immune system. And I promise you, your outward appearance is a direct result of how you take care of the inner you.

The main purpose of your immune system is to distinguish "self" (you) from "nonself" (a host of invaders) through a complex network of antibodies, proteins, and specialized cells. All these cells have a specific duty, which is to keep you healthy at all costs by assaulting and obliterating foreign materials. You can give your cells ammunition to fight foreign matter by following the TLCs in this book. When you neglect to care for yourself or when you expose yourself to environmental toxins, causing your body chemistry to malfunction, your immune system may fail to protect you as it should, resulting in an infection or disease.

TURNAROUND BRAIN CELLS

For years researchers thought that new brain cells do not form later in life, giving little hope to stroke victims or those who had a degenerative disease that impaired the mind. Some new research proves this theory wrong. We now know that our brain continues to produce new cells until we die. And a study published in *Nature* (March 15, 2001) revealed that newly generated nerve cells quickly adapted in forming new memories in the brain. This is good news for all of us who are interested in keeping our brains young and functional.

Five Key Aging and Disease Triggers

I know it's perplexing when you catch every cold that goes around, yet your best friend is always well. And it may seem unfair that your older sister looks ten years younger than you. Perhaps you wonder why two people who eat the same diet and have the same lifestyle develop different diseases. Or why your grandmother is still healthy at ninety-five even though she has a horrible diet and has smoked cigarettes for most of her life, yet there are children dying of cancer at age five.

The "tendency" to have a particular disease is passed on from parents to offspring through a unique genetic code. This is by no means a guarantee that you will get a certain illness. Rather, it means that you have a "weak link" in the genetic chain. If you don't take care of yourself, you may become more susceptible to getting a certain inherited disease. Genetic weaknesses or tendencies grow with each succeeding generation, but only if the parents have negative habits, such as a poor diet, sedentary lifestyle, cigarette smoking, alcohol consumption, and chronic stress, among many others. And you can create a weak link by living a toxic life and passing this genetic message to your offspring—certainly not a gift you'd want to give. The message: you can protect yourself and your children from your genetic tendencies by practicing all eight TLCs.

Let's look at five aging and disease triggers that can increase your chances of illness and premature aging.

1. TOXINS

Conventional Western medicine focuses on defining disease based on measurable symptoms and then eliminating those symptoms using pharmaceuticals or invasive procedures. In contrast, alternative medicine views symptoms as the body's effort to eliminate toxins while it returns to a state of health. These toxins may come in the form of unstable substances and poisonous metabolic products, or they can come from living organisms such as bacteria. Toxins enter the body primarily in two ways:

- Through the digestive system (ingested)
- Through the respiratory system (inhaled)

When you experience optimal health, the body's natural ability to form antibodies destroys many toxins. The liver neutralizes toxic acids before they enter the bloodstream and branch out to the kidneys, lungs, and bowel. If this filtering process did not occur, the blood would become highly acidic and you would die. But over a period of time, as you eat and breathe more toxins, your liver begins to store these and becomes congested, which decreases its filtering efficiency. Then as the liver becomes increasingly overloaded, it starts to release the toxins into the bloodstream, sending them to all your organs, tissues, and cells, where the toxins are stored unless you are fortunate enough to eliminate them through the skin, the body's largest organ. (Or should I say unfortunate, as this is why our skin ages unnecessarily!) As a result of this long-term storage of toxins, the body tissues involved begin to degenerate, which is known as a chronic degenerative disease.

The fewer toxins you take in and the better you are at eliminating them, the healthier you will be. If they are not eliminated and continue to build, they may result in chronic disease. The Total Life Changes showed you how to boost your body's ability to eliminate toxins by eating a high-fiber diet, increasing fluids, and stimulating your lymph system with the H.E.A.R.T. workout.

2. FREE RADICALS

There is great evidence that aging and many diseases may have their origin in oxygen–free radical reactions, chemical processes that change oxygen to free radicals.

In the body, free radicals can damage the proteins and fats that make up the cell membranes and the DNA in cells. Cells may then leak out vital substances or dangerous chemicals that can spread destruction. While cells usually have defense mechanisms to protect themselves from these potentially destructive chemical products, sometimes the rate of production of free radicals is great enough to overwhelm these defenses. However, antioxidants have been shown to tie up these free radicals and take away their destructive power. Eating whole foods that are high in antioxidants (beta-carotene and vitamins C and E) and phytonutrients (healing compounds found in plant-based foods) may help reduce the risk of many chronic diseases and even slow the aging process.

The power of free radicals can also be controlled by exercising at the right intensity. Studies show that the harmful free radical process is increased in those people who exercise at a high intensity. Bringing the intensity down into your Zone One, as explained in TLC 2, will produce all the health benefits of exercise but without the aging side effects.

3. STRESS

It is a fact that emotional stress can trigger a host of health-related problems, ranging from memory loss to impaired immunity, and thanks to extensive research, scientists now have a better understanding of how stress affects the body—inside and out. The fact is, *stress is simply the trigger*. Whether or not there will be health consequences or accelerated aging following exposure to a stressful episode depends on your responses to the external event. These responses involve the immune system, the heart and blood vessels, and how glandular secretion of hormones helps regulate various functions in the body, such as brain function and nerve impulses. All these responses interact and are greatly influenced by your coping style and psychological state, including your attitude and emotions (another key link to disease). You can modify these internal responses by changing your coping strategies, exercising regularly, and practicing meditation, yoga, biofeedback, or deep breathing techniques—all outlined in TLC 8. Stress aging is a very real problem, but it can be halted or even reversed by using natural therapies.

TURNAROUND STRATEGY: ATTITUDE CHECK

D o an attitude check, using the column in your Turnaround Journal (page 19). Make it your goal to stay positive for a 24-hour period. Become "other" directed and give some heart energy to a loved one, a neighbor, or even your pet. Choose anyone or anything (except food). Find a purpose in life and follow it. People who passionately follow their dreams or goals are healthier and live longer. If you're not prepared to choose a lifetime purpose, then find one for today!

4. ATTITUDE AND EMOTIONS

While science has always suspected this, the mechanism of the mind's interplay with the body is just now beginning to be understood through the field of psychoneuroimmunology. We know that our perception—how we view events in our lives—is a key player in our attitudes—the half full vs. half empty scenario. Study after study continues to show that negative emotions such as chronic anger, pessimism, mistrust, cynicism, and depression throw the immune system into a battered state that makes it difficult to resist disease and accelerates aging. Scientists have also found that negative people recover from disease more slowly than their positive counterparts. A weakened immune system will eventually give in to disease and speed up aging.

5. LACK OF KNOWLEDGE

Of all the five links to disease, I believe that ignorance, or what I call lack of knowledge, is probably the most serious. With all the antiaging information available connecting negative lifestyle habits with disease and aging, there is no excuse for hiding your head in the sand when it comes to your health and longevity. The American Institute for Cancer Research (AICR) in a most revealing study found that half of all Americans believe cancer is impossible to prevent and consider it the number one health concern. Less than 50 percent of those questioned realized that they were more susceptible if they ate a diet low in fruits and vegetables; and shockingly, only 35 percent cited obesity or insufficient physical activity as a cause of cancer.

There is clear and convincing evidence that the simple choices we make every 24 hours—like the foods we eat and whether or not we exercise, drink, or smoke—have a dramatic impact on our risk of getting cancer. The AICR also confirms that making the right choices can prevent 70 percent or more of all cancers. I personally believe that statement is conservative.

> The United States is *not* on the list of the top ten countries in terms of longevity—yet we spend the most amount of money on over-the-counter and prescription drugs.

I am grateful for the research that has brought us a better understanding of the aging process. While I wish they had figured it out when I was twenty-five, when our hormonal support begins to diminish, I believe that it is *never* too late to take charge of your biological age. Modern science has given a better understanding of how a proper diet, exercise, sleep, water, no alcohol, and meditation techniques restore youthful levels of hormones.

"An ounce of prevention is worth a pound of cure."

—Benjamin Franklin

Prevention Is Part of the Cure

So is aging inevitable? Reality tells us that no one escapes the subtle changes that come with age—the gray hair, wrinkles, and so on. But these changes are not debilitating and can certainly be delayed or minimized by implementing the eight TLCs. Still, what about those physiological changes associated with chronological aging? Can we take action early enough to change or even avoid altogether the problems associated with getting old? I know we can!

To be most effective, prevention should begin in our younger years. For example, prevention of atherosclerosis (hardening and narrowing of the arteries) actually begins early in life with healthy dietary and exercise habits formed as children, teens, and young adults. The same applies for many other diseases, such as osteoporosis, since bones are built during childhood and adolescence. But if your younger years were not the healthiest, there is still hope. Risk factors can be controlled or even reversed starting today by implementing Total Life Changes within your daily routine.

Early detection of medical problems allows treatment when it is easier, more effective, and less expensive. For example, a simple, painless test can detect blood in the stool, allowing early treatment of colon cancer long before it causes any other signs. Also, a mammogram may detect breast cancer before other signs are present. This allows treatment before the cancer has a chance to spread.

But I want you to go beyond having regular medical checkups. While routine tests may save your life by finding a problem before it is serious, prevention of chronic and terminal illness should be your primary goal.

Take cardiovascular disease, for instance—the number one cause of death for

---

HOW THE 24-HOUR TURNAROUND REDUCES RISK OF DISEASE

DISEASE	YOUR TOTAL LIFE CHANGES
Cancer (many types)	Weight loss, low-fat diet high in key nutrients, the H.E.A.R.T. workout, destressing innercise, no alcohol, healing sleep
High cholesterol levels	Weight loss, a diet low in saturated fats and trans fats, the H.E.A.R.T. workout, no alcohol, destressing, healing sleep
Hypertension	Weight loss, a low-sodium diet filled with fruits and vegetables, the H.E.A.R.T. workout, destressing with innercise, no alcohol, increased water, healing sleep
Obesity	Weight loss, the whole foods Definition Diet low in fat and high in fiber, the H.E.A.R.T. workout, no alcohol, water, healing sleep
Osteoporosis	Diet high in calcium and vitamin D, weight-bearing exercise, the H.E.A.R.T. workout, calcium and vitamin D supplements, no alcohol

---

Halt and Even Reverse Markers of Aging

AGING 101: PHYSIOLOGICAL MARKERS OF HUMAN AGING

DECREASED	INCREASED
Height from bone loss	Weight
Brain function	Blood pressure
Glucose tolerance	Lipid ratios
Muscle mass	Abdominal girth
Aerobic capacity	Wrinkles in skin
Strength	Sagging skin
Reaction time	
Temperature regulation	
Flexibility	
Immune function	
Metabolism	

---

women. Physicians used to believe that atherosclerosis was a normal part of the aging process. *We now know that atherosclerosis is* not *normal.* Doctors were taught that blood pressure naturally increased with age, enabling the heart to pump blood through an elderly person's narrowed arteries. *We now know that to be untrue as well.* You can start to save your life and the lives of your family members by implementing the TLCs in the next 24 hours.

Have you experienced any of these aging markers in the past few years? Perhaps you've noticed your waistline expanding and your height shrinking. Whichever physiological markers of aging you've noticed, you can stop this downward spiral with the 24-Hour Turnaround. By reversing these biological markers, your body can start to look and feel years younger, no matter how many birthdays you have celebrated, and your risk of debilitating illnesses will greatly decrease.

ANTIAGING AND YOUR COLON

I realize not many people relish having an open discussion about their colon or bowels, but this is a vital topic and one that you must understand and consider. We know there is a direct correlation between the condition of the intestinal tract and the overall functioning of the body. When the bowel isn't doing its job releasing all its daily waste, dangerous toxins enter the bloodstream. The bloodstream carries the toxins to key organs (the heart and brain), tissues (the skin and muscles), arteries, veins, lymph, and then all the cells. This toxic condition is believed to contribute to all chronic illness. The other devastating consequence is that any colon blockage prevents nutrient absorption, regardless of the quality of food you eat. Without proper nutrition, your youthfulness will quickly fade. The antiaging equation is not rocket science; it is very simple and is as follows:

nutrition in + waste out = a healthier and younger you

Our quick-and-easy processed American foods have caused the colon to become obstructed, distorted, and engorged with toxic waste matter, resulting in serious stress on the immune system and functions throughout the body. In an interview for *Online Health and Nutrition Newsletter* (November 2001), nutritionist Bernard Jensen, D.C., Ph.D., said, "In the fifty years I've spent helping people to overcome illness, disability, and disease, it has become crystal clear that poor bowel management lies at the root of most people's health problems. In treating over three hundred thousand patients, it is the bowel that invariably has to be cared for before any healing can take place." Regular colon cleansing is essential to good health, yet our Western medical community does not include this practice in preventive or therapeutic care—there's no money in it!

A simple act like cleansing and detoxifying the colon can boost the immediate effectiveness of your Turnaround, helping eliminate toxins, restore normal bowel movements, increase weight loss, and in some cases, flatten your bloated or extended stomach. As I explained in TLC 3, a clean, healthy colon is vital for a healthy life. Normal bowel movements, at least one a day, are essential to stop the clock and halt or even reverse the signs of aging.

The solution is simple: thoroughly cleanse the colon to remove toxic waste, and stop eating processed food that is filled with fat and preservatives. Check

RED FLAG

It is now estimated that the fourth leading cause of death in the United States is adverse drug reactions (ADR). Deaths from ADR are not due to overdoses, as you might guess. They are also not due to mistakes of administration. They are deaths in which a drug was used correctly (according to a pharmaceutical company), but the patient reacted adversely to it. Man has invented a new cause of death that didn't exist before. Just to put this cause into perspective, deaths from ADR are far more common than deaths caused by AIDS, which currently ranks tenth in the United States.

with your local natural food store for a safe and natural colon cleanser. (Also see my website for our 5-star product recommendations.) You might inquire at your health-food store for a list of qualified therapists who do colonics, which is the safe, gentle infusion of water into the colon, and colon therapies using natural herbs.

The Choice Is Yours

Are you ready to *stop the clock and halt or even reverse the signs and symptoms of growing older?*

If you're ready to take the leap, start now to implement the eight Total Life Changes and also incorporate some of the spa secrets discussed in the next chapter. Why not add a pinch of vanity to the Turnaround equation? After all, looking good can mean feeling great! I'll be right here by your side as your TLC personal trainer to help you understand and implement your 24-Hour Turnaround.

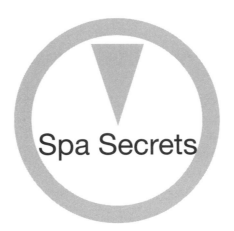

Spa Secrets

A S Y O U H A V E L E A R N E D , the eight Total Life Changes are mandatory to looking and feeling young. But let's face facts—life sometimes gets extremely hurried and the daily routine can get harried. As a busy professional and parent, I know that there is a huge advantage in taking time off away from home and work responsibilities to focus on personal health and fitness. And, as a spa director for more than twenty years, I have seen miraculous changes in people who take the time to visit a spa. Following are the insider secrets from my experiece as a spa director, designer, and consultant that will assure you a healing, relaxing, and antiaging experience.

For centuries Europeans have embraced taking time for a holiday, and a large part of their wellness secret is spa vacation time to pamper themselves and to relax and rejuvenate. In fact, I have many clients from around the world who come to the spa several times each year to be recharged and focus on upgrading their health and fitness program. They consider the money spent a necessary investment in their overall health, youthful good looks, and productivity, both now and in years to come.

The term *spa* is symbolic of wellness, balance, and luxury. A spa and its staff create a haven where people can experience total peace and relaxation and reflect on the things that are most important to them. And the spa industry is growing, as more and more people feel the need to get away and take care of themselves. In fact, according to an International Spa Association (ISA) survey, spas doubled in number between 1994 and 1999. While the ISA reports that a typical spa customer is a woman age thirty-one to fifty-four, men now constitute more than 25 percent of spa clients, up from around 9 percent five years ago.

Perhaps the reason for this incredible growth is the stronger-than-ever urge Americans feel to bypass established medicine and become responsible for their own self-care. In a study of men ages thirty-five to fifty-seven, researchers found that men who took annual vacations were 21 percent less likely to die during the sixteen-year study period than nonvacationers and 32 percent less likely to die of coronary heart disease. And in a twenty-year study of nearly 750 middle-aged women, the Centers for Disease Control and Prevention (CDC) associated lack of vacation time with an increased risk of heart attack and death. The most alarming fact: the United States is considered to be the most vacation-starved nation in the industrialized world.

It does not have to be that way! Taking time away for a spa vacation lets you focus on weight loss, stress reduction, and lowering blood pressure and blood lipids while boosting immune function and rejuvenating aging skin. These are all practical investments in your health—and in your future.

Becoming Spa Savvy

With the number of spas throughout the world growing at an incredible rate, how do you know which spa is best for your needs? The choices seem to grow each year, from destination spas and resort/hotel spas to medical, cruise ship, club, and day spas. You could go to a destination spa for a few days or a week to focus entirely on your mind, body, and spirit with innovative wellness techniques to help you feel young again. Or you might choose a day spa on your lunch hour for a quick fix to your stressful schedule. These "minispas" are popping up in most major cities across the nation and around the world and cater to the busy person who cannot get out of town. Then there are the spa services that first-class resorts have added as part of your family's total vacation experience. These experiences may include a variety of alternative therapies and holistic wellness treatments, including professional nutritional counseling, safe weight-loss programs, and ongoing instruction in ancient disciplines like yoga, tai chi, and qi gong.

To balance the mind and body, replenish your energy sources, and stimulate

Originally intended to describe a mineral spring or a remote resort built around a mineral spring, the word *spa* is now also used to describe products that we can incorporate in our daily hurried lives—from spa candles, incense, and body and face formulas to spa hot tubs (what I tag "wannabe mineral springs")—as well as day spas that you can visit on your lunch hour for a massage or face and body treatment.

your senses, I recommend a spa with natural surroundings. There are many seaside, country, and mountain resort spas that are a perfect choice for active families, couples, close friends, or even coworkers. To help you become more spa savvy, let's look at the optimal choices and the amenities they offer.

DESTINATION SPAS

The essential difference between a destination spa and other spas is focus. At a destination spa there are no distractions, and your stay is devoted to your personal health, relaxation, and education. Destination spas are usually located in spacious and nurturing settings, such as the pristine islands of Hawaii, the mountains of Colorado, a remote country estate in Vermont, or a spacious manor in Europe, where hydrotherapy techniques such as sauna and whirlpool remain popular.

At a destination spa, life focuses exclusively on you—through the various spa programs and activities. Meals are traditionally low in calories and saturated fat but high in healing nutrients; alcohol and caffeine are usually unavailable. If you have a chronic medical condition, such as diabetes or hypertension, destination spas may provide assistance in how to manage your health with specialized diet and exercise. Some offer outdoor activities such as golf, tennis, nature hikes, horseback riding, snow skiing, scuba diving, or sailing, while others focus on mind-body healing with yoga, meditation, and relaxation classes.

RESORT SPAS

If you plan on taking your spouse or the whole family, or if you want a more flexible schedule with time for day trips, shopping, and sightseeing, then a resort spa might be the perfect choice. A resort spa differs from a destination spa in that the spa is an amenity available to guests within the traditional resort setting. Your accommodations and meal service are typically integrated within the hotel and common restaurants. (Make sure to choose a resort that has a special "spa cuisine" menu designed by a qualified nutritionist or at the very least has healthy selections on the regular menu.)

You can often purchase a spa package at a resort, which might include your room, meals, use of fitness facilities, and a few spa treatments. Or guests might pay for these services separately (à la carte). Many resorts offer packages that combine spa treatments with golf, tennis, water sports, skiing, and other activities and are located within easy distance of tourist attractions, restaurants, and specialty shopping districts.

DAY SPAS

If you suffer from daily tension yet have no time for an immediate spa vacation, check out the Yellow Pages in your city for a day spa. Day spas account for 77 percent of all spas in the United States. They cater to the busy man or woman who is low on time and high on stress and offer an easily accessible and relaxing minispa experience. Some day spas focus exclusively on beauty and body treatments; others are located in health clubs or fitness facilities with expanded services that include aerobic exercise classes, toning and conditioning, hatha yoga, and stretching classes.

Most day spas offer a variety of treatments, from a half-hour massage, body wrap, or facial to an herbal bath, hydrotherapy treatment, or reflexology treatment. Offerings vary from à la carte services to half- or full-day packages (with a light lunch included).

SPA PROGRAMS MAY VARY

Some spas, such as weight-loss spas and medical spas, coordinate a treatment schedule for guests prior to arrival. This schedule may include a specific time for massages, exercise, consultation with the spa nutritionist, and educational classes. Be sure to select a spa that customizes the program and cuisine specifically for your personal needs. In other words, make sure the spa is a good fit with your interests and personal health concerns. Also, find out if the spa has a certified nutritionist who works with the chef, rather than an unqualified person who plans the standard menu.

SPA CUISINE

Today's spa cuisine is extremely healthy—low in fat, low in sugar, using fresh, organic, unprocessed ingredients, and quite delicious and sophisticated. As spas have become popular for family vacations and corporate conferences, the menus often showcase the spa chefs' creative talents. It is amazing how both calories and fat can be reduced unbeknownst to the discerning eye of the guest. Make sure that the spa you choose has the cuisine options clearly marked on the menus and has calorie, fat, and fiber content listed or available for your review.

PACKAGES AND PRICES

An all-inclusive package at a destination spa generally includes everything: your food, room, exercise classes, use of the fitness facilities, fitness/nutrition consultations, and several spa treatments. Resort spa fees are more flexible and can be designed with your schedule and choices in mind. Many spas plan designated weeks with reduced rates to accommodate a group. (In Hawaii, we do our 24-Hour Turnaround spa package for individuals or corporate groups.)

Spa Bodywork Offerings

You can find endless wellness experiences at a spa, but bodywork remains the most requested therapy. *Bodywork* is an umbrella term that encompasses body manipulation therapies used for relaxation, stimulation, and pain and injury relief. This form of touch therapy is a reliable and well-accepted approach to healing, as it relaxes muscles, slows breathing, lowers blood pressure, and increases circulation.

MASSAGE THERAPY

Of all the types of bodywork offered at spas, massage therapy, the hands-on manipulation of the body's soft tissues, is perhaps the most popular. For centuries people have used massage as a healing art; the first reference to it dates back four thousand years to ancient China. Throughout history, the "laying on of hands" to enhance healing has been valued among spiritual traditions. Even Hippocrates, the Father of Medicine, included massage as a form of healing in his writings, saying, "The physician must be experienced in many things, but most assuredly in rubbing."

The basic philosophy of massage therapy is to affect the musculoskeletal, circulatory-lymphatic, nervous, and other systems of the body, so that the body heals itself. Massage stimulates the flow of lymph, a bodily fluid that carries wastes and impurities away from tissues and that relies on muscle contractions to move efficiently throughout the body. A sedentary lifestyle may result in stagnant lymph flow.

Human touch is the basic medium of massage therapy. In order to apply pressure without hurting you, the massage therapist uses sensitivity and intuition to find the degree of pressure that is safe for you. The therapist assesses your skeleton, muscle tension and tone, painful trigger or tender points, and any soft-tissue problems you may have and becomes a healing artist, using different hands-on techniques, such as rubbing, kneading, holding, pressing, vibrating, and gliding, among others. Be prepared: depending on the treatment, your therapist may use her forearms, elbows, or even her feet! Before your treatment begins, communicate with your therapist regarding past or current injuries or health concerns, current medications, and the type of treatment or intensity of pressure you prefer. And communicate during the treatment if the intensity is too much or not enough.

Swedish massage. Swedish massage, the most common massage technique, helps flush the tissue of lactic and uric acids and other metabolic wastes as well as improve circulation without increasing the load on the heart. The therapist uses a system of long strokes, kneading, and friction techniques to massage the more superficial layers of the muscles. The therapist applies pressure and rubs the muscles in the same direction as the flow of blood returning to the heart.

Deep-tissue massage. Deep-tissue massage is applied with greater pressure and at deeper layers of the muscle than basic Swedish massage. The therapist may do hands-on movements across the grain of your muscles, using slow strokes or direct pressure with fingers, thumbs, or even elbows to get the expected result.

Sports/athletic massage. Sports massage is another popular type of bodywork provided at spas. This therapy targets the muscles used in athletic activities, and the deep-tissue therapeutic application helps increase muscle tone and range of motion as well as blood flow to the site of soreness or injury (shoulders, upper back, calves) to promote faster healing. Golfer's massage is a popular hands-on sports therapy for the husbands that come to our Couples Spa Week. Sports massage also helps those who suffer from tennis elbow or other recreational injuries.

Neuromuscular therapy massage. Neuromuscular therapy helps relax soft tissue and tense muscles, releases entrapped nerves, and restores the body's natural flow of energy. This massage therapy combines the basic principles of Asian pressure therapies with a specific hands-on deep-tissue therapy to help reduce chronic muscle or myofascial (soft-tissue) pain. This massage is ideal for relieving the stress-tension-pain syndrome and restoring neurological balance.

Myofascial release. Myofascial release is a great way to relieve muscle and fascia tension and ease chronic pain or tender points. In its natural state, the fascia gives strength and support to the body as it wraps and encases the muscles. But when the fascia becomes constricted due to illness or trauma, it can pull muscles or bones out of alignment. During a myofascial release session, the therapist palpates different areas of the body to find the places of restriction. Then, using long strokes, the tissues are gently stretched along the direction of the muscle fibers until the therapist feels resistance. This tension or resistance is held until the soft tissues relax, with the goal of elongating the tissue.

The Trager method. With the Trager method of bodywork, the deeply relaxed feelings you experience resonate through the nervous system, ultimately benefiting tissues and organs deep within your body. Trager therapists believe that many physical ailments are caused by patterns of tightness that are held in the unconscious mind as much as in the tissues. In contrast with massage, the therapist avoids using pressure, relying instead on gentle, rhythmic rocking to release tension and loosen joints. The therapist's goal is to help you experience true relaxation and serenity—a goal consistent with the spa experience! The results from this technique are lasting.

Lymphatic drainage massage. With this therapeutic massage, the practitioner uses light rhythmic strokes to improve the flow of lymph, a fluid that circulates throughout the body carrying away debris and bringing white blood cells to sites of infection. The gentle pumping technique helps drain pockets of water retention and trapped toxins and is designed to help stimulate circulation and boost the body's ability to eliminate wastes and absorb nutrients. This technique is used as part of a cellulite treatment and can be used for conditions related to poor lymph flow, including lymphedema (which sometimes afflicts women after a mastectomy), types of edema (swelling), situational water retention, and certain kinds of nerve pain.

Cranio-sacral therapy. Because the cerebral spinal fluid has a circulation and rhythm all its own and operates separately from the body's blood and lymph flow, many therapists incorporate this technique into their massage treatment. The therapist strives to determine and obtain a balance of the cerebral spinal fluid by releasing restrictions using very light touch. The work is extremely gentle, involving very slight pressure on specific parts of the body, including the skull and the feet.

Cryotherapy (ice massage) and back pain. While the heating pad or the hot tub sounds great, cold is the proper treatment to soothe a muscle spasm. The Texas Back Institute recommends ice massage as an excellent treatment option for back or neck spasms or discomfort. At our spa we have a treatment called *cryotherapy,* for those who suffer from chronic pain. Many therapists are experienced in this technique and can add it to your treatment.

You can replicate this cryotherapy relief at home by freezing water in a paper cup, peeling down the top of the cup a few inches, and having someone use the exposed ice to gently massage your back on either side of your spine while you lie on your stomach. Keep a pillow under your stomach to help support your back, and remember not to rub the bones of your spine with the ice. Do this for no more than 7 minutes. This action will numb the afflicted area, decrease pain, and reduce inflammation, allowing the injury to resolve itself. Cryotherapy can also interrupt the pain-spasm cycle.

After an ice massage, follow up with a few gentle back stretches if there is no pain. Over-the-counter anti-inflammatory medications, such as aspirin or ibuprofen, can also help alleviate both inflammation and the subsequent pain. This easy home-care method of treating minor back pain may not have you doing back flips, but it could get you back on your feet a little faster.

Reflexology. While a foot massage is a rare treat for most of us, spa reflexologists use this healing art to resolve many physical ailments. Reflexologists believe that specific *reflex zones* on the feet reflect every organ and every single area of the

nstead of just having a "feel-good" massage, try to schedule a series of massage treatments that work together to produce a specific result, whether to reduce muscle tension in your neck and shoulders, alleviate back pain, or ease chronic stress. Drink at
least 2 cups of water immediately after the massage therapy, followed by 1 cup each hour
according to your hydration schedule

body as well as its corresponding energy level. When pressure is applied to these
zones, you will experience increased circulation as well as removal of any energy
blocks in the body.

Treatment of reflex zones stimulates the blood flow to or surrounding the
organs or area, stimulates the body's production of endorphins, and stimulates the
elimination of waste materials. Reflexology will help revive your energy flow and
bring your body back into homeostasis, or a state of balance. Here is a chart of the
zones so that you can see how this alternative healing therapy might work for you.

REFLEXOLOGY CHART

REFLEX POINT	CORRESPONDING BODY ZONE
Metatarsal area (balls of the feet)	Chest, lung, and shoulder area
Toes	Head and neck
Upper arch	Diaphragm, upper abdominal organs
Lower arch (toward heel)	Pelvic and lower abdominal organs
Heel	Pelvic and sciatic nerve
Outer foot	Arm, shoulder, hip, leg, knee, lower back
Inner foot	Spine
Ankle area	Reproductive organs and pelvic region

HEAT THERAPY

Heated stones are now being integrated into therapeutic massage in some spas. Practitioners believe the stones help turn positive ions (representing congested areas) into negative ions throughout the body. When used with massage therapy, stones help open and warm the underlying tissues of the skin for optimal healing.

ASIAN MERIDIAN BODYWORK

Asian meridian bodywork, another popular spa offering, is based on the belief that *ch'i* is an energy force that is common to all living matter and that the smooth flow of this energy is essential to good health. It's believed that improving the flow of energy along particular pathways through the body, called meridians, enhances the body's natural recuperative powers, relaxing the muscles and improving the flow of blood and lymph. To keep *ch'i* flowing smoothly and dislodge blockages, various touch-based systems are used, including the following:

Acupuncture. Natural energy or *ch'i* travels along fourteen meridians in the body to keep your body nourished. These meridians are connected to specific organs and bodily functions. When *ch'i* is blocked or thrown off balance, illness or symptoms result. The acupuncturist stimulates the points along these meridians, using tiny needles to remove the energy block and restore the balance and flow of energy along the pathway. When one portion of the body is stimulated, an effect is obtained in the same or another portion of the body. It is also believed that acupuncture causes the body to release endorphins—your body's natural pain relievers. Acupuncture may also trigger the release of serotonin, a chemical in the brain that makes you feel calm and serene.

Acupressure. First introduced in China centuries ago, this finger massage works on the same principle as acupuncture in that applying pressure to specific points or meridians in the body triggers natural healing and the release of muscle tension.

Shiatsu. This Japanese therapy also draws on the Chinese notion of *ch'i*. Shiatsu sessions focus on relieving pain and helping the body rid itself of any toxins

WHAT'S ACUPUNCTURE GOOD FOR?

Acupuncture is approved by the National Institutes of Health for the following uses:

- Nausea during pregnancy
- Nausea and vomiting associated with surgery or chemotherapy
- Postoperative dental pain

The World Health Organization has compiled the following list of ailments that may respond well to acupuncture:

- Arthritis
- Asthma
- Bladder dysfunction
- Bronchitis
- Cervicobrachial syndrome
- Colitis
- Constipation
- Diarrhea
- Duodenal and peptic ulcer
- Facial or Bell's palsy
- Frozen shoulder
- Gastric hyperacidity
- Gastritis
- Headache and migraine
- Hiccups
- Hypertension
- Intercostal neuralgia
- Lower back pain
- Ménière's disease
- Nausea
- Paralysis following a stroke
- Paralytic ileum
- Peripheral neuropathy
- PMS and irregular menstruation
- Rhinitis
- Sciatica
- Sinusitis
- Spasm of esophagus
- Tennis elbow
- Torticollis
- Trigeminal neuralgia

before they develop into illness. The therapist applies firm, rhythmic pressure on specific points for 3 to 10 seconds in order to wake up the meridians or healing channels of the body. The pressure may help stimulate the body's endorphins to produce a tranquilizing effect, or it may help by loosening up muscles and improving blood circulation. Shiatsu is said to help ease or eliminate back pain and sciat-

SOFT TISSUE RELEASE

Soft Tissue Release (STR) is a powerful injury treatment technique developed by Stuart Taws while working with the British athletic team. Also referred to as British Sports Therapy or the Taws Technique, this therapy deals directly with the reasons for soft tissue dysfunctions and subsequent referred pain and nerve entrapment. In acute situations, STR affects the way scar tissue is formed, and in chronic conditions STR breaks up the fibrotic and adhered mass of scar tissue to quickly allow the muscle to return to its natural resting length. For more information, you can reach Stuart Taws through www.24hourturnaround.com.

ica, digestive problems, headaches, insomnia, leg and menstrual cramps, respiratory problems, and shoulder stiffness.

> "The doctor of the future will give no medicine but will interest his patient in the care of the human frame, in diet, and in the cause and prevention of disease."
>
> —Thomas Edison

AROMATHERAPY AND HEALING ESSENTIAL OILS

Aromatherapy also plays a tremendous role in spa therapies. This use of essential and absolute oils and other substances is intended to enhance the physical and psychological benefits of bodywork. The aroma from the scented candles, bath oils, or fragrances also stimulates a pleasure response.

Essential oils are highly concentrated substances extracted from a variety of different parts of a plant, including the flower, bark, roots, leaves, wood, resin, seeds, and rind. The oils contain natural healing vitamins, antibiotics, and antiseptics and represent the "life force" of the plant.

Comprising hundreds of organic constituents, including hormones, vitamins, and other natural elements, essential oils work on many levels. They can be sedative or stimulating; some are antispasmodic, and most are antibacterial.

When aromatherapy is used with massage, therapists believe that the essential oils are absorbed and used by the skin and carried by body fluids to the main body systems, such as the nervous and muscular systems, for a healing effect.

You can use the following oils at home with massage, self-massage, or a soothing aromatherapy bath.

Essential Oil	Healing Benefits
Lavender	Heals burns and cuts; destroys bacteria; relieves inflammation, spasms, headaches, respiratory allergies, muscle aches, nausea, menstrual cramps
Peppermint	Alleviates digestive problems; cleans wounds; decongests the chest; relieves headache, neuralgia, and muscle pain
Eucalyptus	Clears sinuses; has antibacterial and antiviral properties; relieves coughs
Rosemary	Relieves pain; increases circulation; decongests the chest; reduces swelling
Chamomile	Reduces swelling; treats allergic symptoms; relieves stress, insomnia, and depression; useful in treating digestive problems
Thyme	Lessens laryngitis and coughs; fights skin infections; relieves pain in the joints
Tarragon	Stimulates digestion; calms nervous system and digestive tract; relieves menstrual symptoms and stress
Everlasting	Heals scars; reduces swelling after injuries; relieves sunburn; treats pain from arthritis, muscle injuries, sprains and strains, and tendonitis

Best Spa Body Treatments

As I've discussed in the Total Life Changes, stress, the effects of improper diet, and alcohol consumption show on your skin as well as your face. Yet no matter what your past diet and drinking history may be, there are excellent spa body treatments that are both relaxing and therapeutic and can turn around the health and appearance of your skin very quickly.

- Sea salt treatments are used on the body for exfoliation. The Hawaiian sea salt treatment is unforgettable and prepares your skin for an essential oil massage.

- Seaweed treatments calm the nervous system, help to remove toxins from the body, hydrate the skin, and feed it with vitamins and minerals, producing a smooth and soft feeling.

- Mud treatments (sometimes called *Fango* treatments) are some of the most detoxifying treatments on a spa menu. It's important to use the right variety of mud, and one of the best is Neyharting Moor, which is filled with beneficial nutrients. Neyharting Moor is used extensively in Germany to treat illness. Mud can relieve arthritic pain and rheumatism and is therapeutic for people with dermatitis and psoriasis.

DESTRESS WITH HYDROTHERAPY

Floating in warm salt water induces the relaxation response, resulting in fewer stress hormones, a lower heart rate, and relaxed muscles. Relaxing in the ocean gives optimal healing from life's stressors. If you are doing a hydro-treatment indoors, make sure the water is filtered, as chlorine will have a negative effect on your system.

FIVE-STEP ANTICELLULITE PROGRAM

One of the most common questions that arises during a spa consultation or seminar is "How can I get rid of cellulite?" Cellulite, the lumpy fat that is commonly found on the thighs, stom-

AYURVEDIC TREATMENTS

Ayurveda, the oldest system of medicine in the world, is incorporated in many types of spa offerings—healing aromas, herbs, foods, therapeutic massage, and meditation. Ayurveda is based on the belief that diseases begin with an imbalance or stress in the person's consciousness. This imbalance is treated with lifestyle interventions that take into account your environment, diet, work, and family.

According to Ayurvedic belief, the body's functions are composed of combinations of five elements: air, fire, space, water, and earth. There are three other physiological forces called *doshas* (*vata, pitta,* and *kapha*) in which the five elements are manifest. All of us are made of a combination of *doshas* that give us a particular metabolic type yet have one *dosha* that dominates. *Vata* people are thin and energetic, *pittas* are hot-tempered, and *kaphas* are slow and solid. Ayurvedic spa therapies are customized according to your particular body type and lifestyle.

ach, and buttocks, is just a fancy name for fat cells that lie directly beneath your skin and the fibrous connective tissue that pulls on them, creating a honeycomb appearance. The amount of cellulite you see is determined by the percentage of fat on your body, your age, the thickness of your skin, and the health of your connective tissue, not the weight on the scale.

While there are no miracle products, treatments, or medicines that can eliminate cellulite, there is still some good news: you can reduce and in many cases eliminate cellulite with the proven five-step program below. Body treatments, or endermologie, are helpful in reducing the dimpled appearance and carrying the toxins and fluids away from the cells as part of the program but are not mandatory. A spa trip is the optimal time to start an anticellulite program.

The complete five-step anticellulite program includes:

1. Increased hydration to carry toxins, extra fluids, and fat away from the area and out of the body. Water and green tea are the best sources of hydration.

2. A low-fat diet with plenty of whole grains to thicken your skin.

BEAUTY AND BODY TREATMENTS

*B*eauty and cosmetic treatments include facials, image consultation, makeovers, manicure/pedicure, and waxing.

Body treatments include massage, cellulite treatments, herbal wraps, salt glow, seaweed wraps, and various forms of hydrotherapy.

3. H.E.A.R.T. workouts to metabolize the fat.

4. Dry brushing the skin daily with a soft dry brush made of natural vegetable bristles to help stimulate the lymph system. Dry brushing of the skin removes dead layers and impurities while stimulating circulation. At home you can use a brush purchased from the health-food store. Starting from the knees, brush the skin in a circular motion up toward the thighs. Finish with the buttocks and stomach area, if needed.

5. Spa cellulite treatments to encourage removal of waste from the area. At home, you can use a stimulation gel on the area after your daily dry brushing. A stimulation gel can be purchased at most health-food stores and day spas, or check my website for recommendations.

When you check into a spa, advise the spa director or programmer that fat loss and cellulite reduction are your goals. Your spa experience can help speed up your metabolism and develop the extra enzymes necessary to burn stubborn fat. Be aware that a take-home program is mandatory for continued success in ridding your body of cellulite. Note: you can reduce the fat in the cellulite fat cell, but often the connective tissue remains the same. Your yoga practice will help improve the elasticity of the connective tissue, reducing the appearance of the cellulite.

I am often asked in client consultations, "And what about cosmetic surgery?" Due to the ever-growing emphasis in our society on maintaining a youthful appearance and the continued aging of the baby boomer population, there has been an explosive growth in noninvasive cosmetic surgery. Treatments not requiring significant recuperation time comprise both the largest and fastest-growing categories of procedures. These mini- or superficial procedures have little downtime and discomfort and lower risk of disfiguring side effects. The new advanced techniques can provide many of the benefits of the invasive surgical procedure without the risks (excessive bleeding, infection, allergic reactions, and scarring) and expense. The techniques include peels, resurfacing, photo facials, hair removal, lightening, injections of your own cells, and even a 72-Hour Noninvasive Face Lift. (For more information, visit www.gregorykeller.com.) My best advice is to use your TLCs first to be the best you can be. You can take years off your looks naturally. If you decide to do any cosmetic procedures, make an informed decision!

Spa Skin Therapies

The condition of your skin is not just a cosmetic concern. The skin is also the window to your internal world, providing a clue to the speed at which you are aging.

Your skin is part of your immune system and a front-line fighter of disease. It's laced with Langerhans cells, which capture bacteria, viruses, and toxins and keep them from entering the body. Chronic exposure to the sun reduces the efficiency of the Langerhans cells.

We know that a large part of skin aging involves structural changes in the dermis, which is the sensitive vascular inner layer of the skin, and in particular the structural proteins (collagen and elastin) that maintain its flexibility. Wrinkled skin is a combination of reduced collagen synthesis and free radical–induced cross-linking of collagen fibers. This also occurs in the elastin fibers, generating a lack of elasticity in the skin. How are collagen and elastin enhanced? Good diet, exercise, plenty of water, no alcohol, and healing sleep.

As we age, the rate of new skin cell synthesis can drop by nearly 50 percent, but the good news is that we make billions of brand-new cells every day (the reason why the 24-Hour Turnaround works). The amount of time between the birth of a new skin cell and its appearance on the skin's outer layer is approximately fifteen to thirty days. Therefore, in two to four weeks you can have a younger appearance if you religiously follow your Turnaround, and that process can start today. Note: for a 24-Hour Turnaround, eliminate your evening cocktail and stay on your hydration schedule to plump up your skin cells.

The vibrant complexion that's usually associated with good health can be credited to improved blood flow (vasodilatation action) and improved nutrient delivery to the skin, which is essential for the synthesis of new structural protein. If you have a sallow skin tone, it usually indicates that blood flow is constricted in the skin and also in the cardiovascular system. Your H.E.A.R.T. workout will turn this around.

ENZYME TREATMENT

A good way to measure your skin's vitality and estimate the amount of free radical damage is to perform the *skin elasticity test*. Grasp the skin on the back of your hand between the thumb and index finger. Now raise the skin and then release it. The skin fold should immediately flatten. If a ridge remains, the skin has been damaged by cross-linking or free radicals.

Enzymes are important in your battle against aging skin and can help prevent or treat skin damage by fighting deleterious free radicals and reducing stress on the body's systems. Enzymes also improve nutrient content in the skin's blood supply. When used as exfoliants, enzymes rejuvenate the skin, stimulate new cell growth, and improve skin tone and texture. An exfoliant or facial peel that contains papain, the enzyme from young green papaya (the most potent), can

---

SIX SKIN SUPERSTARS

1. Fresh vegetables high in antioxidants
2. Legumes
3. Prunes
4. Apples
5. Fish
6. Tea (green or black)

digest dead protein cells from the skin's outer layer without harming the younger, living cells. There is empirical evidence suggesting that papain enzymes help heal uneven pigmentation, fine lines, and brown spots in addition to exfoliating skin.

Several other enzymes are also effective when applied topically. For instance, bromelain, from pineapple, is used as a skin exfoliant, while trypsin, from animal sources, and amylase and lipase, both from microbial sources, break down and dissolve dead skin cells.

Taken orally, enzymes fight free radicals and improve digestion, thereby increasing nutrient absorption—all important steps in improving skin quality and appearance. By taking digestive and antioxidant enzyme supplements and using topical antioxidant enzymes, you can improve the health of your skin and prevent a variety of skin conditions. Anyone with dull skin, acne, eczema, skin cancer, wrinkles, scars, stretch marks, or brown spots would be wise to explore enzyme therapy. Most spas provide this treatment.

ZAPPING WRINKLES

Science is just now confirming what Angelika, our skin specialist, and other professionals have known for years: a healthy diet helps prevent wrinkles. Angelika has repeatedly told our clients that great skin comes from what you put inside your body, not what you put on the outside. In a study published in February 2001 in the *Journal of the American College of Nutrition,* researchers found that those who had diets abundant in vegetables and legumes experienced less skin wrinkling as they aged than people who consumed more animal products, dairy, and butter.

DID YOU KNOW THAT . . .

- If you have dry, flaking skin, the essential fatty acids found in Definition Diet foods like salmon, sardines, walnuts, and flaxseed can restore a youthful appearance quickly?

- Dehydration ages you? Aim to consume at least 10 cups of either bottled or filtered water per day (especially if you are over forty) to assist in achieving a smooth, glowing appearance.

- A rosacea skin condition is exacerbated by drinking alcohol or eating meat and dairy products? Stick with your Definition Diet for healthy, younger-looking skin.

- A large number of skin diseases, including atopic dermatitis and psoriasis, appear to be precipitated or exacerbated by stress? Keep doing your mind-body innercise, as explained in TLC 8.

ANTIOXIDANTS ARE ANTIAGING

Eating foods high in antioxidants increases the skin's cell renewal rate, normalizes cell growth, and stimulates collagen formation. Synthetic forms of vitamin A have been proved to aid in the treatment of cancer, precancerous skin growths, wrinkles, and acne, and vitamins A, C, and E are known to reduce harmful damage to the skin from sun exposure. Good sources of vitamin A include fresh fruit and vegetables, while nuts and seeds provide excellent sources of vitamin E. Vitamin C is found in citrus fruits, potatoes, broccoli, and brussels sprouts.

The best way to take antioxidants in supplemental form is within your multivitamin—three times a day. Check www.24hourturnaround.com for supplement recommendations.

AT-HOME TECHNIQUE: GET A NATURAL EVENING GLOW

For naturally glowing skin, exfoliate with a sea salt paste and a blend of calming oils. Measure ½ cup of coarse sea salt (or kosher salt); mix with a few tablespoons of olive oil and 3 drops of lavender oil. Massage the salt mixture over your entire body from the neck down, rubbing in a circular motion, and be sure to include your feet. Immediately shower the mixture off in warm water. Pat dry, and finish with a light body moisturizer.

FACIALS

Upon arriving for your spa skin treatment, give information about your health, skin products used, diet and water intake, hormones and other medications, smoking, alcohol, and any surgeries or chemical peels that you may have had. For any skin treatment, always request a licensed esthetician (not a cosmetologist!) who has been out of school for at least one year. All facials should include manual (by hand) extractions. Never ever let anyone use a comedome for your extractions. A comedome is a small tool used to extract debris from your pores. Always request an enzyme peel to digest the dead protein off the skin. The treatment will be more effective, and your new cells will have an easier time making it to the surface! Consider having acupressure and some lymphatic drainage on certain points of the face to increase circulation and decrease puffiness.

Spa Skin Care Products

Most women's skins are on product overload. In fact, new research confirms that the overuse of moisturizers can increase the penetration of irritants, and there are a host of irritants in many skin products, including harmful petrochemicals.

Your skin's needs are simple: cleansing, nourishing, and protecting. As you shop for skin care products, keep in mind that approximately 60 percent of what we put on our skin is absorbed into the bloodstream. That fact was my inspiration

SEVEN BODY, SKIN, AND HAIR PRODUCT INGREDIENTS TO AVOID

1. *Sodium lauryl sulfate.* This detergent and emulsifier can combine with other unnatural ingredients to form nitrogen compounds that are not good for the inner and outer layers of your skin. This chemical additive is drying, irritating, and interferes with the skin's barrier.

2. *Propylene glycol.* This petroleum derivative is the most common moisture-carrying component in skin care—but stay away from it, as it can become toxic in the body.

3. *Formaldehyde.* This preservative is not only an irritant but a neurotoxin and a carcinogen. In its derivative form, formaldehyde may be called imidazolidinyl urea, which causes dermatitis, or diazolidinyl urea. Be sure to check for all these names on product labels.

4. *Parabens.* This widely used preservative causes irritation and is a xenoestrogen, a chemical that acts like estrogen in the body. On a product label parabens may read as methyl-, butyl-, ethyl-, and propylparaben.

5. *Artificial colors.* Avoid artificial colors since they can be carcinogenic and are completely unnecessary in skin care.

6. *Isopropyl alcohol.* This solvent is derived from petroleum and can dry out your skin, leaving it flaky and irritated.

7. *Paraffin.* This additive is derived from petroleum or coal and is used in some creams, hair removers, and eyebrow pencils.

to look for natural products to put on my skin! If you want to cut down on your exposure to chemicals, check out the labels on skin care products. The wording on packaging can be complicated, so I've provided you with a list of seven ingredients you do *not* want in your skin care products, both face and body. When absorbed into your skin, these ingredients can wreak havoc on your hormones and may cause long-term health problems, not to mention immediate skin irritation.

I want you to head for the health-food store (or ask your esthetician) for natural skin care products. You will need a natu-

CHOOSING A SUNSCREEN

As you select a sunscreen that works with your skin type, be on the alert for damaging chemicals in the list of ingredients. I highly recommend checking at the health-food store, or ask your dermatologist or esthetician to recommend a natural product. Zinc oxide is a natural and effective sunscreen, especially for those with sensitive skin.

ral skin cleanser, a light moisturizer (depending on your skin type and the age of your skin), and sun protection. A skin freshener or balancer is optional.

Many companies that make natural products have made it simple for you. They will state "no petrochemical ingredients" and "natural fragrance." Fragrance-free just means that you can't smell the artificial ingredients.

If you have time and are a bit ambitious, you may want to try making your own natural skin, body care, and hair care products. There are excellent resources available that can teach you how. I've listed these books and products on my website and will continue to keep you informed on the companies that provide natural products for skin and body.

Ten Spa Therapies to Use at Home

1. Try milk as a natural cleanser. Wet a cotton ball or tissue with skim milk if your skin is oily, whole milk if it's dry; wipe it across the face, and do not wash off. The result? A natural sheen, with no after-smell.

2. Use egg white to tighten facial pores. Lightly beat one egg white; rub on skin and leave for 20 minutes. Wash clean and pat dry. Add ¼ teaspoon

freshly squeezed lemon juice to the beaten egg white for oily skin. For dry skin, use a lightweight natural oil (lavender or tea tree) on your face before applying the egg white.

3. Boost circulation with a facial massage. Apply a facial moisturizer to your hands and lightly rub your cheeks, working from the middle of the face to the earlobes. Massage your forehead and temples, to the middle of the forehead and hairline. Use the same pressure to firmly press the chin area and up the jawline to the earlobes. Lightly pinch the earlobes for an invigorating touch therapy.

4. Increase alertness with essential oil. If you are fatigued yet have a big deadline looming, boost alertness and concentration by putting several drops of oil of peppermint or oil of lemon on a tissue. Wave it under your nose for a quick pick-me-up.

5. Ease computer eyestrain. Fill a small zippered sandwich bag about halfway full with uncooked dried beans. Place in the freezer to chill. Whenever your eyes burn from overuse, place the bag over your eyes and relax.

6. Treat your feet. Representing only about 2 percent of your weight, your feet must bear 98 percent of your body weight, so it makes sense to treat them with great kindness. Fill a zippered sandwich bag with half ice cubes and half water. Rub each bare foot with the icy refreshment. Then mix a solution of tea tree and lemon oil in distilled water and mist the bare feet. Towel dry and elevate your feet for a few minutes.

7. Try the healing yoga lift shown on page 56. Lie on the floor on your back with your legs raised and propped against a wall (form a 90-degree angle). Place your arms in a comfortable position, and then slowly breathe through your nose by using your diaphragm. Let the air expand your belly, and keep your chest quiet. Once your lungs are full, hold your breath (comfortably) to fully

TWO TIPS FOR TENSION RELIEF

1. Tension headache? Take two tennis balls and put them in a sock. Lie down on a firm surface and put the balls behind your neck, just beneath the shelf of the skull. Close your eyes and breath deeply, then gradually reposition the balls further down your neck.

2. Muscle tension or pain? Lie on the floor or back up against a wall and position a tennis ball where you find intense soreness. The ball will add pressure to painful trigger points, similar to the way acupressure or acupuncture works. Exercise caution until you define your pressure limits.

oxygenate the blood. Exhale for twice as long as your inhalation count. This position drains pooled blood from your lower legs and ankles, and the breathing clears your head. The blood and oxygen are great for your facial skin.

8. Whiten your nails naturally. If your nails are discolored or yellow, try a milk-and-lemon bath to bring back their sparkling beauty. First bleach the nails by soaking in a small saucer of freshly squeezed lemon juice. Then moisturize the cuticles in a bowl of warm milk for 5 minutes. Rinse and pat dry.

9. Get healing sleep. Just when you figured I had said enough on the topic, here are some more important benefits to getting at least 8 hours of sleep each night: shiny hair, supple skin, and strong nails. Sleep deprivation can reduce the body's store of vitamin B and make you look dried out and old.

10. Be a moon worshiper. The sun is your worst enemy when you want to have young-looking skin. Even in the wintertime, the sun can cause UV damage, leaving your skin dry, flaky, and rough. Make sure you slather on sunscreen before you leave your home each day—even on cloudy days, when the sun does hidden damage. If you don't like sunscreen, well, become a moon worshiper!

Take Time for You

Teach your family members the importance of self-care and time-out, and consider booking the next family vacation at a resort spa—so you can take advantage of the healing spa therapies while your kids enjoy the variety of activities and programs. But be sure to do your homework. Think ahead about the kind of spa experience you desire. Do you want to go alone to be pampered and treated like royalty? Do you want to go with your spouse and have couples' activities? Do you want to take your kids sightseeing and be outdoors most of the time? Do you want a spa that caters to women? Whether you choose a destination spa, a day spa, a resort spa, or even implement some of the spa secrets in the privacy of your home, I urge you to stop the busyness of your life and take time for the inner and outer you. The R&R (regeneration and rejuvenation) will optimize your antiaging turnaround.

Recipes for
Your 24-Hour Turnaround

I ENCOURAGE YOU to look for recipes in natural health magazines, cook-books, and on the Internet. You now know which foods are "in" and which need to be left out, so modify your favorite recipes or replace them with upgraded versions. Use fresh or canned veggie broth or a pump or spray of oil to sauté, and save the calories for some real food.

These recipes are some of my favorites—they're easy, satisfying, great for your skin, and kid-compatible. They're also low in fat, high in fiber, antiaging, and hormone-friendly.

Many of the recipes that follow were created for the Definition Diet by Luiz Ratto. I first met Luiz when I did an in-home consultation with a client in New York. We worked together to create a low-fat, high-fiber menu that was delicious. These are just a few of the many creative dishes that will be published in his forthcoming book, *Luiz Ratto's Healthy Table*.

Breakfast

Here are some suggestions for breakfast foods that fill you up and keep you going.

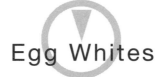

Egg Whites

Substituting egg whites for whole eggs is a great way to get the protein without the fat or cholesterol. An egg white contains 17 calories and 4 grams of protein. Buy hormone-free, antibiotic-free eggs when you can. Use them in scrambled eggs, omelets, and Ezekiel French toast. My favorite is cinnamon-raisin Ezekiel bread soaked in egg whites, cooked on both sides, and served with a tablespoon of maple syrup and lots of berries on top.

Maple Oatmeal with Prunes

1 cup water
1½ cups soy milk
2 cups rolled oats
1 cup prunes, diced
4 tablespoons maple syrup
¼ teaspoon ground cinnamon

Bring the water and soy milk to a simmer in a medium saucepan. Stir in the oats and simmer, covered, for 5 minutes. Turn off the heat and stir in the prunes, maple syrup, and cinnamon. Cover for 3 minutes and serve. For a creamier texture add extra soy milk. *Serves 4*

Per serving: 220 calories, 3 g fat, 9 g protein, 42 g carbohydrate, 6 g fiber

Angelika's Skin Antiaging Cereal

Angelika swears that uncooked raw grains are best—and it's working for me!

½ cup quinoa
½ cup whole rye
½ cup whole barley
½ cup whole oats
½ cup whole millet
½ cup whole spelt
½ cup amaranth
6 tablespoons plus ½ cup water
½ cup low-fat vanilla soy milk
Chopped apricots, dates, nuts, and seeds to taste

All these whole-grain ingredients can be found at a health-food store (check the bulk-food bins). Combine the grains and store in a glass jar in the refrigerator. The evening before, put ½ cup of the grains in a food processor or your Champ blender and pulse until the grains are broken down but not powdered. Put the grains in a bowl with enough water (about 6 tablespoons) to moisten the grains, cover, and return to the refrigerator. In the morning the grains can be served raw with soy milk (or nonfat cow's milk), nuts, seeds, and dried or fresh fruit. Or, in a saucepan, combine the grains, ½ cup water, ½ cup soy milk, and the dried fruits, nuts, or seeds. Cook over medium heat for 5 minutes, covered (add water if needed). Remove from the heat and let sit for another 5 minutes.

Serves 2

Per serving: 255 calories, 3 g fat, 8 g protein, 50 g carbohydrate, 7 g fiber

Veggie Dreams

Incorporating vegetables into your day can be easy. Your goal is to eat them raw, lightly steamed, or seared/grilled. The following recipes are some ideas to get you started.

Salad Bowl (Jay's Trough)

1 cup spinach leaves, washed and chopped
1 cup alfalfa sprouts
1 medium tomato, diced
¼ cup chopped raw carrots
¼ cup raw cauliflower florets
¼ cup raw or crisp-steamed broccoli florets
¼ cup chopped raw purple cabbage
3 small olives, chopped
2 medium radishes, chopped
¼ cup garbanzo beans, rinsed

In a large bowl, combine all the ingredients. Toss with a Spectrum fat-free salad dressing.

Serves 1

Per serving: 262 calories, 5 g fat, 14 g protein, 45 g carbohydrate, 14 g fiber

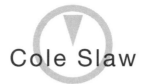

Cole Slaw

Both recipes from the forthcoming book *Luiz Ratto's Healthy Table*

2 cups each thin-sliced green and red cabbage
2 cups grated carrots
2 tablespoons nonfat plain yogurt
1 tablespoon each white vinegar, chopped Vidalia onion,
 minced garlic, minced ginger, and honey
5 tablespoons chopped parsley
Salt and pepper to taste

In a large mixing bowl, combine all the ingredients. Cover and refrigerate for 1 hour. Serve as a salad, under a piece of fish, or as a side dish.   *Serves 4*

Per serving: 83 calories, trace fat, 3 g protein, 19 g carbohydrate, 4 g fiber

Salad Dressings

1 cup blueberries	1 cup cherries, pitted	1 cup pineapple chunks	1 cup papaya chunks
1 clove garlic, minced	¼ Vidalia onion, minced	1 Tbsp. minced ginger	¼ red onion, minced
1 Tbsp. minced parsley	1 Tbsp. minced thyme	2 Tbsp. minced cilantro	4 basil leaves,
¾ cup balsamic vinegar	½ cup red wine vinegar	½ cup lime juice	½ cup white vinegar

Fruit breaks the acidity of vinegar and adds a lot of flavor to dressings. Choose a column, combine the four ingredients in a blender, and correct the seasoning to your taste (salt and pepper are optional). Mix and match the ingredients to make your own creative dressings.

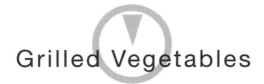

Grilled Vegetables

From the forthcoming book *Luiz Ratto's Healthy Table*

3 cloves garlic, minced

12 sprigs thyme, stems removed and leaves minced

1½ cups balsamic vinegar

Salt and pepper to taste

1 tablespoon Spectrum fat-free marinade (Toasted Sesame or
Honey Dijon)

1 medium eggplant, cut into 1¼-inch-thick diagonal slices

1 large zucchini, cut into 1¼-inch-thick diagonal slices

1 large yellow squash, cut into 1¼-inch-thick diagonal slices

2 large red bell peppers, cut into 1½-inch-thick slices

In a large mixing bowl combine the seasonings with the marinade. Whisk well.
Add the vegetables and marinate for 20 minutes. Grill the vegetables to taste
and serve with the marinade. Save the leftovers for lunch the next day, or chop
them and include them in your egg white omelet for breakfast.   *Serves 4*

Per serving: 132 calories, 5 g fat, 4 g protein, 24 g carbohydrate, 10 g fiber

Garbanzo Bean, Spinach, and Shiitake Mushroom Tart

From the forthcoming book *Luiz Ratto's Healthy Table*

If you're looking for an alternative vegetable side dish, these tarts are high in nutrition and low in fat. Place them on a bed of greens or right on the dinner plate.

One 14½-ounce can organic garbanzo beans
6 pumps olive oil spray
½ medium Vidalia onion, minced
3 cloves garlic, minced
1 cup shiitake mushrooms, sliced
3 cups baby spinach
Salt and pepper to taste
½ cup minced chives
Sesame oil to taste (4 to 12 drops)
1 small Thai pepper, minced
Olive oil and seasoned bread crumbs for coating ramekins
4 egg whites

Puree the garbanzo beans in a food processor and reserve. Preheat the oven to 350 degrees. Spray a large skillet with olive oil. Add the onions and sauté over medium heat until they're golden brown. Add the garlic and sauté for 1 minute. Add the mushrooms and sauté for 3 minutes, always shaking the pan so they don't burn. Add the spinach and sauté for 2 minutes. Season with some salt so the mushrooms release some water. Add the garbanzo bean puree and mix well. Season with pepper, chives, sesame oil, and Thai pepper. Transfer into a bowl and let cool. Grease 6 small ramekins with some olive oil and coat them lightly with seasoned bread crumbs. Beat the egg whites until they're firm, and fold them gently into the garbanzo bean mixture, little by little, using a rubber spatula. Fold the whole mixture into the ramekins. Bake for 10 minutes on the lower rack of the oven. Let cool for 2 minutes and invert onto the serving plate.   *Serves 6*

Per serving: 208 calories, 1 g fat, 9 g protein, 46 g carbohydrate, 8 g fiber

Soups

Soup is a great way to fill you up (not out) and make a quick and easy lunch or dinner. The following recipes also cover your bean requirement for the day. High in fiber and low in calories and fat, they're a five-star Definition Diet choice. Soups make great leftovers.

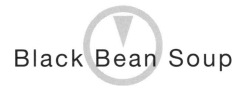

Black Bean Soup

From the forthcoming book *Luiz Ratto's Healthy Table*

Olive oil spray
1 medium Spanish onion, minced
4 cloves garlic, minced
2 cans black beans, rinsed and drained (or cooked dried beans)
1 teaspoon cumin
1 teaspoon cayenne pepper
1 cup vegetable broth
2 bay leaves
1 cup water
Salt and pepper to taste
Minced chives for garnish

Spray a saucepan with olive oil and sauté the onions over medium heat for 3 minutes. Add the garlic and sauté for 1 minute. Add the beans, cumin, and cayenne pepper and sauté for 2 more minutes. Add the vegetable broth. Transfer everything to a blender and liquefy. Transfer back to the pan, and add the bay leaves and water. Season with salt and pepper. Cook for 10 minutes. Remove the bay leaves. Serve in a bowl with chives sprinkled on top.   *Serves 4*

Per serving: 119 calories, 2 g fat, 6 g protein, 20 g carbohydrate, 5 g fiber

---

Vegetable Barley Soup

From the forthcoming book *Luiz Ratto's Healthy Table*

¼ cup barley
10 cups vegetable stock (fresh or canned)
2 cups corn kernels, fresh or frozen
One 14½-ounce can low-sodium diced tomatoes, including juice
4 large carrots, cubed
2 cups lima beans
1 large baking potato, peeled and cubed
⅛ teaspoon sea salt
2 cups green beans

Rinse the barley and drain. Place all ingredients except the green beans in a pot. Bring to a boil, then turn down to a simmer. Cook for 30 minutes, stirring occasionally. Add the green beans and cook until potatoes are tender and barley is soft, about 15 minutes more. Add water if needed. Serve with a toasted piece of Ezekiel sesame bread.   *Serves 12*

Per serving: 112 calories, 0.3 g fat, 3.1 g protein, 26 g carbohydrate, 4.4 g fiber

Dips

Dips are an A+ snack that will make your raw veggie snacks more interesting. Quick and easy to make, they store in the refrigerator for days. When you are standing (and starving) in front of the open refrigerator, they are a no-brainer answer to a nutritious snack or lunch. They also make great sandwich spreads.

Low-Fat Hummus

One 15-ounce can chickpeas (garbanzo beans)
1 tablespoon fresh lemon juice
¼ teaspoon ground cumin
1 small clove garlic, minced
Pinch cayenne pepper
2 tablespoons minced parsley
2 tablespoons minced red onion

Drain the chickpeas, reserving juice. Do not rinse. Transfer the chickpeas to a food processor or blender and blend with ½ cup reserved chickpea juice, the lemon juice, cumin, garlic, and cayenne. Add the parsley and red onion and pulse briefly just to mix. Serve with raw veggies or baked chips. Refrigerate and use with roll-ups.

Serves 4

Per serving: 130 calories, 2.1 g fat, 7.2 g protein, 22.5 g carbohydrate, 7 g fiber

Carrot and Apple Roll-Up with Low-Fat Hummus

1 sprouted-wheat tortilla
¼ cup low-fat hummus
½ cup grated carrots
½ red apple, chopped
½ cup arugula leaves

Warm the tortilla so that it is pliable. Spread the hummus over the entire tortilla. Layer with carrots, apple, and arugula. Roll tightly and refrigerate.   *Serves 1*

Per serving: 210 calories, 2.5 g fat, 8 g protein, 32 g carbohydrate, 9 g fiber

Roasted Garlic and Tofu Spread

From the forthcoming book *Luiz Ratto's Healthy Table*

1 garlic bulb
Olive oil spray
1 teaspoon dried oregano
Salt and pepper to taste
1½ cups chopped chives
One 12- to 16-ounce tofu block (Mori-Nu organic lite is my favorite)

Preheat the oven to 400 degrees. Cut the top off the garlic bulb so the cloves are exposed, and spray with olive oil, then sprinkle with oregano, salt, and pepper. Roast for about 20 minutes in a garlic roaster or in aluminum foil. Using a spatula, squeeze the garlic out of the papery cover into a bowl; it should have the consistency of a paste. Add the chives and tofu and mix well with a fork until smooth. Reseason with salt and pepper. Serve with raw veggies at snack time or refrigerate and use with roll-ups. I use this on my sandwiches instead of mayonnaise.

Serves 8

Per serving: 46 calories, 2 g fat, 4 g protein, 3 g carbohydrate, 1 g fiber

Tempeh Burger Roll-Up with Roasted Garlic and Tofu Spread

From the forthcoming book *Luiz Ratto's Healthy Table*

1 tempeh burger, diced small (a soy product that's available
   in health-food stores)
¼ cup vegetable broth
1 sprouted-wheat tortilla
Roasted Garlic and Tofu Spread (see page 379)
1 tomato, sliced
1½ cups baby spinach

Sauté the tempeh in the veggie broth. Warm the tortilla so that it is pliable. Cover the entire surface with the garlic and tofu spread. Layer the tempeh, tomato, and spinach. Roll the tortilla and refrigerate. Great for snacks or lunches.

Serves 1

Per serving: 260 calories, 6 g fat, 7 g protein, 46 g carbohydrate, 4 g fiber

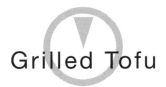

Grilled Tofu

From the forthcoming book *Luiz Ratto's Healthy Table*

1 tablespoon balsamic vinegar

1 tablespoon teriyaki sauce

2 cloves garlic, minced

10 sprigs thyme, stems removed and leaves minced

1¼ tablespoons dried oregano

5 tablespoons lemon juice

1 firm tofu block (20 ounces), cut into 1½-inch slices

Olive oil spray

2 red bell peppers, cut into strips

8 basil leaves

2 cups spinach leaves

In a mixing bowl, combine the first six ingredients. Arrange the tofu slices in a shallow baking dish. Pour the marinade over the tofu and refrigerate for 1 hour, turning the slices once. Lightly spray a very hot grill with olive oil and brown the tofu slices on both sides. Be careful not to burn them. Brown the red peppers. Layer the tofu, basil, and roasted peppers over the greens.   *Serves 4*

Per serving: 55 calories, 1 g fat, 2 g protein, 13 g carbohydrate, 5 g fiber

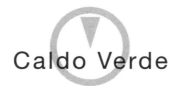

Caldo Verde

From the forthcoming book *Luiz Ratto's Healthy Table*

Olive oil spray
1 small Spanish onion, diced
6 cloves garlic, minced
2 Idaho potatoes, cut into ½-inch cubes
6 cups vegetable stock (fresh or canned)
1 cup sliced savoy cabbage
2 cups chopped spinach
1 cup chopped kale
1 cup chopped watercress
Salt and pepper to taste

In a nonstick pan with a light spray of olive oil, sauté the onions and garlic until soft. Add the potatoes and stock and cook for 5 minutes. Add the cabbage and cook for 5 minutes more. Add the spinach, kale, and watercress and cook for an additional 5 to 8 minutes. Season to taste. Serve with croutons.

Serves 6

Per serving: 215 calories, 4 g fat, 8 g protein, 38 g carbohydrate, 5 g fiber

Hawaiian Tempeh Chili

This chili can be made in advance and is amazing for lunch the next day. Serve over short-grain brown rice.

1 large onion, chopped
2 medium cloves garlic, minced
4 tablespoons vegetable broth
One 8-ounce package tempeh, cut into ½-inch cubes
    (a soy product that's available in health-food stores)
One 4-ounce can whole green or jalapeño chilies,
    drained and chopped
⅛ cup chili powder
1 teaspoon ground cumin
1 teaspoon dried oregano
One 28-ounce can low-sodium tomatoes, diced
½ cup chopped fresh cilantro leaves

In a heavy skillet or Dutch oven over medium-high heat, sauté the onion and garlic until soft in the vegetable broth. Add the tempeh and cook until lightly brown, about 2 minutes. Stir in the chilies, chili powder, cumin, and oregano. Cook until the chilies and spices are fragrant, about 1 minute. Add the tomatoes with their liquid, and cilantro. Bring to a boil, reduce heat, and simmer, uncovered, until the chili is thick, about 10 minutes. Season to taste. *Serves 4*

Per serving: 232 calories, 4 g fat, 14 g protein, 22 g carbohydrate, 9 g fiber

Rice and Soybean Salad

1 tablespoon sesame seeds

1 cup brown rice

2 cups boiling water

2 carrots, peeled, quartered lengthwise, and cut into ½-inch sections

1 cup broccoli florets

⅛ cup brown rice vinegar

1 teaspoon honey

½ teaspoon salt

1 cup soybeans, steamed and popped (shelled edamame
  can be purchased frozen)

6 scallions, cut into 1-inch strips

2 sheets nori (dried seaweed), cut into 2-inch strips with scissors

1 teaspoon wasabi powder (Japanese green horseradish)

½ tablespoon hot water

1 tablespoon cold water

1 tablespoon soy sauce

1 teaspoon finely grated fresh ginger

In a sauté pan, toast the sesame seeds over moderate heat until golden. Set aside. Toast the rice for 2 minutes. Add the boiling water, cover, and simmer for 20 minutes. Steam the carrots and broccoli lightly for 2 minutes, then dice. In a saucepan, bring the vinegar to a boil. Add the honey and salt and remove from heat. In a large bowl combine the sesame seeds, rice, carrots, broccoli, vinegar mixture, soybeans, scallions, and nori. Refrigerate for 20 minutes or store until the next day. Stir the wasabi powder into the hot water, then stir in the cold water, soy sauce, and ginger. Toss the rice and vegetable mixture with the wasabi dressing.

Serves 4

Per serving: 226 calories, 5 g fat, 9 g protein, 39 g carbohydrate, 4 g fiber

Quinoa Risotto with Sun-Dried Tomatoes

1 cup quinoa

1½ cups water

1½ cups vegetable stock (fresh or canned)

Olive oil spray

½ medium onion, minced

2 cloves garlic, minced

½ cup chopped sun-dried tomatoes

¼ cup Parmesan cheese (or soy Parmesan)

½ teaspoon salt

¼ cup minced parsley

In a sauté pan, toast the quinoa for 2 to 3 minutes, or until it starts to pop. Add the water and 1 cup of the vegetable stock and bring to a boil. Cover and cook on low for 10 minutes; add more vegetable stock as needed. In a nonstick pan lightly sprayed with olive oil, sauté the onion and garlic until tender. Add the garlic, onion, and tomatoes to the quinoa and continue to cook on low for another 10 minutes. Add the Parmesan, salt, and parsley and serve. Great for lunch leftovers.

Serves 6

Per serving: 178 calories, 4 g fat, 7 g protein, 30 g carbohydrate, 3 g fiber

Brown Rice with Almonds and Cranberries

From the forthcoming book *Luiz Ratto's Healthy Table*

1 cup brown rice

2½ cups water

½ medium Spanish onion, minced

2 cloves garlic, minced

¼ cup vegetable broth

½ cup almond slivers

1 cup dried cranberries

½ cup minced parsley

3 scallions, sliced

Salt to taste

In a large skillet, toast the rice for 2 minutes. It will start to crackle. Add the water and bring to a boil. Cover, reduce the heat to low, and simmer for 20 minutes. Sauté the onion and garlic in the vegetable broth for 1 minute. Add the almonds and cranberries and sauté for 2 minutes more. Add the onion mixture to the rice. Stir and add water if needed. Cover and cook for 5 more minutes. Remove from the heat and add the parsley, scallions, and salt. Serve immediately.   *Serves 6*

Per serving: 198 calories, 7 g fat, 5 g protein, 29 g carbohydrate, 2 g fiber

Salmon Asian Style

From the forthcoming book *Luiz Ratto's Healthy Table*

- 3 tablespoons soy sauce
- 3 tablespoons balsamic vinegar
- 3 tablespoons fresh lemon juice
- 2 tablespoons minced fresh ginger
- 2 tablespoons chopped cilantro leaves
- 3 scallions, sliced
- Four 3-ounce salmon fillets

To make the marinade, blend all the ingredients except the salmon in a shallow baking dish. Lay the salmon fillets in the dish and marinate for 15 minutes; turn and marinate for another 15 minutes or more. Grill the salmon to your taste.

Serves 4

Per serving: 158 calories, 4 g fat, 24 g protein, 6 g carbohydrate, 1 g fiber

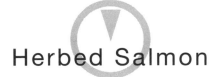

Herbed Salmon

¼ cup fat-free Spectrum marinade

2 teaspoons white wine vinegar

2 tablespoons finely minced fresh rosemary
(or tarragon, thyme, sage, or dill)

1 teaspoon salt

1 teaspoon freshly ground pepper

Four 3-ounce salmon fillets

4 lemon wedges

To make the marinade, blend all the ingredients except the salmon and lemon wedges in a shallow baking dish. Place the salmon in the dish skin side up and turn to coat. Cover and marinate in the refrigerator for 1 to 2 hours. Preheat the grill. Remove the salmon from the marinade and place the fillets in the center of the grill. Cook 7 to 8 minutes on each side, or until fish is opaque throughout. Garnish with lemon wedges. *Serves 4*

Per serving: 165 calories, 4 g fat, 24 g protein, 2 g carbohydrate, 1 g fiber

Sardine Spread

One 3½-ounce can sardines in water
½ cup plain nonfat yogurt
¼ cup green (or black) olives, pitted and chopped
1 tablespoon minced garlic
Salt and pepper to taste

In a food processor, blend all the ingredients well. Use the spread in roll-ups or on whole-grain crackers for a snack that's high in omega-3 oils and great for your skin, brain, and heart. *Serves 2*

Per serving: 64 calories, 3 g fat, 5 g protein, 2 g carbohydrate, 1 g fiber

Sardine Apple Salad

Two 3½-ounce cans sardines
1 cup unpeeled, diced red apple
1 tablespoon fresh lemon juice
½ cup chopped celery
⅓ cup Spectrum Toasted Sesame or your favorite fat-free dressing
1 cup chopped romaine lettuce

Drain the sardines and cut into chunks. Sprinkle the apple cubes with the lemon juice to keep the color bright. Combine the sardines, apple, celery, and dressing. Serve over the lettuce with a side of brown rice or quinoa. *Serves 2*

Per serving: 68 calories, 2 g fat, 4 g protein, 11 g carbohydrate, 3 g fiber

Desserts

Desserts do not have to be made with sinful ingredients; they can be high in fiber and low in calories and still taste delicious.

Riley's Cinnamon-Raisin Bread Pudding

This bread pudding is my twelve-year-old daughter, Riley's, favorite. I've been known to have it for breakfast.

1 apple, peeled and diced
4 slices Ezekiel cinnamon-raisin bread, torn into small pieces
2 egg yolks
5 egg whites
¾ cup maple syrup
1 cup nonfat vanilla soy milk
1½ teaspoons vanilla extract
1¼ teaspoons cinnamon

Preheat the oven to 350 degrees. Place the apple and bread pieces in an 8-inch square glass baking dish that's been wiped with oil. In a bowl, combine the egg yolks and egg whites and beat slightly. Add the syrup, soy milk, vanilla, and cinnamon and mix well. Pour the egg mixture over the bread and apple mixture; let rest for 15 minutes. Stir the mixture gently. Place the baking dish in a water bath (a larger baking dish containing ½ inch water). Bake for 45 to 50 minutes or until set.

Serves 8

Per serving: 137 calories, 2 g fat, 4 g protein, 23 g carbohydrate, 4 g fiber

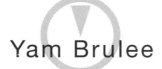

Yam Brulee

4 medium yams, peeled and cut into 8 pieces each

2 teaspoons maple syrup

¼ teaspoon vanilla extract

2 tablespoons maple or natural cane sugar

Steam the yams in a large covered pot until soft, about 20 minutes. Preheat the broiler. Transfer the yams to a food processor or the bowl of an electric mixer and puree for about 2 minutes or until smooth. Add the maple syrup and vanilla extract and puree for 30 seconds more. Divide the yam mixture among 6 individual custard dishes. Coat the surface of each with sugar. Place the custard dishes on a baking sheet and set under the broiler until the sugar melts and bubbles, about 5 minutes. Watch carefully and remove before the sugar starts to burn.
Serves 6

Per serving: 100 calories, 0.1 g fat, 1.3 g protein, 24 g carbohydrate, 2.3 g fiber

Smoothies for You and the Kids

Smoothies are a quick and easy way to cover snack time for you and the kids and to integrate soy and fruit into your diet. Many children have not developed a taste for soy products; this is an easy way to get these important phytonutrients into their bodies at an early age. But not all smoothies are created equal—those found at "smoothie shops" can contain lots of sugar, nonorganic dairy products, and sweetened fruit, adding tons of wasted calories.

This is Riley's favorite smoothie recipe. Just throw everything into a blender. This recipe serves two, but Riley drinks the whole thing, filling her fruit and soy requirements for the day.

8 ounces lite vanilla soy milk
1 medium banana
1 cup frozen berries (strawberries, raspberries, or blueberries)
Small handful of ice cubes

Per serving: 136 calories, 1.5 g fat, 4.5 g protein, 26 g carbohydrate, 4 g fiber

Zip-Lock Snacks

Snacks are a very important part of your Definition Diet. They fill in the nutrition gaps between meals. They help maintain normal blood sugar levels, reduce hunger, increase energy, and improve mood. They help your hormonal environment, and they help you lose weight. Here is a list of what I call zip-lock snacks because they can survive in a zip-lock bag or container for at least 4 hours—many of them all day. Make three or four and throw them in your backpack, purse, or briefcase. Some of the snacks come in snack-size packages of their own. If your lunch plans get canceled and you are stuck in the office, have two snacks instead of cafeteria food. I recommend buying a reusable cold pack and a thermal lunch box.

They're soft and small and can fit in your purse. This allows you to bring leftovers that require refrigeration.

All fruits

Cut-up raw veggies with
- 1 ounce bean dip
- 1 ounce Spectrum fat-free dips
- 1 ounce hummus

1 piece of Ezekiel cinnamon-raisin bread with a teaspoon of almond butter, folded in half (can go 6 hours without refrigeration)

Teriyaki, barbeque, or smoked tofu bars (individually packaged in the tofu section of the health-food store; can go 4 hours without refrigeration)

Bearitos snack-size bean dip (in a pop-top can) with a zip-lock of baked chips

½ ounce toasted almonds with dried apricots

½ ounce walnuts with raisins

Dates and a couple of whole-wheat crackers

2 cups air-popped corn

2 large Mi-Del whole-grain graham crackers with 1 teaspoon cashew butter in between

½ ounce toasted soy nuts and raisins

4 to 6 tablespoons low-fat hummus with rice crackers

1 cup nonfat organic yogurt with ½ cup frozen raspberries (or other berries; no refrigeration needed; the berries will keep the yogurt cold)

½ cup nonfat organic cottage cheese with Guiltless Gourmet Mucho Nacho chips—1 ounce only

Dr. McDougall's Split Pea with Barley Soup (just add hot water)

Leftover anything from the night before

Shopping List for Your 24-Hour Turnaround

I advise you to shop at a natural food store for the majority of your food. Read the labels on *everything* you buy. Buy organic when you can. Remember, you may think that these products are more expensive, but in the long run the dollars you save by staying healthy will pay off. Besides, there is nothing more important than your health and the health of your family, especially growing children.

VEGGIES AND FRUIT

The one and only rule for going food shopping is that you leave the store with more fresh food than packaged food. In other words, the majority of the shopping cart will be filled with fresh veggies and fruits. When you look at your lunch and dinner plate, the same will hold true—fruits, veggies, or both will take up the majority of the space on the plate. So head for the produce and pick your favorites, try a new one, and go for color.

SOY PRODUCTS

Soybeans (edamame) can be found fresh and frozen. They come in a pod (like peas) and require steaming and shelling, an easy and fun thing for kids to do. Soybeans are the only beans that contain more protein than carbs. Edamame are excellent in soups, salads, rice and pasta dishes, or plain.

Tempeh is made from soybeans and used as a meat substitute. It's great in spaghetti sauce, casseroles, sandwiches, and on rice. I love Lean Green Foods tempeh burgers (especially the ginger teriyaki flavor).

Tofu can be purchased in aseptic packages or fresh. I prefer fresh. Firm is easiest to cook with.

Soy milk comes in plain and vanilla, high and low fat. Buy the light versions. Vanilla is best in coffee, on cereal, and in smoothies.

FISH, EGGS, AND NONFAT ORGANIC DAIRY

Fresh salmon and tuna are available in most markets. Go ahead! Buy a can of sardines and try one of our sardine recipes.

Egg whites are a great fat-free source of protein. Buy free-range eggs (from hormone- and antibiotic-free hens fed a vegetarian diet) for omelets, egg salad, pancakes, and baking.

If organic, hormone-free dairy is not available in your market, try your health-food store. They also have dairy-free products that are a must to try. Soyco Foods makes a low-fat Veggie Parmesan. But watch the fat content—there are many high-fat food choices at the health-food store.

FROZEN FOODS

Berries: strawberries, blueberries, and raspberries (highest in fiber)—great for desserts and smoothies.

Veggies: keep on hand corn, peas, and baby lima beans for a great last-minute veggie dish, when fresh is unavailable.

Veggie burgers: Amy's California Burgers, Boca Burgers, Gardenburger (low-fat), and Yves hot dogs, ham, and salami substitutes.

Frozen entrées: Amy's pizza, lasagna, and assorted entrées; Natural Sea fish sticks; Gloria's Kitchen dinners.

BREADS, BAGELS, TORTILLAS, BURGER BUNS, AND ENGLISH MUFFINS

Food for Life (makers of Ezekiel bread) makes the best sprouted-grain (flourless) bread, burger buns, tortillas, and 7-grain English muffins. They're high in fiber and protein and low in fat. Check the frozen food section. Alvarado St. Bakery makes sprouted-wheat bagels in all flavors. Mana breads are sprouted grains with the addition of nuts, seeds, and dried fruits. These selections are the only Definition Diet breads, but you'll love them!

CEREALS AND GRAINS

Low-fat granola: Back to Nature (several flavors), bulk granola (usually found in bins—look for low fat without added oil or sugar).

Boxed (prepared) cereals: Barbara's O's, Star's and Puffins. Boxed cereals are not my favorite, but they are a good transition from Kellogg's to whole grain.

Oatmeal, nine-grain, and spelt flakes: Quaker Oats (slow cooking), U.S. Mills, Arrowhead Mills, and bulk cereals (found in bins). Spelt flakes look, cook, and taste similar to oatmeal but are considerably higher in protein.

Brown rice, quinoa, barley, rye: All grains are carried in bulk, and many come in packaged side dishes or entrées made by Fantastic Foods, Arrowhead Mills, and Lundberg Family Farms.

PASTA

Whole durum wheat and whole-grain kamut and spelt pastas: high in fiber and protein, eggless, and low-fat; Eden Foods, Vita Spelt, and DeBoles are excellent brands. Annie's macaroni and cheese is Riley's favorite. Westbrae Natural makes a line of ramen noodles.

Pasta sauces: Muir Glen and Amy's.

Other sauces: Ayla's Organics Curry, Szechwan, and Thai.

OTHER PACKAGED FOODS

Instant soups and rice dinners: These are easy for lunches and quick snacks. Dr. McDougall's are high in fiber and low in calories and fat. Fantastic Foods makes soups and instant rice meals in a box.

Tofu entrée mixes: These easy-to-use quick tofu "helpers" are tasty and healthy. Mori-Nu tofu hero and Hain taco seasoning mix are a couple of the good ones.

Salad dressings: I love Spectrum low- and nonfat organic dressings. Ayla's Organics makes oil-free dressings in many varieties. Hain Pure Foods makes an Italian and Herb Mix that is a perfect marinade.

Jams and jellies (fruit spreads): Buy all flavors and use on toast, bagels, and pancakes. My favorites are Cascadian Farm and Knudsen.

Beans: Check out Bearitos refried beans and minicans of bean dip; Westbrae Natural black, pinto, navy.

Snacks and desserts: Mi-Del Graham crackers, San J rice crackers, Guiltless Gourmet chips and bean dips, Santa Cruz applesauce, Imagine Foods puddings, Panda Licorice.

Vegetable broth: Use for sautéing instead of oil or as an excellent base for soups.

Nuts and nut butters: Have on hand almonds, walnuts, and flaxseeds. Try peanut, almond, and cashew butters from Maranatha Natural Foods.

Teas: Celestial Seasonings herbal teas are an interesting alternative to water.

Drinks: Knudsen Spritzers are the only "soda" that I would give to my kids. All the flavors are good.

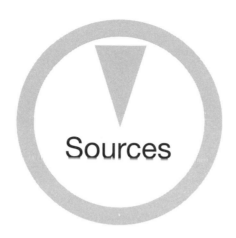

Sources

Introduction

Titan, S. M., et al. 2001. Frequency of eating and concentrations of serum cholesterol in the Norfolk population of the European Prospective Investigation into Cancer (EPIC-Norfolk): Cross sectional study. *British Medical Journal* 323:1286–88.

Total Life Change 1

Benson, Herbert, M.D. *The Relaxation Response.* New York: Avon, 1990.

Bloch, George J. *Elements of Human Biology, Behavior, and Health.* Los Altos, Calif.: William Kaufman, Inc., 1985.

Braun, D. L., and S. R. Sunday. 1999. Bright light therapy decreases winter binge frequency in women with bulimia nervosa: A double-blind, placebo-controlled study. *Comprehensive Psychiatry* 40(6):442–48.

Hafen, Brent, et al. *The Effects of Attitudes, Emotions, and Relationships.* Boston: Addison-Wesley Publishing, 1995.

Itami, J., et al. 1994. Laughter and immunity. *Japanese Journal of Psychosomatic Medicine* 34:565–71.

Jacobs, Donald Trenton. *Patient Communication for First Responders and EMS Personnel: The First Hour of Trauma.* Englewood Cliffs, N.J.: Prentice-Hall, 1988.

Jones-Webb, R., et al. 1996. Relationships between depressive symptoms, anxiety, alcohol consumption, and blood pressure: Results from the CARDIA study. *Alcoholism Clinical and Experimental Research* 20(3):420–27.

Neuhaus, I. M., et al. 1999. Gender differences in glycosylated hemoglobin levels in seasonal affective disorder patients and controls. *Comprehensive Psychiatry* 40(3):234–37.

Ostir, G. V., et al. 2001. The association between emotional well-being and the incidence of stroke in older adults. *Psychosomatic Medicine* 63(2):210–15.

Rossi, Ernest L. *The Psychobiology of Mind-Body Healing.* New York: W. W. Norton, 1993.

Theodorakis, Y., et al. 2001. Self-talk in a basketball-shooting task. *Perceptual and Motor Skills* 92(1):309–15.

Unger, J. B., and C. A. Johnson. 1995. Social relationships and physical activity in health club members. *American Journal of Health Promotion* 9(5):340–43.

Wooten, P. 1996. Humor: An antidote for stress. *Holistic Nursing Practice* 19(2):49–56.

Total Life Change 2

Bloomfield, Harold, and Robert Cooper. *The Power of Five: Hundreds of 5-Second to 5-Minute Scientific Shortcuts to Ignite Your Energy, Burn Fat, Stop Aging, and Revitalize Your Love Life.* Emmaus, Pa.: Rodale Press, 1996.

Braun, B., et al. 1995. Effects of exercise intensity on insulin sensitivity in women with non-insulin-dependent diabetes mellitus. *Journal of Applied Physiology* 78:300–306.

Evans, W. J., and J. G. Cannon. 1991. The metabolic effects of exercise-induced muscle damage. *Exercise and Sports Sciences Review* 19:99–125.

Kronenberg, F., et al. 2000. Influence of leisure time physical activity and television watching on atherosclerosis risk factors in the NHLBI Family Heart Study. *Atherosclerosis* 153(2):433–43.

Lee, I. M., et al. 2001. Physical activity and coronary heart disease in women: Is no pain, no gain passé? *Journal of the American Medical Association* 285(11):1447–54.

Leeuwenburgh, Jill et al. 1998. Oxidative stress and aging: Role of exercise and its influences on antioxidant systems. *Annals of the New York Academy of Sciences* 854:102–17.

Lehmann, R., et al. 2001. Alterations of lipolytic enzymes and high-density lipoprotein subfractions induced by physical activity in type 2 diabetes mellitus. *European Journal of Clinical Investigation* 31:37–44.

MacDonald, J. R., et al. 1999. Bouts of mild- to moderate-intensity exercise may be beneficial in the control of hypertension: The effects of exercise intensity on post exercise hypotension. *Journal of Human Hypertension* 13:527–31.

Mangione, K. K., et al. 1999. The effects of high-intensity and low-intensity cycle ergometry in older adults with knee osteoarthritis. *Journal of Gerontology* 54A:M184–90.

Mayer-Davis, E. J., et al. 1998. Intensity and amount of physical activity in relation to insulin sensitivity: The Insulin Resistance Atherosclerosis Study. *Journal of the American Medical Association* 279:669–74.

McBride, J. M., et al. 1998. Effect of resistance exercise on free radical production. *Medicine and Science in Sports and Exercise* 30(1):67–72.

Moreira, W. D., et al. 1999. Exercising at a low intensity lowered blood pressure as effectively as high-intensity training. *Journal of Clinical Epidemiology* 52(7):637–42.

Pedersen, B. K., and A. D. Toft. 2000. Effects of exercise on lymphocytes and cytokines. *British Journal of Sports Medicine* 34(4):246–51.

Total Life Change 3

Arts, I. C., et al. 2001. Catechin intake might explain the inverse relation between tea consumption and ischemic heart disease: The Zutphen Elderly Study. *American Journal of Clinical Nutrition* 74(2):227–32.

Barnard, N. D., et al. 2000. Effectiveness of a low-fat vegetarian diet in altering serum lipids in healthy premenopausal women: Antimicrobial and antioxidant activities of unripe papaya. *American Journal of Cardiology* 85(8):969–72.

Boyd, N. F., et al. 1996. Long-term effects of participation in a randomized trial of a low-fat, high-carbohydrate diet. *Cancer, Epidemiology Biomarkers and Prevention* 5(3):217–22.

Campbell, D. R., and M. D. Gross. 1994. Plasma carotenoids as biomarkers of vegetable and fruit intake. *Cancer, Epidemiology Biomarkers and Prevention* 3(6):493–500.

Challier, B., et al. 1998. Garlic, onion and cereal fiber as protective factors for breast cancer: A French case-control study. *European Journal of Epidemiology* 14(8):737–47.

de Meester, C., and G. B. Gerber. 1995. The role of cooked food mutagens as possible etiological agents in human cancer: A critical appraisal of recent epidemiological investigations. *Revue d'Épidémiologie et de Santé Publique* 43(2):147–61.

De Roos, N. M., et al. 2001. Replacement of dietary saturated fatty acids by trans fatty acids lowers serum HDL cholesterol and impairs endothelial function in healthy men and women. *Arteriosclerosis, Thrombosis, and Vascular Biology* 21(7):1233–37.

De Stefani, E., et al. 1997. Dietary fiber and risk of breast cancer: A case-control study in Uruguay. *Nutrition and Cancer* 28(1):14–19.

Goodman, Marc T., et al. 1997. Soy and fiber consumption and the risk of endometrial cancer. *American Journal of Epidemiology* 146:294–306.

Green, S. M., and J. E. Blundell. 1996. Effect of fat- and sucrose-containing foods on the size of eating episodes and energy intake in lean dietary restrained and unrestrained females: Potential for causing overconsumption. *European Journal of Clinical Nutrition* 50(9):625–35.

Green, S. M., et al. 2000. Comparison of high-fat and high-carbohydrate foods in a meal or snack on short-term fat and energy intakes in obese women. *British Journal of Nutrition* 84(4):521–30.

Hubert, P., et al. 1998. Uncoupling the effects of energy expenditure and energy intake: Appetite response to short-term energy deficit induced by meal omission and physical activity. *Appetite* 21(1):9–19.

Jacobs, D. R., et al. 2000. Fiber in whole grains vs. refined grains reduces chronic disease. *Journal of the American College of Nutrition* 19(3):326S–30S.

Koutsari, C., et al. 2001. Exercise prevents the accumulation of triglyceride-rich lipoproteins and their remnants seen when changing to a high-carbohydrate diet. *Arteriosclerosis, Thrombosis, and Vascular Biology* 21(9):1520–25.

Leyenaar, J., et al. 1998. Self-reported physical and emotional health of women in a low-fat, high-carbohydrate dietary trial (Canada). *Cancer Causes and Control* 9(6):601–10.

Liu, S., et al. 2001. Dietary glycemic load assessed by food-frequency questionnaire in relation to plasma high-density-lipoprotein cholesterol and fasting plasma triacylglycerols in postmenopausal women. *American Journal of Clinical Nutrition* 73:560–66.

Ludwig, David S., et al. 1999. High glycemic index foods, overeating, and obesity. *Pediatrics* 103(3):e26.

Ludwig, D. S., et al. 2000. Dietary fiber, weight gain, and cardiovascular disease risk factors in young adults. *Journal of the American Medical Association* 283(14):1821.

Manson, J. E., et al. 1999. A prospective study of walking as compared with vigorous exercise in the prevention of coronary heart disease in women. *New England Journal of Medicine* 341(9):650–58.

McCarty, M. F. 1999. Vegan proteins may reduce risk of cancer, obesity, and cardiovascular disease by promoting increased glucagon activity. *Medical Hypotheses* 53(6):459–85.

Nieman, D. C. 1997. Immune response to heavy exertion. *Journal of Applied Physiology* 82:1385–94.

Ong, P. J., et al. 1999. Effect of fat and carbohydrate consumption on endothelial function. *The Lancet* 354(9196):2134.

Robbins, John. *The Food Revolution: How Your Diet Can Help Save Your Life and Our World.* Berkeley: Conari Press, 2001.

Roodenburg, A. J., et al. 2000. Amount of fat in the diet affects bioavailability of lutein esters but not of alpha-carotene, beta-carotene, and vitamin E in humans. *American Journal of Clinical Nutrition* 71(5):1029–30.

Slattery, M. L., et al. 2000. Carotenoids and colon cancer. *American Journal of Clinical Nutrition* 71(2):575–82.

Slattery, M. L., et al. 1997. Plant foods and colon cancer: An assessment of specific foods and their related nutrients (United States). *Cancer Causes and Control* 8(4):575–90.

Smith, C. F., and L. E. Burke. 2000. Vegetarian and weight-loss diets among young adults. *Obesity Research* 8(2):123–29.

Speechly, D. P., and R. Buffenstein. 1999. Greater appetite control associated with an increased frequency of eating in lean males. *Appetite* 33(3):285–97.

Spiller, G. A., et al. 1998. Nuts and plasma lipids: An almond-based diet lowers LDL-C while preserving HDL-C. *Journal of the American College of Nutrition* 17(3):1285–90.

St. Jeor, S., et al. 2001. AHA advises against high-protein diets. *Circulation* 104:1869–74.

Walton, P., and E. C. Rhodes. 1997. Glycaemic index and optimal performance. *Sports Medicine* 23(3):164–72.

Williams, M. J., et al. 1999. Impaired endothelial function following a meal rich in used cooking fat. *Journal of the American College of Cardiology* 33(4):1050–55.

Wing, R. R., et al. 2001. Behavioral science research in diabetes: Lifestyle changes related to obesity, eating behavior, and physical activity. *Diabetes Care* 24:117–23.

Zandstra, E. H. et al. 2000. Short- and long-term effects of changes in pleasantness on food intake. *Appetite* 34(3):253–60.

Total Life Change 4

Batmanghelidj, Walter F., M.D. *Your Body's Many Cries for Water.* Vienna, Va: Global Health Solutions, 1995.

Global Health Solutions: http://www.watercure.com.

Total Life Change 5

Cornuz, J., and W. A. Ghali. 2000. Physicians' attitudes towards prevention: Importance of intervention-specific barriers and physicians' health habits. *Family Practitioner* 17(6):535–40.

Freedman, J. E., et al. 2001. Select flavonoids and whole juice from purple grapes inhibit platelet function and enhance nitric oxide release. *Circulation* 103(23):2792–98.

Total Life Change 6

King, A. C., et al. 1997. Moderate-intensity exercise and self-rated quality of sleep in older adults. *Journal of the American Medical Association* 277(1):32–37.

Montplaisir, J., et al. 2001. Sleep in menopause: Differential effects of two forms of hormone replacement therapy. *Menopause* 8:10–16.

Shochat, T., et al. 2000. Illumination levels in nursing home patients: Effects on sleep and activity rhythms. *Journal of Sleep Research* 9(4):373–79.

Stickgold, R., et al. 2000. Visual discrimination learning requires sleep after training. *Nature Neuroscience* 3(12):1237–38.

Zhdanova, I.V., and R. J. Wurtman. 2001. Melatonin treatment for age-related insomnia. *Journal of Clinical Endocrinology and Metabolism* 86(10):4727–30.

Total Life Change 7

Alekel, D. L., et al. 2000. Isoflavone-rich soy protein isolate attenuates bone loss in the lumbar spine of perimenopausal women. *American Journal of Clinical Nutrition* 72:844–52.

Arjmandi, B. H., et al. 1998. Role of soy protein with normal or reduced isoflavone content in reversing bone loss induced by ovarian deficiency in rats. *American Journal of Clinical Nutrition* 6:1358S–63S.

Duncan, A. M., and K. E. Underhill. 1999. The modest hormonal effects of soy isoflavones in postmenopausal women. *Journal of Clinical Endocrinology and Metabolism* 84:3479–84.

Erdman, J. W., Jr., and R. J. Stillman. 2000. Provocative relation between soy and bone maintenance. *American Journal of Clinical Nutrition* 2:679–80.

2001. Familial breast cancer: Collaborative reanalysis of individual data from 52 epidemiological studies including 58,209 women with breast cancer and 101,986 women without the disease. *The Lancet* 358:1389–99.

Mosca, Lori, M.D., and Peter Collins, M.D. 2001. Hormone replacement therapy and cardiovascular disease. *Circulation* 104:499.

Potter, S. M., et al. 1998. Soy protein and isoflavones: Their effects on blood lipids and bone density in postmenopausal women. *American Journal of Clinical Nutrition* 68:1375S–79S.

Ricca, T. A., et al. 2001. Energy restriction and bone resorption. *American Journal of Nutrition* 73:347–52.

Total Life Change 8

Chopra, Deepak, M.D. *Ageless Body, Timeless Mind: The Quantum Alternative to Growing Old*. New York: Harmony Books, 1998.

Epel, E., and R. Lapidus. 2001. Stress may add bite to appetite in women: A laboratory study of stress-induced cortisol and eating behavior. *Psychoneuroendocrinology* 26(1):37–49.

Garg, A., and M. M. Chren. 2001. Psychological stress perturbs epidermal permeability barrier homeostasis: Implications for the pathogenesis of stress-associated skin disorders. *Archives of Dermatology* 137(1):53–59.

Manchanda S. C., et al. 2000. Retardation of coronary arteriosclerosis with yoga lifestyle intervention. *Journal of the Association of Physicians of India* 48:687–94.

Mockel, M., et al. 1994. Immediate physiological responses to different types of music: Cardiovascular, hormonal and mental changes. *European Journal of Applied Physiology* 68:451–59.

Ostir, G. V., and K. S. Markides. 2001. The association between emotional well-being and the incidence of stroke in older adults. *Psychosomatic Medicine* 63(2):210–15

Reibel, D. K., and J. M. Greeson. 2001. Mindfulness-based stress reduction and health-related quality of life in a heterogeneous patient population. *General Hospital Psychiatry* 23(4):183–92.

Restak, Richard. *The Longevity Strategy*. New York: John Wiley and Sons, 1998.

Rosmond, R., et al. 2000. Food-induced cortisol secretion. *International Journal of Obesity* 24:416–22.

Simonson, M. 1990. Obesity may be linked to poor management of stress. *Obesity 90 Update* (September–October):3.

Takkouche, B., et al. 2001. A cohort study of stress and the common cold. *Epidemiology* 12(3):345–49.

William, K. A., and M. M. Kolar. 2001. Evaluation of a wellness-based mindfulness stress reduction intervention: A controlled trial. *American Journal of Health Promotion* 15(6):422–32.

You *Can* Turn Back the Clock

Blackburn, G. L. 2001. The public health implications of the Dietary Approaches to Stop Hypertension trial. *American Journal of Clinical Nutrition* 74(1):1–2.

Bush, David E. 2001. Even mild depression increases risk of death after acute MI (controlled through exercise). *American Journal of Cardiology* 88:337–41.

Bushinsky, David. 1999. High protein diet's link to bone loss. *Journal of Physiology*.

de Jong, N., et al. 2000. Dietary supplements and physical exercise affecting bone and body composition in frail elderly persons. *American Journal of Public Health* 90(6):947–54.

Hakim, I. A., et al. 2000. Citrus peel use is associated with reduced risk of squamous cell carcinoma of the skin. *Nutrition and Cancer* 37(2):161–68.

Hermansen, K. 2000. Diet, blood pressure and hypertension. *British Journal of Nutrition* 83:S113–19.

Hirsch, K., et al. 2000. Effect of purified allicin, the major ingredient of freshly crushed garlic, on cancer cell proliferation. *Nutrition and Cancer* 38(2):245–54.

Joshipura, K. J., et al. 2001. The effect of fruit and vegetable intake on risk for coronary heart disease. *Annals of Internal Medicine* 134(12):1106–14.

Laurin, D., et al. 2001. Physical activity and risk of cognitive impairment and dementia in elderly persons. *Archives of Neurology* 58(3):498–504.

Millen, B. E., and P. A. Quatromoni. 2001. Nutritional research within the Framingham Heart Study. *Journal of Nutrition, Health, and Aging* 5(3):139–43.

Paw, M. J., et al. 2000. Immunity in frail elderly: A randomized controlled trial of exercise and enriched foods. *Medicine and Science in Sports and Exercise* 32(12):2005–11.

Slavin, J. L., et al. 2001. The role of whole grains in disease prevention. *Journal of the American Dietetics Association* 101(7):780–85.

Tymchuk, C. N., et al. 2001. Evidence of an inhibitory effect of diet and exercise on prostate cancer cell growth. *Journal of Urology* 166(3):1185–89.

Wynder, E. L., et al. 1994. Prostate cancer: A proposal for dietary intervention. *Nutrition and Cancer* 22(1):1–10.

Yaffe, K., et al. 2001. A prospective study of physical activity and cognitive decline in elderly women: Women who walk. *Archives of Internal Medicine* 61(14):1703–8.

Spa Secrets

Garg, A., and M. M. Chren. 2001. Psychological stress perturbs epidermal permeability barrier homeostasis: Implications for the pathogenesis of stress-associated skin disorders. *Archives of Dermatology* 137(1):53–59.

Held, E., and T. Agner. 2001. Effect of moisturizers on skin susceptibility to irritants. *Acta Dermato-Venereologica* 81(2):104–7.

Klaschka, F. *Oral Enzymes: New Approach to Cancer Treatment.* Munich, Germany: Forum-Medizin, 1996.

Landis, S. H., et al. 1998. Cancer statistics—1998. *CA-A Cancer Journal for Clinicians* 48(1):6–30.

Osato, J. A., L. A. Santiago, and G. M. Remo. 1993. Antimicrobial and antioxidant activities of unripe papaya. *Life Sciences* 53:1383–89.

Purba, M. B. et al. 2001. Skin wrinkling: Can food make a difference? *Journal of the American College of Nutrition* 20(1):71–80.

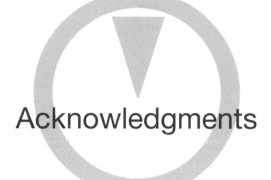

Acknowledgments

T O B E H O N E S T, my favorite way to work with clients to achieve weight loss and prevent aging is to have them check into the spa and spend a week with me. I can personally hold their hand and give them the valuable antiaging information you've read in this book. I can train them, teach them to meditate, and encourage and inspire them to be the best that they can be. And I have spent the last twenty-six years of my life doing just that.

One day I was having lunch with my friend and client Michael Milken, and he asked me, "Jay, what is your ultimate goal in your work?" My answer: "To heal the world, of course!" Michael pointed out that working with one person at a time was going to make that goal somewhat difficult. Yet my innermost philosophy is aligned with that of the Chinese, who believe that when you heal one, you heal the world because it is all the same energy. Nonetheless, I was inspired that day to reach out to as many as I could.

Michael Fuchs, the genius who created HBO, came to me as a client while he was building an empire. I took care of his health and training program and watched him become leaner, stronger, and younger. We have since become great friends and now take care of each other. Michael sent me a friend of his, Judith Regan, president and publisher of ReganBooks. Judith has the brilliance, conviction, and guts that many publishers lack. She truly believes that if you want to offer something that works to help people, you can't always conform to what is popular at the moment. Judith is an amazing, gifted woman who has inspired many to share their beliefs with the world. Thank you, Judith. Now I can go forward with my goal and take on the world.

I would also like to acknowledge the help of three very important people: John Zulli, Ph.D., for contributing his amazing technique for motivation; Debra Fulghum Bruce, for her outstanding and expeditious work on the book; and the most incredible editor in the business, Cassie Jones. Her sense of humor kept me going.